Recent Advances in Therapeutic Strategies for the Treatment of Pediatric Diseases

Recent Advances in Therapeutic Strategies for the Treatment of Pediatric Diseases

Guest Editors

Mariaevelina Alfieri
Peppino Mirabelli

MDPI

Basel • Beijing • Wuhan • Barcelona • Belgrade • Novi Sad • Cluj • Manchester

Guest Editors
Mariaevelina Alfieri
Clinical Pathology
A.O.R.N.
Santobono-Pausilipon
Naples
Italy

Peppino Mirabelli
Clinical and Translational
Research Unit
Santobono-Pausilipon
Children's Hospital
Naples
Italy

Editorial Office
MDPI AG
Grosspeteranlage 5
4052 Basel, Switzerland

This is a reprint of the Special Issue, published open access by the journal *Pharmaceutics* (ISSN 1999-4923), freely accessible at: https://www.mdpi.com/journal/pharmaceutics/special_issues/7T4U4JZZCS.

For citation purposes, cite each article independently as indicated on the article page online and as indicated below:

Lastname, A.A.; Lastname, B.B. Article Title. *Journal Name* **Year**, *Volume Number*, Page Range.

ISBN 978-3-7258-5017-4 (Hbk)
ISBN 978-3-7258-5018-1 (PDF)
https://doi.org/10.3390/books978-3-7258-5018-1

Contents

About the Editors

Mariaevelina Alfieri

Mariaevelina Alfieri, PhD, is currently a Senior Clinical Biologist at the UOC of Clinical Pathology, P.O. Pausilipon (Naples), where she leads the Clinical Biochemistry Unit. She has a strong background in molecular biology, genomics, and translational research, developed over more than 15 years of experience in both academic and clinical settings. Dr. Alfieri earned her PhD in Systems Biology from the University of Salerno and holds a specialization in Medical Genetics from the University of Naples Federico II. She has carried out research at prestigious institutions including TIGEM and the University of Salerno, focusing on topics ranging from ciliopathies and gene regulation to plant-derived nanovesicles and cancer biomarkers. She has authored numerous peer-reviewed publications that have been published in international journals, and her current research explores innovative approaches to precision oncology, including 3D bioprinting technologies. In parallel, she actively contributes to academic teaching and mentoring in the fields of biochemistry, molecular genetics, and biotechnology. Dr. Alfieri continues to bridge basic research with clinical applications, with a focus on pediatric care, omics sciences, and biomarker discovery, aiming to enhance diagnostic and therapeutic strategies through personalized medicine.

Peppino Mirabelli

Peppino Mirabelli earned a PhD in Biotechnologies from the Università degli Studi dell'Aquila, Napoli, Campania, Italy, in 2007. He currently works for the Azienda Ospedaliera di Rilievo Nazionale Santobono Pausilipon, Clinical and Translational Research Unit (Naples). He has 79 publications with 2537 citations and an h-index of 27 (Scopus, 29 July 2025).

pharmaceutics MDPI

Editorial

Recent Advances in Therapeutic Strategies for the Treatment of Pediatric Diseases

Peppino Mirabelli [1] and Mariaevelina Alfieri [2,*]

1 Clinical and Translational Research Unit, Santobono-Pausilipon Children's Hospital, 80129 Naples, Italy; p.mirabelli@santobonopausilipon.it
2 Clinical Pathology, Santobono-Pausilipon Children's Hospital, 80129 Naples, Italy
* Correspondence: m.alfieri@santobonopausilipon.it

Medical research has been traditionally focused on diseases that primarily affect adults, often due to their greater impact on life expectancy and economic productivity. However, in recent years, there has been growing recognition of the importance of pediatric diseases. These conditions often differ significantly from those in adults in terms of causes and underlying mechanisms, necessitating more specialized and complex research approaches. Moreover, enrolling children in clinical trials can be particularly challenging, requiring tailored methodologies and the involvement of specially trained personnel.

Pediatric diseases also have a significant impact on public health. Indeed, beyond the medical aspects, pediatric diseases often place a significant emotional and practical burden on families. When a child becomes ill (especially in the case of chronic or life-threatening disease), parents or caregivers may need to take extended time off work or even leave their jobs entirely to provide care, leading to financial strain and disruption of daily life. Despite this, medical research on pediatric diseases remains less common than that on adult conditions.

More importantly, the research on pediatric diseases can lead to the development of new treatments and cures for diseases that affect children.

In recent years, gene therapy, biological drugs, and innovative treatments are opening new opportunities for diagnosis and treatment of children affected by different diseases such as immunodeficiencies, tumors, hematological disorders, and genetic diseases. Numerous studies on pediatric diseases have been initiated, and many of them have led to important advances in the understanding and treatment of these diseases.

Some drugs, such as biologicals and gene therapy, are changing the natural history and long-term fate of patients who until a few years ago were considered incurable. Precision medicine allows us to make individualized diagnoses and to guarantee increasingly personalized therapies: not only the most suitable, most effective, and safest drug or treatment, but also the "tailor-made" dosage.

Pediatric therapies usually rely on previous clinical experience in adults. However, there exists scientific evidence that drug pharmacokinetics and pharmacodynamics in children differ from those in adults. For example, the interaction of specific drugs with their target receptors undergoes changes over the maturation of the different organs and systems. A similar phenomenon is observed for toxicity and adverse effects. Thus, it is clear that the treatment of disease in children cannot be simplified to the direct adjustment of the dose to the body weight/surface [1].

Children cannot be considered "miniature adults". There are important anatomical, physiological, and developmental differences in the various organs between these two populations, including between different pediatric age groups. The ways in which the body and drugs interact with each other (pharmacokinetics and pharmacodynamics) change, particularly comparing infants (even more so if premature) and adults. Differences in the absorption, metabolism, distribution, and elimination of drugs can cause the so-called half-life (a pharmacokinetic indicator expressing the time interval required for the plasma concentration of the drug to decrease by 50 percent) in the newborn to be about twice that observed in the adult. This means that at the same dose normalized for body weight, the concentration of the drug in the infant decreases more slowly than in the adult [2].

For this reason, drugs should be properly studied in the pediatric population before they are administered, which, even today, despite advances, is still not guaranteed.

Over the past fifty years, pharmaceutical research has made great progress in the area of treatment for adults, but the same cannot be said in the case of pediatric medicines. About 50 percent of pediatric medicines, as mentioned above, are administered without first being tested on children. While it is true that the new figures attest to some progress, many medicines continue to be used "off-label" [3], while others are even used unlicensed, that is, without authorization. Overall, it appears that the use of medicaments for pediatric use is an area that has so far not been sufficiently studied and is worthy of further investigation, and that a large number of medicaments newly introduced to the market are not tested in the various pediatric age groups. This fact led Harry Shirkey to use as early as the late 1960s the definition, referring to children, of therapeutic orphans [4]. Regarding the side effects of medicines, the absence of pediatric authorization poses a higher risk for children than for adults.

In this Special Issue, titled "Recent Advances in Therapeutic Strategies for the Treatment of Pediatric Diseases", we proposed to collect original research reports, reviews, and perspectives regarding the treatment of pediatric diseases. In fact, although to date several pediatric diseases are efficiently treated, any efforts in the development of new therapeutic strategies are appreciated to reduce side effects and ameliorate the life styles of affected children.

The Special Issue consists of eight published papers (four research articles, three review articles, and one systematic review) presenting different and significant advances in this field.

In contribution 1, Adamiszak and colleagues evaluated fluconazole dosing regimens for Candida spp. prophylaxis in hemato-oncologic pediatric patients. Although the results shown require clinical validation by assessing a larger number of patients, the authors conclude that hemato-oncologic pediatric patients require increased fluconazole doses to obtain the therapeutic efficacy.

Zuccari et al. (contribution 2) investigated the colloidal stability of the liposomes and the chemical stability of amphotericin B over time at storage conditions, demonstrating that the most diluted formulation (addressed to the more vulnerable patients), kept at room temperature, showed marked changes in the aggregation state and high cytotoxicity. For these results, the authors concluded that the centralization of the dilution of AmBisome® at the pharmacy in the G. Gaslini children hospital is extremely relevant for patient safety.

It is known that oral forms (capsules) of drugs are not adapted for use in children. However, in contribution 3 Caroline Lemarchand and colleagues demonstrated that mixing Temozolomide (TMZ, a drug used in managing pediatric cancers) capsule content with food may result in significant underexposure, as it is likely that children will not complete their meals. The study presented in contribution 4 showed that oral TMZ suspension and TMZ oral capsule treatment are bioequivalent medicines without unexpected safety signals or local toxicity.

Heart disease represents the main cause of death in children with cancer due to the cardiotoxicity induced by chemotherapy treatments. So, the early detection of the cardiac damage is crucial. In contribution 5, the authors reviewed the main biomarkers for the monitoring of chemotherapy-induced cardiotoxicity, highlighting the importance of the high-sensitivity method for the detection of cardiac troponin to further improve the effectiveness of risk stratification and monitoring of cardiotoxicity during chemotherapy treatment cycles.

As mentioned above, many drugs never tested on children are prescribed by pediatricians. In contribution 6, authors examined in a comprehensive review the prevalence of off-label drug use in pediatrics by conducting a literature search and including studies from 2012 to 2022 that assessed the prevalence of off-label medications in various pediatric patient populations.

Gene therapies offer incredible potential. In contribution 7 authors provided background for a recent trial exploring the use of a fixed-dose onasemnogene abeparvovec (a self-complementary AAV serotype 9 vector that encodes a functional copy of SMN1, whose mutation is responsible for spinal muscular atrophy) in children up to 5 years of age through intrathecal administration. Marco Zaffanelli and colleagues (contribution 8) presented a systematic review in which clinical evidence on the efficacy and safety of intranasal corticosteroids and oral montelukast was evaluated for treating sleep-disordered breathing and adenoid hypertrophy. They concluded that the combination of intranasal corticosteroids and oral montelukast effectively and safely treats adenoid hypertrophy and mild-to-moderate OSA symptoms in children, although larger prospective trials with standardized protocols are necessary to provide robust conclusions.

There are numerous difficulties underlying the small number of pediatric trials, which can be summarily identified as organizational–managerial, economic, and ethical.

From the organizational point of view, pediatric trials have a greater complexity, also considering the need to minimize all procedures that involve stress and pain for the subject.

Fortunately, children in most cases represent a healthy population that mainly needs a limited number of drugs (painkillers/antifebriles, antibiotics, and respirators) for acute illnesses that resolve in a few days, such as airway infections, and pharmaceutical spending concerning children and adolescents. The poor economic return, therefore, does not encourage pharmaceutical industries from studying drugs with pediatric indication, particularly if the drug is already on the pharmaceutical market for adults.

From an ethical point of view, children are not able to choose for themselves whether to participate in a trial, and consent must be provided by parents. The fact that a child, especially a young child, will receive treatment that could cause as yet unknown side effects and be subjected to invasive or painful procedures as part of the study may be of concern to parents and a brake on participation.

On the other hand, however, using drugs that have not been properly designed for that age group could pose greater health risks to the child than a clinical trial.

In conclusion, the landscape of pediatrics is rapidly evolving due to continued advances in genetics, biological therapies, and the understanding of inflammatory and infectious diseases. These advances not only improve our ability to treat rare and complex diseases but also offer new hope and possibilities to our youngest patients and their families. In the future, the further integration of biotechnology with daily clinical practice promises to radically transform pediatrics, leading to increasingly personalized care based on the individual needs of the child.

Conflicts of Interest: The authors declare no conflict of interest.

List of Contributions:

1. Adamiszak, A.; Derwich, K.; Bartkowska-Śniatkowska, A.; Pietrzkiewicz, K.; Niewiadomska-Wojnałowicz, I.; Czyrski, A.; Jusko, W.J.; Bienert, A. Fluconazole Dosing for the Prevention of Candida spp. Infections in Hemato-Oncologic Pediatric Patients: Population Pharmacokinetic Modeling and Probability of Target Attainment Simulations. *Pharmaceutics* **2025**, *17*, 488. https://doi.org/10.3390/pharmaceutics17040488
2. Zuccari, G.; Villa, C.; Iurilli, V.; Barabino, P.; Zorzoli, A.; Marimpietri, D.; Caviglia, D.; Russo, E. AmBisome® Formulations for Pediatrics: Stability, Cytotoxicity, and Cost-Effectiveness Studies. *Pharmaceutics* **2024**, *16*, 466. https://doi.org/10.3390/pharmaceutics16040466
3. Lemarchand, C.; Bienaymé, H.; Rieutord, A.; Abbou, S.; Annereau, M.; Bastid, J. Dispensing Oral Temozolomide in Children: Precision and Stability of a Novel and Ready to Use Liquid Formulation in Comparison with Capsule Derived Mixtures. *Pharmaceutics* **2023**, *15*, 2711. https://doi.org/10.3390/pharmaceutics15122711
4. Ducray, F.; Ramirez, C.; Robert, M.; Fontanilles, M.; Bronnimann, C.; Chinot, O.; Estrade, F.; Durando, X.; Cartalat, S.; Bastid, J.; et al. A Multicenter Randomized Bioequivalence Study of a Novel Ready-to-Use Temozolomide Oral Suspension vs. Temozolomide Capsules. *Pharmaceutics* **2023**, *15*, 2664. https://doi.org/10.3390/pharmaceutics15122664
5. Meo, L.; Savarese, M.; Munno, C.; Mirabelli, P.; Ragno, P.; Leone, O.; Alfieri, M. Circulating Biomarkers for Monitoring Chemotherapy-Induced Cardiotoxicity in Children. *Pharmaceutics* **2023**, *15*, 2712. https://doi.org/10.3390/pharmaceutics15122712
6. Petkova, V.; Georgieva, D.; Dimitrov, M.; Nikolova, I. Off-Label Prescribing in Pediatric Population—Literature Review for 2012–2022. *Pharmaceutics* **2023**, *15*, 2652. https://doi.org/10.3390/pharmaceutics15122652
7. René, C.A.; Parks, R.J. Expanding the Availability of Onasemnogene Abeparvovec to Older Patients: The Evolving Treatment Landscape for Spinal Muscular Atrophy. *Pharmaceutics* **2023**, *15*, 1764. https://doi.org/10.3390/pharmaceutics15061764
8. Zaffanello, M.; Pietrobelli, A.; Nosetti, L.; Antoniazzi, F.; Frassoldati, R.; Piacentini, G. Intranasal Corticosteroids and Oral Montelukast for Paediatric Obstructive Sleep Apnoea: A Systematic Review. *Pharmaceutics* **2025**, *17*, 588. https://doi.org/10.3390/pharmaceutics17050588

References

1. Alrasheed, M.M.; Alakeel, Y.S. Developmental Pharmacokinetics. In *Manual of Pediatric Cardiac Care*; Yelbuz, T.M., Bin-Moallim, M.A., Husain, W.J.M., Alakeel, Y.S., Kabbani, M.S., Alghamdi, A.A., Eds.; Springer: Singapore, 2024. [CrossRef]
2. Kimland, E.; Odlind, V. Off-label drug use in pediatric patients. *Clin. Pharmacol. Ther.* **2012**, *91*, 5. [CrossRef] [PubMed]
3. Conroy, S.; Choonara, I.; Impicciatore, P.; Mohn, A.; Arnell, H.; Rane, A.; Knoeppel, C.; Seyberth, H.; Pandolfini, C.; Raffaelli, M.P.; et al. Survey of unlicensed and off label drug use in paediatric wards in European countries. *BMJ* **2000**, *320*, 79–82. [CrossRef] [PubMed]
4. Shirkey, H. Therapeutic orphans. *J. Pediatr.* **1968**, *72*, 119–120. [CrossRef] [PubMed]

pharmaceutics

MDPI

Article

Fluconazole Dosing for the Prevention of *Candida* spp. Infections in Hemato-Oncologic Pediatric Patients: Population Pharmacokinetic Modeling and Probability of Target Attainment Simulations

Arkadiusz Adamiszak [1,2,*], Katarzyna Derwich [3], Alicja Bartkowska-Śniatkowska [4], Krzysztof Pietrzkiewicz [4], Izabela Niewiadomska-Wojnałowicz [3], Andrzej Czyrski [5], William J. Jusko [6] and Agnieszka Bienert [1]

1. Department of Pharmacology, Poznan University of Medical Sciences, 60-806 Poznan, Poland; agbienert@ump.edu.pl
2. Doctoral School, Poznan University of Medical Sciences, 60-812 Poznan, Poland
3. Department of Pediatric Oncology, Hematology and Transplantology, Poznan University of Medical Sciences, 60-572 Poznan, Poland; kderwich@ump.edu.pl (K.D.); izabela.niewiadomskawojnalowicz@ump.edu.pl (I.N.-W.)
4. Department of Paediatric Anaesthesiology and Intensive Therapy, Poznan University of Medical Sciences, 60-572 Poznan, Poland; asniatko@ump.edu.pl (A.B.-Ś.); kpietrzkiewicz@ump.edu.pl (K.P.)
5. Department of Physical Pharmacy and Pharmacokinetics, Poznan University of Medical Sciences, 60-806 Poznan, Poland; aczyrski@ump.edu.pl
6. Department of Pharmaceutical Sciences, School of Pharmacy and Pharmaceutical Sciences, State University of New York at Buffalo, Buffalo, NY 14214, USA; wjjusko@buffalo.edu

* Correspondence: arkadiusz.adamiszak@student.ump.edu.pl

Abstract: Objectives: A population pharmacokinetic (popPK) model was used to evaluate fluconazole dosing regimens for *Candida* spp. prophylaxis in hemato-oncologic pediatric patients. **Methods**: Data were collected from patients receiving 3–12 mg/kg of fluconazole once daily as a 0.5 or 1 h infusion. Fluconazole concentrations were determined using a validated HPLC-UV method. The popPK model employed non-linear mixed effects modeling using the FOCEI algorithm implemented in nlmixr2. Monte Carlo simulations and probability of target attainment (PTA) analysis were performed in the rxode2 package to investigate dosing recommendations. **Results**: Concentration time data from nine patients, aged 7 months to 18 years, with 35 samples, were described by a one-compartment model with first-order elimination and allometric scaling of body weight. Assuming a *Candida* spp. MIC = 2 mg/L and the ratio of the area under the unbound concentration–time curve at a steady state to the MIC (fAUC/MIC) $\geq$ 100 as the pharmacokinetic/pharmacodynamic (PK/PD) target, the standard dosing regimens reported in the Summary of Product Characteristics (SmPC) did not achieve the target for patients treated with doses < 6 mg/kg. **Conclusions**: Hemato-oncologic pediatric patients require increased fluconazole doses to attain therapeutic efficacy. These results warrant clinical validation and should be confirmed by assessing a larger number of patients.

Keywords: fluconazole; population pharmacokinetics; Monte Carlo simulations; probability of target attainment; *Candida* spp. prophylaxis

1. Introduction

Fluconazole (FLU) is a triazole group antifungal drug widely used in clinical conditions and outpatient treatment [1–3]. In the pediatric population, FLU is indicated to treat invasive and mucosal candidiasis, cryptococcal meningitis, and prophylaxis of *Candida* spp. infections in immunocompromised and other high-risk patients [2,4,5].

An oral dose of FLU has ~90% bioavailability and a comparable plasma concentration as intravenous (IV) administration [4,6–9]. The volume of distribution (V) of FLU is similar to the total body water of adult patients (0.7 L/kg) [4,6,10,11]. In turn, in children aged 0.25–12 years, the V is 33% higher (0.95 L/kg) [10,11]. The plasma protein binding is relatively low and reported as 11–12% [4,6,8,10]. Approximately 80% of the administered FLU dose is eliminated unchanged in urine [4,8,10,12,13]. The half-life in adults is about 30 h and in children is about 22 h, perhaps necessitating higher doses in children [10,11].

The activity and efficacy of FLU are related to the ratio of the area under the free drug concentration–time curve (fAUC) over 24 h at a steady state to the pathogen's minimum inhibitory concentration (MIC) [14–16]. The higher pharmacokinetic/pharmacodynamic (PK/PD) target was established as an fAUC/MIC $\geq$ 100 [2,13,16,17]. For *Candida* spp. considered susceptible to FLU treatment (MIC $\leq$ 2 mg/L) [18], the fAUC must reach at least 200 mg $\times$ h/L [2,15]. The less rigorous PK/PD target is fAUC/MIC $\geq$ 50; when assuming MIC $\leq$ 2 mg/L, the fAUC is thus at least 100 mg $\times$ h/L [17,19]. Although attaining the PK/PD targets improves treatment outcomes, therapeutic drug monitoring (TDM) is not a clinical routine mainly because of the broad FLU therapeutic index, favorable safety profile, and linear dose–concentration correlation [14,17,20–22]. Lack of routine TDM combined with limited knowledge of the PK of azoles in the pediatric population results in subtherapeutic FLU dosages in almost 40% of patients [3,14,15,17,22].

Since underexposure to FLU during treatment of the pediatric population has been suggested in the literature, our study aimed to investigate the efficacy of registered FLU doses used as a prophylaxis of *Candida* spp. infections.

2. Materials and Methods

2.1. Study Population and Data Collection

This study was performed in accordance with the Declaration of Helsinki, approved by the local ethics committee (the Poznan University of Medical Sciences Bioethics Committee, decision number: KB-820/21, 3 November 2021), and registered at ClinicalTrials.gov (NCT05426499). Written informed consent was obtained from patients and their legal representatives before inclusion. This study was conducted at the Poznan University of Medical Sciences (PUMS) Karol Jonscher Teaching Hospital: Department of Pediatric Oncology, Hematology and Transplantology, and Department of Paediatric Anaesthesiology and Intensive Therapy. Patients were recruited between December 2022 and October 2024.

Inclusion criteria for the study were age <18 years and treatment or prophylaxis with IV FLU administered according to the Summary of Product Characteristics (SmPC). The sampling procedure involved minimizing patient risk by collecting most of the blood samples at the time of scheduled biochemical assays (like complete blood count or CRP), routinely performed during hospitalization. Consequently, sampling times varied for all patients. Baseline demographic, biological, and clinical data were collected from medical patient records and included sex, age, body weight, height, body surface area (DuBois Method), the serum creatinine estimated glomerular filtration rate (eGFR) calculated using the Bedside Schwartz equation [23], eGFR calculated using the Schartz 2012 equation [24], bilirubin, total proteins, aspartate aminotransferase (AST), alanine aminotransferase (ALT), C-reactive protein (CRP), and procalcitonin (PCT).

2.2. Bioanalytical Methods

Blood samples (0.5 mL) were collected into lithium heparin tubes (BD Vacutainer®, Becton, Dickinson and Company, Franklin Lakes, NJ, USA) and then immediately centrifuged at 3000× g for 15 min to harvest plasma. Collected plasma samples were stored at −25 °C pending analysis. Fluconazole plasma concentrations were determined using our previously developed and validated method involving high-performance liquid chromatography with ultraviolet detection (HPLC-UV) [25]. The determination range was 0.5–100.0 mg/L.

2.3. Population Pharmacokinetic Analysis

Fluconazole concentration–time data were analyzed using PopPK modeling using the first-order conditional estimation with interaction (FOCEI) algorithm for non-linear mixed effects models implemented in the nlmixr2 R package [26]. One- and two-compartment structural compartment models with linear clearance (*Cl*) from the central compartment were tested. The interindividual variability (IIV) of PK parameters was assumed to follow a log-normal distribution. Proportional and combined error models were tested to describe the residual unexplained variability. Allometric scaling of the parameters was implemented according to the following:

$$CL = CL_T \times \left(\frac{WT}{70}\right)^{0.75} \tag{1}$$

and

$$V = V_T \times \left(\frac{WT}{70}\right)^{1} \tag{2}$$

where CL and V are the clearance and volume of distribution, CL_T and V_T are typical values for a 70 kg adult, and WT is body weight expressed in kilograms.

The covariate model was investigated according to the classic stepwise covariate modeling method [27]. Pearson's correlation test was performed to check for any relationships between random effects and covariates and whether they should be added to the model. Additionally, the mlcov R package was used to investigate possible covariates that should be considered during model development [28]. The effect of covariates was evaluated using the following equations.

For continuous covariates

$$\theta_i = \theta_{pop} \times \left(\frac{COV_i}{median_{COV_i}}\right)^{\theta_{cov}} \times e^{\eta_i} \tag{3}$$

For categorical covariates

$$\theta_i = \theta_{pop} \times e^{\theta_{cov}} \times e^{\eta_i} \tag{4}$$

where θ_i represents the individual parameter estimate, θ_{pop} is the population estimated value for this parameter, COV_i corresponds to the individual value of a covariate, θ_{cov} is the estimated effect of that covariate on the parameter, and η_i is equal to the individual value of the random effect associated with the parameter describing the difference between the population value of the parameter and the individual value of that parameter for the ith subject.

Model selection was based on a decrease of at least 3.84 points ($p < 0.05$) for 1 degree of freedom in the Bayesian Information Criteria (BIC), objective function value (OFV), the stability of the model, the precision of the parameter estimates, and the goodness-of-fit

(GOF) diagnostic plots evaluated at each step of the building process. The final model was assessed using Visual Predictive Checks (VPCs).

2.4. Simulations

Simulations of *f*AUC after the 6th dose (between 144 and 168 h) and dosing regimens based on the final model were performed in the rxode2 R package [29]. We tested 3–12 mg/kg in a 30 min infusion daily according to the dosages proposed in SmPC for prophylaxis of *Candida* spp. infections. Additionally, we tested alternatively higher 15 and 18 mg/kg doses. For each combination, 2500 virtual patients were simulated as 50 patients per group replicated 50 times, accounting for the same individuals among the simulated groups. An *f*AUC/MIC ≥ 100 was the PK/PD target, according to the European Committee on Antimicrobial Susceptibility Testing (EUCAST) [12,16]. Alternatively, a less rigorous PK/PD target (*f*AUC/MIC ≥ 50) was also investigated [17,19]. According to the EUCAST breakpoints for antifungals, we assumed an MIC = 2 mg/L for FLU as the highest MIC value of susceptible *Candida* spp. strains. [18]. The probability of target attainment (PTA) > 90% was considered an acceptable probability of success [30]. Assuming an FLU half-life of about 30 h and at least 5 half-lives to reach a steady state, for the PTA analysis we simulated the *f*AUC after the 6th dose (between 144 and 168 h) [4,18]. The free fraction of FLU was calculated based on the ~11% protein binding in the SmPC [4]. In addition, simulations for standard SmPC doses and the *f*AUC/MIC ≥ 100 PK/PD target with MIC values from 0.125 to 2 mg/L were performed.

3. Results

3.1. Study Population

A total of 35 plasma concentrations from nine patients were used. The average number of samples per patient was four, with a range of two and five. All concentrations were above the lower limit of quantification (0.5 mg/L) [25]. Patients received FLU in doses of 3–11 mg per kg of body weight as 0.5–1 h infusions once daily. The baseline characteristics of the studied population are presented in Table 1.

Table 1. Patients' characteristics (n = 9).

Characteristics	Number (%) or Median [Range]
Sex	
Female/Male (%)	6 (66.7%), 3 (33%)
Age (years)	9.75 [0.50–18.00]
Weight (kg)	28.50 [6.00–58.50]
Height (cm)	28.50 [74.00–178.00]
Body surface area, BSA (m^2)	1.14 [0.35–1.73]
Serum creatinine, S_{Cr} (mg/dL)	0.31 [0.18–0.59]
Bedside Schwartz eGFR (mL/min/1.73 m^2)	151.0 [115.5–240.3]
Schwartz 2012 eGFR (mL/min/1.73 m^2)	117.77 [95.31–170.03]
Bilirubin (mg/dL)	0.50 [0.19–1.55]
Total proteins (g/dL)	5.70 [4.80–6.87]
Alanine aminotransferase, AST (IU/L)	26.0 [14.0–77.0]
Aspartate aminotransferase, ALT (IU/L)	44.0 [8.0–139.0]
C-reactive protein, CRP (mg/dL)	0.34 [0.02–6.71]
Procalcitonin, PCT (ng/mL)	0.30 [0.04–1.92]

3.2. Population Pharmacokinetic Model

Plasma FLU concentrations are described by the one-compartment model with clearance from plasma. The allometric scaling, according to Equations (1) and (2), enabled the model to fit well. The proportional error model resulted in the best data fit. The final model estimates are presented in Table 2. The range of estimated *CL* values normalized for body weight is 0.31 mL/min/kg for a 58.5 kg patient to 0.55 mL/min/kg for a 6 kg patient. The estimated *V* value normalized for body weight is 1.49 L/kg.

The individual PK profiles of dose-normalized concentrations in time are presented in Figure 1. Similar regular and log-scaled graphs clustered according to dose group are presented in Figures S1 and S2. The VPC and GOF plots for the final model indicated a good description of the data and no major model misspecification. The points in the observed vs. predicted plots are symmetrically clustered around the line, indicating no evident trends. The residuals are distributed around zero, and most points are within the range of −2 and 2 (Figure S3). The VPC showed that most observed concentrations were within the predicted intervals (Figure S4). The nlmixr2 code of the final model along with graphs of the distribution of the residuals (Figure S5), the distribution of the individual parameters (Figure S6), the distribution of the standardized random effects (Figure S7), and the correlation between random effects (Figures S8 and S9) are presented in the Supplementary Materials.

Table 2. Estimates for the base and final population pharmacokinetic models for fluconazole.

Parameters	Mean Estimate (%RSE)
	A One-Compartment Model with Allometric Scaling (Final Model)
Clearance, *CL* (L/h)	1.24 (23.23)
Weight (kg), WT on *CL*	fixed 0.75
IIV on *CL* (CV%)	88.54
Volume, *V* (L)	104.07 (21.59)
Weight (kg), WT on *V*	fixed 1.00
IIV on *V* (CV%)	55.85
Proportional residual error (CV%)	25.19
BIC	208.82
OFV	126.72

BIC, Bayesian Information Criteria; CV%, coefficient of variation calculated as $\sqrt{\exp(\omega^2)-1} \times 100\%$; *IIV*, interindividual variability; OFV, objective function value.

In accordance with the assumptions of allometric scaling, the values of clearance normalized by body weight significantly decrease with increasing body weight, which best explains the course of the log-log regression curve. In contrast, the lack of significant correlation when *CL* is normalized based on body weight to the power of 0.75 indicates the validity of using allometric scaling of *CL* according to Equation (1) and compensating for the effect of body weight on *CL* (Figure 2).

A post hoc analysis of the effect of age on the *CL* of fluconazole showed a statistically significant decrease in *CL* with increasing age. The median *CL* for patients aged below the median age is 0.68 mL/min/kg, while for older patients it is 0.32 mL/min/kg. The effect of eGFR on fluconazole *CL* was not significant; however, differences in *CL* were observed according to an eGFR above or below the median. Patients with an eGFR below 117.9 mL/min/1.73 m^2 showed a median *CL* of 0.32 mL/min/kg, while patients with a higher eGFR had a *CL* of 0.56 mL/min/kg (Figure 3).

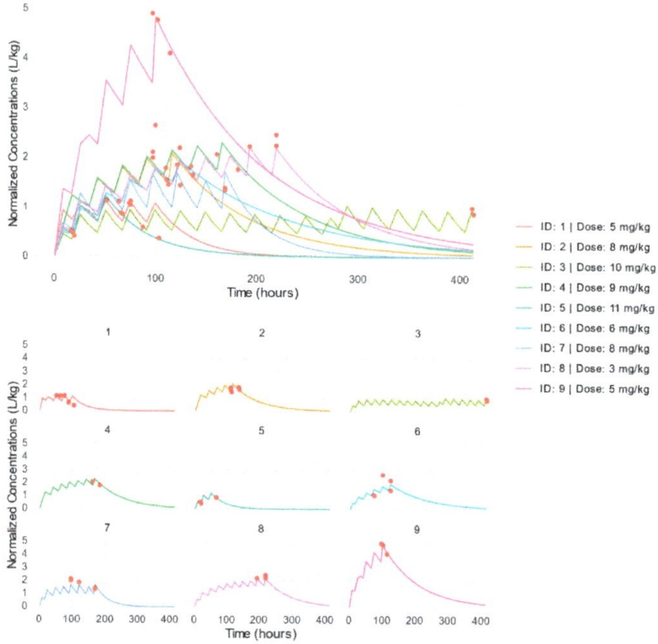

Figure 1. Clustered (**Top**) and separate (**bottom**) individual PK profiles of dose-normalized FLU concentrations versus time. Red dots indicate individual patient concentrations.

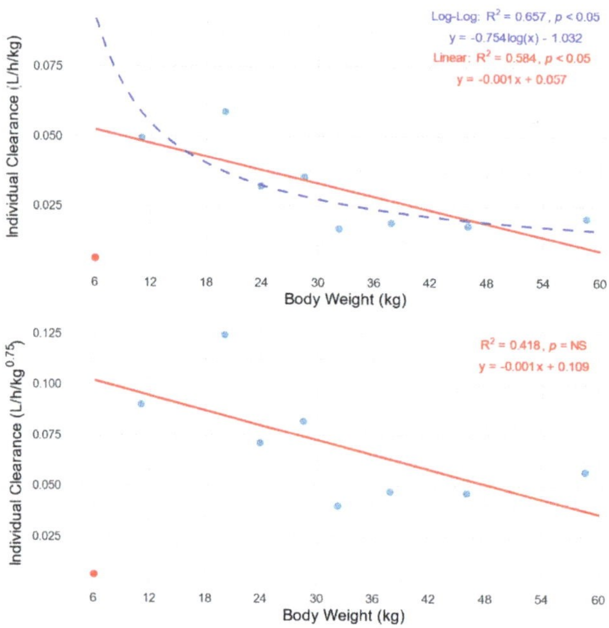

Figure 2. Relationship of body-weight-normalized clearances (CL/BW **top** and $CL/\text{BW}^{0.75}$ **bottom**) versus patients' body weight. The red lines represent linear regression analysis, while the blue dashed line corresponds to the log-log regression analysis. The blue dots indicate individual patients' values, while the red dot represents an outlier patient ID: 9.

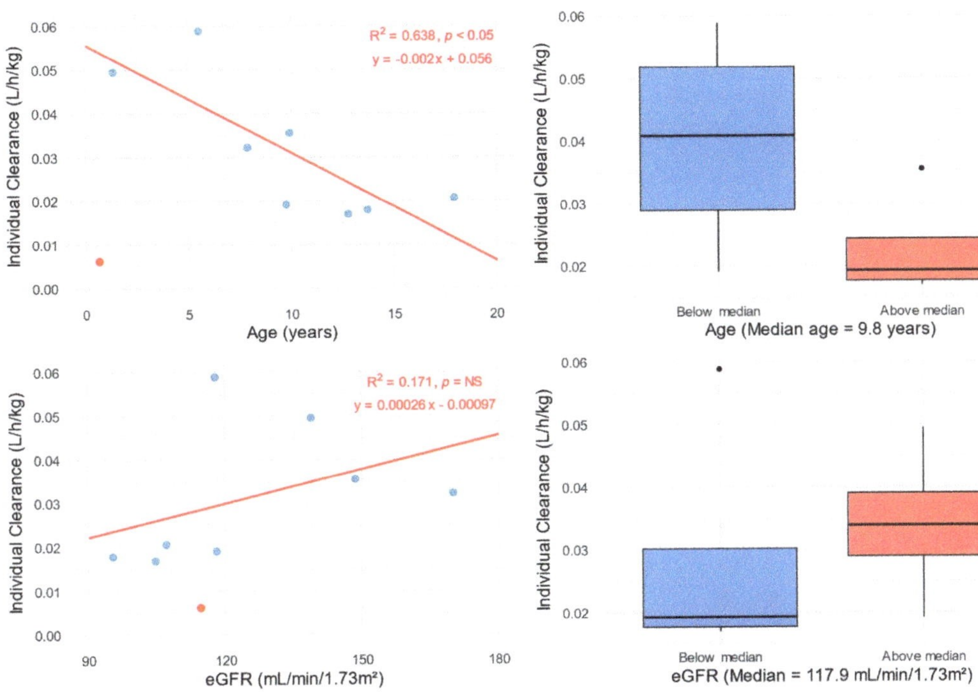

Figure 3. Total FLU clearance estimated from the popPK analysis and normalized for body weight versus age (**left top**) and calculated using the Schwartz 2012 equation eGFR (**left bottom**). Total FLU clearance estimated from the popPK analysis and normalized for body weight in relation to age group (**top right**) and eGFR group (**bottom right**). Patient ID: 9 was excluded from the analysis as an outlier (marked with a red dot). The blue dots indicate individual patients' values. Solid red lines represent linear regressions with fit (R^2), *p*-value, and equation values shown in the right corners of the graphs. The division into groups was based on the median of the analyzed variables.

3.3. Simulations and Probability of Target Attainment Analysis

The evaluation of the *f*AUC at a steady state indicates that children treated with low doses of FLU (3–5 mg/kg) were not able to achieve the intended therapeutic target (*f*AUC/MIC > 100, assuming *Canida* spp. MIC = 2 mg/L). Patients treated with intermediate (6–8 mg/kg) and high (9–11 mg/kg) FLU doses achieved an average of 256 and 328 mg × h × L^{-1} (Figure 4).

According to the dosing simulations, for the *f*AUC/MIC ≥ 100 target, already registered FLU dosages exceed the assumed 90% of PTA in the case of 48–60 kg patients treated with 12 mg/kg FLU dose. For the *f*AUC/MIC ≥ 50 target, the higher SmPC doses (9–12 mg/kg) enable the target PTA to be achieved. The simulation results for both PK/PD targets and MIC = 2 mg/L are presented in Figure S10. The PTA analysis of different MIC values of susceptible *Candida* spp. (0.125–2 mg/L) showed that at MIC values ≤ 1 mg/L, the FLU doses indicated in the SmPC are sufficient to achieve the target *f*AUC/MIC ≥ 100 (Figure S11).

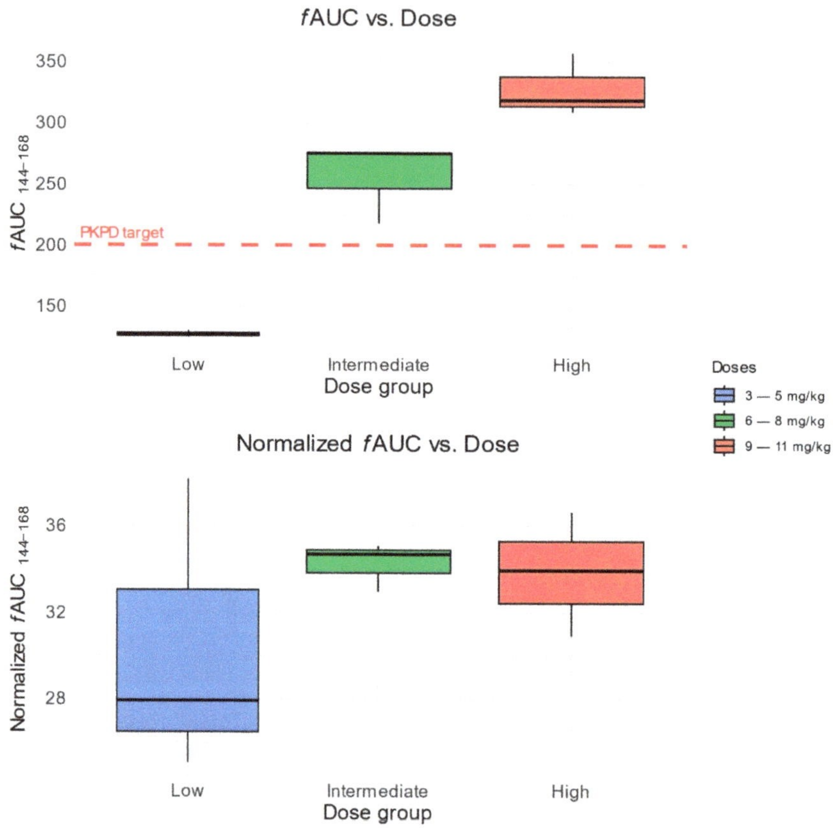

Figure 4. Predicted *f*AUC (**Top**) and dose-normalized *f*AUC (**Bottom**) in FLU dose groups. The red dashed line indicates the assumed PK/PD target (fAUC/MIC $\geq$ 100) for *Candida* spp. MIC = 2 mg/L.

4. Discussion

This may be one of the first FLU popPK models devoted to *Candida* spp. prophylaxis in hemato-oncologic pediatric patients. In addition to providing PK assessment, the PK model served as a tool to evaluate the effectiveness of FLU doses registered for the prophylaxis of *Candida* spp. infections. We found that the registered FLU doses < 6 mg/kg appear to be of limited value owing to resultant subtherapeutic concentrations. Consequently, higher doses (6–12 mg/kg) appear necessary in children.

The one-compartment model appeared adequate for our limited data. Adding a second compartment did not show a statistically significant improvement and even decreased the stability of the estimated parameters. The relatively small number of samples per patient and the unsystematized sample collection timing explained this. The opportunistic approach to sample collection limited sampling, and so increasing the number of recruited patients was not feasible in our study [31,32]. Nonetheless, given its implementation in most published FLU popPK models in different populations, the one-compartment model was sufficient to analyze FLU PK [2,7,15,30,33–40]. The estimated *CL* calculated per kg of body weight (0.018 L/h/kg for 70 kg adult) is consistent with previously published FLU pop models [30,34]. In turn, the estimated *V* per kg (1.49 L/kg) is higher (~50%) than published values for children or adults [3,30,34]. This may be a result of the underlying illness, administered chemotherapy, and/or hyper-hydration [14,41]. The increased *V* in pediatric oncology patients could explain the reduced FLU exposure observed in the Van Der Elst et al. study compared to other pediatric populations [14]. Nonetheless, the observed *V* needs to be confirmed in future FLU PK studies in similar patients.

The slope coefficient of log-log regression for the body-weight-normalized *CL* versus body weight equal to −0.754 is consistent with the assumptions of allometric scaling and the use of *CL* per kg scaling to the power of 0.75. Additional confirmation of the discussed assumption is the lack of a significant relationship between $CL/BW^{0.75}$ and body weight (Figure 2). This is in line with existing knowledge of allometric *CL* scaling in the pediatric population [42,43].

In general, according to the SmPC and FLU Product Label, children have a higher FLU *CL* than adults [4,44]. This is consistent with our results, where patients, especially those younger than the median age, showed a *CL* equal to 0.65 mL/min/kg. In the case of pediatric patients older than the mentioned median (9.8 years), the *CL* was lower (0.32 mL/min/kg) and closer to the *CL* for adults (0.23 mL/min/kg) reported in the Product Label [44]. Some trends were observed in the relationship between the body-weight-normalized *CL* and eGFR (Figure 3). In general, patients with an eGFR lower than 117.9 mL/min/1.73 m^2 (population median calculated using Schwartz et al. equation [24]) showed a lower *CL*/BW (0.32 mL/min/kg) than patients with a higher eGFR (0.56 mL/min/kg). The effect of the eGFR on *CL* is primarily due to the significant elimination of FLU via the renal route [4,44]. Indirect confirmation of our observation is also provided by previous PK FLU studies indicating serum creatinine as a covariate of *CL* [30,37,39,45].

The results of the *f*AUC simulations showed that low doses of FLU (3–5 mg/kg) are insufficient to achieve the intended PK/PD target and thus show unsatisfactory efficacy in the prophylaxis of *Candida* spp. infections. The PTA analysis results indicated the limited utility of the doses in the SmPC when it is necessary to achieve *f*AUC/MIC $\geq$ 100, assuming a *Candida* spp. MIC = 2 mg/L. In the case of a lesser PK/PD target (*f*AUC/MIC $\geq$ 50), the doses between 6 and 12 mg/kg were sufficient to achieve a PTA $\geq$ 90%. The need for higher dosages in the pediatric cancer patient population is consistent with the observations of Van Der Elst et al., resulting in recommendations for usage of 12 mg/kg doses in their hospital [14]. According to the PTA analysis, the MIC values > 2 mg/L make it impossible to achieve the PK/PD target (*f*AUC/MIC $\geq$ 100) with the FLU doses included in the SmPC. This observation is consistent with the data for *Candida* spp. susceptibility to FLU treatment presented in the latest "Breakpoint tables for interpretation of MICs for antifungal agents" established by the EUCAST [16,18].

The individual PK of patient ID: 9 stands out (Figure 1). The explanation most notably for the low *CL* (0.006 L/h/kg) was the patient's young age of 6 months. This is supported by the Fluconazole Product Label and pharmacokinetic studies conducted in infants [3,30,44,46]. The median *CL* reported by Watt et al. for non-ECMO patients aged 31 days to 2 years was 0.017 L/h/kg with a range of 0.008 to 0.029 L/h/kg. Thus, patient ID: 9 was excluded from the fitting analysis and is presented in the graphs as a red dot (Figures 2 and 3).

Our main limitation is the small number of patients and plasma samples per patient. This is due to difficulties in recruiting pediatric patients, which resulted in high refusal rates. A less critical limitation is the inability to determine the free fraction of FLU. However, binding to proteins at ~11% would have a minor impact on the PK of FLU. Given the above, we recommend caution in the clinical implementation of our study results. The raw data listed in the Supplementary Materials may help expand the knowledge of PK FLU in the search for optimal FLU therapy in the pediatric population.

5. Conclusions

Body weight implemented as allometric scaling influences the elimination of FLU, leading to the need for tailoring dosages to achieve the assumed PK/PD target for *Candida* spp. infection prophylaxis. As a rule, decreased weight (correlated with younger age) requires increased FLU doses per kg of body weight. Although the eGFR was not included as one of the covariates in the popPK model, indirect analysis confirmed its effect on fluconazole's CL as observed in studies to date. In general, doses < 6 mg/kg pose a risk of subtherapeutic concentrations and, as a consequence, higher (6–12 mg/kg) doses are recommended for hemato-oncologic pediatric patients. In turn, even higher than registered FLU dosages might be required to reach an fAUC/MIC $\geq$ 100; however, its safety has not yet been studied. The described approach does not apply to *Candida glabrata*, for which the MIC determining susceptible strains is < 0.001 mg/L [18].

Supplementary Materials: The following supporting information can be downloaded at https://www.mdpi.com/article/10.3390/pharmaceutics17040488/s1, Figure S1: Dose-normalized concentrations for each dose group versus time; Figure S2: Dose-normalized concentrations (logarithmic scale) for each dose group versus time; Figure S3: Goodness-of-fit plots of the final fluconazole one-compartment model; Figure S4: VPC plot of the final fluconazole one-compartment model; Figure S5: Distribution of residuals; Figure S6: Model parameter distribution; Figure S7: Random effects plots; Figure S8: Correlations of random effects; Figure S9: Correlations of random effects excluding outlier (marked in red); Figure S10: Probability of target attainment charts for fluconazole dosages 3–18 mg/kg, body weight 6–60 kg, and fAUC/MIC $\geq$ 100 (top) or fAUC/MIC $\geq$ 50 (bottom) assuming *Candida* spp MIC = 2 mg/L; Figure S11: Probability of target attainment charts for fluconazole doses 3–12 mg/kg, body weight 6–60 kg, and fAUC/MIC $\geq$ 100, assuming different *Candid*a spp MICs; nlmixr2 final model code; GitHub repository hyperlink.

Author Contributions: Conceptualization, A.A., K.D., A.B.-Ś., K.P., I.N.-W., A.C., W.J.J. and A.B.; methodology, A.A., W.J.J. and A.B.; software, A.A., W.J.J. and A.B.; validation, A.A., K.D., A.B.-Ś., K.P., I.N.-W., A.C., W.J.J. and A.B.; formal analysis, A.A. and A.B.; investigation, A.A., K.D., A.B.-Ś., K.P., I.N.-W., A.C., W.J.J. and A.B.; resources, A.A., A.C. and A.B.; data curation, A.A. and W.J.J.; writing—original draft preparation, A.A.; writing—review and editing, K.D., A.B.-Ś., K.P., I.N.-W., A.C., W.J.J. and A.B.; visualization, A.A. and W.J.J.; supervision, A.B.; project administration, A.A. and A.B.; funding acquisition, A.A., A.C., and A.B. All authors have read and agreed to the published version of the manuscript.

Funding: This research was funded by the Doctoral School of Poznan University of Medical Sciences in Poznan, Poland (grant number SDUM-DGB 01/04/2023).

Institutional Review Board Statement: This study was performed in accordance with the Declaration of Helsinki, approved by the local ethics committee (the Poznan University of Medical Sciences Bio-ethics Committee, decision number: KB-820/21, 3 November 2021), and registered at ClinicalTrials.gov (NCT05426499).

Informed Consent Statement: Informed consent was obtained from all subjects involved in the study.

Data Availability Statement: Data are contained within the article and Supplementary Materials.

Acknowledgments: Arkadiusz Adamiszak is a participant of the STER Internationalisation of Doctoral Schools Programme from the NAWA Polish National Agency for Academic Exchange No. PPI/STE/2020/1/00014/DEC/02.

Conflicts of Interest: The authors declare no conflicts of interest.

Abbreviations

The following abbreviations are used in this manuscript:

ALT	Alanine aminotransferase
AST	Aspartate aminotransferase
BIC	Bayesian Information Criteria
BW	Body weight
CL	Clearance
COVi	Individual value of a covariate
CRP	C-reactive protein
CV%	Coefficient of variation
CWRES	Conditional weighted residuals
eGFR	Estimated glomerular filtration rate
EUCAST	The European Committee on Antimicrobial Susceptibility Testing
*f*AUC	Area under the free drug concentration–time curve
FLU	Fluconazole
FOCEI	First-order conditional estimation with interaction
GOF	Goodness of fit
HPLC-UV	High-performance liquid chromatography with ultraviolet detection
IIV	Interindividual variability
MIC	Minimum inhibitory concentration
OFV	Objective function value
PCT	Procalcitonin
PK	Pharmacokinetic
PK/PD	Pharmacokinetic/pharmacodynamic
popPK	Population pharmacokinetic
PTA	Probability of target attainment
SCr	Creatinine serum
SmPC	Summary of Product Characteristics
TDM	Therapeutic drug monitoring
V	Volume of distribution
VPC	Visual Predictive Checks
WT	Body weight
ηi	Random effect
θcov	Estimated effect of the covariate on the parameter
θi	Individual parameter estimate
θpop	Population estimated value for the parameter

References

1. Janowski, M.; Demchuk, O.M.; Wujec, M. Fluconazole Analogs and Derivatives: An Overview of Synthesis, Chemical Transformations, and Biological Activity. *Molecules* **2024**, *29*, 2855. [CrossRef] [PubMed]
2. Chen, L.; van Rhee, K.P.; Wasmann, R.E.; Krekels, E.H.J.; Wiezer, M.J.; van Dongen, E.P.A.; Verweij, P.E.; van der Linden, P.D.; Brüggemann, R.J.; Knibbe, C.A.J. Total Bodyweight and Sex Both Drive Pharmacokinetic Variability of Fluconazole in Obese Adults. *J. Antimicrob. Chemother.* **2022**, *77*, 2217–2226. [CrossRef] [PubMed]
3. Bury, D.; Tissing, W.J.E.; Muilwijk, E.W.; Wolfs, T.F.W.; Brüggemann, R.J. Clinical Pharmacokinetics of Triazoles in Pediatric Patients. *Clin. Pharmacokinet.* **2021**, *60*, 1103–1147. [CrossRef] [PubMed]
4. Diflucan—Referral | European Medicines Agency (EMA). Available online: https://www.ema.europa.eu/en/medicines/human/referrals/diflucan (accessed on 4 January 2025).
5. Zhang, T.; Bai, J.; Huang, M.; Li, R.; Liu, Y.; Liu, A.; Liu, J. Posaconazole and Fluconazole Prophylaxis during Induction Therapy for Pediatric Acute Lymphoblastic Leukemia. *J. Microbiol. Immunol. Infect.* **2021**, *54*, 1139–1146. [CrossRef]
6. Carrasco-Portugal, M.d.C.; Flores-Murrieta, F.J. Gender Differences in the Oral Pharmacokinetics of Fluconazole. *Clin. Drug Investig.* **2007**, *27*, 851–855. [CrossRef]

7. Seay, R.E.; Larson, T.A.; Toscano, J.P.; Bostrom, B.C.; O'Leary, M.C.; Uden, D.L. Pharmacokinetics of Fluconazole in Immune-Compromised Children With Leukemia or Other Hematologic Disease. *Pharmacotherapy* **1995**, *15*, 52–58. [CrossRef]
8. Lee, J.W.; Seibel, N.L.; Amantea, M.; Whitcomb, P.; Pizzo, P.A.; Walsh, T.J. Safety and Pharmacokinetics of Fluconazole in Children with Neoplastic Diseases. *J. Pediatr.* **1992**, *120*, 987–993. [CrossRef]
9. Rajagopalan, P.; Pelz, R.K.; Lipsett, P.A.; Swoboda, S.M.; Rinaldi, M.G.; Hendrix, C.W. Enteral Fluconazole Population Pharmacokinetics in Patients in the Surgical Intensive Care Unit. *Pharmacotherapy* **2003**, *23*, 592–602. [CrossRef]
10. Turner, K.; Manzoni, P.; Benjamin, D.K.; Cohen-Wolkowiez, M.; Smith, P.B.; Laughon, M.M. Fluconazole Pharmacokinetics and Safety in Premature Infants. *Curr. Med. Chem.* **2012**, *19*, 4617–4620. [CrossRef]
11. Brammer, K.W.; Coates, P.E. Pharmacokinetics of Fluconazole in Pediatric Patients. European journal of clinical microbiology & infectious diseases. *Eur. Soc. Clin. Microbiol.* **1994**, *13*, 325–329. [CrossRef]
12. Patel, K.; Roberts, J.A.; Lipman, J.; Tett, S.E.; Deldot, M.E.; Kirkpatrick, C.M. Population Pharmacokinetics of Fluconazole in Critically Ill Patients Receiving Continuous Venovenous Hemodiafiltration: Using Monte Carlo Simulations To Predict Doses for Specified Pharmacodynamic Targets. *Antimicrob. Agents Chemother.* **2011**, *55*, 5868–5873. [CrossRef] [PubMed]
13. Van Daele, R.; Wauters, J.; Lagrou, K.; Denooz, R.; Hayette, M.-P.; Gijsen, M.; Brüggemann, R.J.; Debaveye, Y.; Spriet, I. Pharmacokinetic Variability and Target Attainment of Fluconazole in Critically Ill Patients. *Microorganisms* **2021**, *9*, 2068. [CrossRef] [PubMed]
14. Van Der Elst, K.C.M.; Pereboom, M.; Van Den Heuvel, E.R.; Kosterink, J.G.W.; Schölvinck, E.H.; Alffenaar, J.W.C. Insufficient Fluconazole Exposure in Pediatric Cancer Patients and the Need for Therapeutic Drug Monitoring in Critically Ill Children. *Clin. Infect. Dis. Off. Publ. Infect. Dis. Soc. Am.* **2014**, *59*, 1527–1533. [CrossRef]
15. Boonstra, J.M.; Märtson, A.G.; Sandaradura, I.; Kosterink, J.G.W.; van der Werf, T.S.; Marriott, D.J.E.; Zijlstra, J.G.; Touw, D.J.; Alffenaar, J.W.C. Optimization of Fluconazole Dosing for the Prevention and Treatment of Invasive Candidiasis Based on the Pharmacokinetics of Fluconazole in Critically Ill Patients. *Antimicrob. Agents Chemother.* **2021**, *65*, aac.01554-20. [CrossRef]
16. Brown, D. *Rationale for the EUCAST Clinical Breakpoints*; EUCAST: Växjö, Sweden, 2012.
17. McCreary, E.K.; Davis, M.R.; Narayanan, N.; Andes, D.R.; Cattaneo, D.; Christian, R.; Lewis, R.E.; Watt, K.M.; Wiederhold, N.P.; Johnson, M.D. Utility of Triazole Antifungal Therapeutic Drug Monitoring: Insights from the Society of Infectious Diseases Pharmacists. *Pharmacother. J. Hum. Pharmacol. Drug Ther.* **2023**, *43*, 1043–1050. [CrossRef]
18. Eucast: Breakpoints for Antifungals. Available online: https://www.eucast.org/astoffungi/clinicalbreakpointsforantifungals (accessed on 18 February 2025).
19. Pea, F.; Lewis, R.E. Overview of Antifungal Dosing in Invasive Candidiasis. *J. Antimicrob. Chemother.* **2018**, *73*, i33–i43. [CrossRef]
20. Andes, D.; Pascual, A.; Marchetti, O. Antifungal Therapeutic Drug Monitoring: Established and Emerging Indications. *Antimicrob. Agents Chemother.* **2009**, *53*, 24–34. [CrossRef]
21. Pappas, P.G.; Kauffman, C.A.; Andes, D.; Benjamin, D.K., Jr.; Calandra, T.F.; Edwards, J.E., Jr.; Filler, S.G.; Fisher, J.F.; Kullberg, B.-J.; Zeichner, L.O.; et al. Clinical Practice Guidelines for the Management Candidiasis: 2009 Update by the Infectious Diseases Society of America. *Clin. Infect. Dis.* **2009**, *48*, 503–535. [CrossRef]
22. Ashbee, H.R.; Barnes, R.A.; Johnson, E.M.; Richardson, M.D.; Gorton, R.; Hope, W.W. Therapeutic Drug Monitoring (TDM) of Antifungal Agents: Guidelines from the British Society for Medical Mycology. *J. Antimicrob. Chemother.* **2014**, *69*, 1162–1176. [CrossRef]
23. Schwartz, G.J.; Muñoz, A.; Schneider, M.F.; Mak, R.H.; Kaskel, F.; Warady, B.A.; Furth, S.L. New Equations to Estimate GFR in Children with CKD. *J. Am. Soc. Nephrol.* **2009**, *20*, 629–637. [CrossRef]
24. Schwartz, G.J.; Schneider, M.F.; Maier, P.S.; Moxey-Mims, M.; Dharnidharka, V.R.; Warady, B.; Furth, S.L.; Muñoz, A. Improved Equations Estimating GFR in Children with Chronic Kidney Disease Using an Immunonephelometric Determination of Cystatin C. *Kidney Int.* **2012**, *82*, 445–453. [CrossRef] [PubMed]
25. Adamiszak, A.; Czyrski, A.; Sznek, B.; Grześkowiak, E.; Bienert, A. The Application of the Design of Experiments and Artificial Neural Networks in the Development of a Fast and Straightforward HPLC-UV Method for Fluconazole Determination in Hemato-Oncologic Pediatric Patients and Its Adaptation to Therapeutic Drug Monitoring. *Pharmaceuticals* **2024**, *17*, 1679. [CrossRef] [PubMed]
26. Fidler, M.; Xiong, Y.; Schoemaker, R.; Wilkins, J.; Wang, W.; Trame, M.; Xu, H.; Harrold, J.; Denney, B.; Papathanasiou, T.; et al. Nlmixr2: Nonlinear Mixed Effects Models in Population PK/PD. 2024. Available online: https://nlmixr2.org/ (accessed on 6 December 2024).
27. Svensson, R.J.; Jonsson, E.N. Efficient and Relevant Stepwise Covariate Model Building for Pharmacometrics. *CPT Pharmacomet. Syst. Pharmacol.* **2022**, *11*, 1210–1222. [CrossRef]
28. Rebai, I.; Duval, V.; Akil, A.; Craig, J.; Talley, M.; Largajolli, A.; Fauchet, F. Mlcov: R Package for Covariate Selection Using Machine Learning. Available online: https://www.page-meeting.org/pdf_assets/10996-abstract.pdf (accessed on 17 February 2025).

29. Fidler, M.L.; Wang, W.; Hindmarsh, A.; Srinivasan, A.; Al-Mohy, A.H.; Denney, B.; Moler, C.; Cooley, D.; Schmidt, D.; Hairer, E.; et al. Rxode2: Facilities for Simulating from ODE-Based Models. 2025. Available online: https://nlmixr2.github.io/rxode2/ (accessed on 9 December 2024).
30. Watt, K.M.; Gonzalez, D.; Benjamin, D.K.; Brouwer, K.L.R.; Wade, K.C.; Capparelli, E.; Barrett, J.; Cohen-Wolkowiez, M. Fluconazole Population Pharmacokinetics and Dosing for Prevention and Treatment of Invasive Candidiasis in Children Supported with Extracorporeal Membrane Oxygenation. *Antimicrob. Agents Chemother.* **2015**, *59*, 3935–3943. [CrossRef]
31. El Hassani, M.; Liebchen, U.; Marsot, A. Does Sample Size, Sampling Strategy, or Handling of Concentrations Below the Lower Limit of Quantification Matter When Externally Evaluating Population Pharmacokinetic Models? *Eur. J. Drug Metab. Pharmacokinet.* **2024**, *49*, 419–436. [CrossRef]
32. Yan, D.; Wu, X.; Li, J.; Tang, S. Statistical Analysis of Two-Compartment Pharmacokinetic Models with Drug Non-Adherence. *Bull. Math. Biol.* **2023**, *85*, 65. [CrossRef]
33. Han, S.; Kim, J.; Yim, H.; Hur, J.; Song, W.; Lee, J.; Jeon, S.; Hong, T.; Woo, H.; Yim, D.S. Population Pharmacokinetic Analysis of Fluconazole to Predict Therapeutic Outcome in Burn Patients with Candida Infection. *Antimicrob. Agents Chemother.* **2013**, *57*, 1006–1011. [CrossRef]
34. Aoyama, T.; Hirata, K.; Hirata, R.; Yamazaki, H.; Yamamoto, Y.; Hayashi, H.; Matsumoto, Y. Population Pharmacokinetics of Fluconazole after Administration of Fosfluconazole and Fluconazole in Critically Ill Patients: Pharmacokinetics of Fluconazole in Critically Ill Patients. *J. Clin. Pharm. Ther.* **2012**, *37*, 356–363. [CrossRef]
35. Piper, L.; Smith, P.B.; Hornik, C.P.; Cheifetz, I.M.; Barrett, J.S.; Moorthy, G.; Hope, W.W.; Wade, K.C.; Cohen-Wolkowiez, M.; Benjamin, D.K. Fluconazole Loading Dose Pharmacokinetics and Safety in Infants. *Pediatr. Infect. Dis. J.* **2011**, *30*, 375–378. [CrossRef]
36. Leroux, S.; Jacqz-Aigrain, E.; Elie, V.; Legrand, F.; Barin-Le Guellec, C.; Aurich, B.; Biran, V.; Dusang, B.; Goudjil, S.; Coopman, S.; et al. Pharmacokinetics and Safety of Fluconazole and Micafungin in Neonates with Systemic Candidiasis: A Randomized, Open-Label Clinical Trial. *Br. J. Clin. Pharmacol.* **2018**, *84*, 1989–1999. [CrossRef]
37. Watt, K.M.; Benjamin, D.K.; Cheifetz, I.M.; Moorthy, G.; Wade, K.C.; Smith, P.B.; Brouwer, K.L.R.; Capparelli, E.V.; Cohen-Wolkowiez, M. Pharmacokinetics and Safety of Fluconazole in Young Infants Supported with Extracorporeal Membrane Oxygenation. *Pediatr. Infect. Dis. J.* **2012**, *31*, 1042–1047. [CrossRef] [PubMed]
38. Kim, Y.K.; Lee, J.; Oh, J.; Rhee, S.J.; Shin, S.H.; Yoon, S.H.; Lee, S.H.; Kim, H.S.; Yu, K.S. Population Pharmacokinetic Study of Prophylactic Fluconazole in Preterm Infants for Prevention of Invasive Candidiasis. *Antimicrob. Agents Chemother.* **2019**, *63*, aac.01960-18. [CrossRef]
39. Wade, K.C.; Wu, D.; Kaufman, D.A.; Ward, R.M.; Benjamin, D.K.; Sullivan, J.E.; Ramey, N.; Jayaraman, B.; Hoppu, K.; Adamson, P.C.; et al. Population Pharmacokinetics of Fluconazole in Young Infants. *Antimicrob. Agents Chemother.* **2008**, *52*, 4043–4049. [CrossRef]
40. Krzeska, I.; Yeates, R.A.; Pfaff, G. Single Dose Intravenous Pharmacokinetics of Fluconazole in Infants. *Drugs Exp. Clin. Res.* **1993**, *19*, 267–271.
41. Theuretzbacher, U. Pharmacokinetic and Pharmacodynamic Issues for Antimicrobial Therapy in Patients with Cancer. *Clin. Infect. Dis.* **2012**, *54*, 1785–1792. [CrossRef]
42. Germovsek, E.; Barker, C.I.S.; Sharland, M.; Standing, J.F. Scaling Clearance in Paediatric Pharmacokinetics: All Models Are Wrong, Which Are Useful? *Brit J. Clin. Pharm.* **2017**, *83*, 777–790. [CrossRef]
43. Meibohm, B.; Läer, S.; Panetta, J.C.; Barrett, J.S. Population Pharmacokinetic Studies in Pediatrics: Issues in Design and Analysis. *AAPS J.* **2005**, *7*, E475–E487. [CrossRef]
44. Diflucan—Product Label | U.S. Food and Drug Administration. Available online: https://www.accessdata.fda.gov/drugsatfda_docs/label/2011/019950s056lbl.pdf (accessed on 9 March 2025).
45. Momper, J.D.; Capparelli, E.V.; Wade, K.C.; Kantak, A.; Dhanireddy, R.; Cummings, J.J.; Nedrelow, J.H.; Hudak, M.L.; Mundakel, G.T.; Natarajan, G.; et al. Population Pharmacokinetics of Fluconazole in Premature Infants with Birth Weights Less than 750 Grams. *Antimicrob. Agents Chemother.* **2016**, *60*, 5539–5545. [CrossRef]
46. Nahata, M.C.; Tallian, K.B.; Force, R.W. Pharmacokinetics of Fluconazole in Young Infants. *Eur. J. Drug Metab. Pharmacokinet.* **1999**, *24*, 155–157. [CrossRef]

pharmaceutics

MDPI

Article

AmBisome® Formulations for Pediatrics: Stability, Cytotoxicity, and Cost-Effectiveness Studies

Guendalina Zuccari [1,*], Carla Villa [1], Valentina Iurilli [2], Paola Barabino [2], Alessia Zorzoli [3], Danilo Marimpietri [3], Debora Caviglia [1] and Eleonora Russo [1,*]

1 Department of Pharmacy, University of Genoa, Viale Benedetto XV, 16132 Genoa, Italy; carla.villa@unige.it (C.V.); debora.caviglia@edu.unige.it (D.C.)
2 UOC—Unità Operativa Complessa, IRCCS Istituto Giannina Gaslini, via Gerolamo Gaslini 5, 16147 Genoa, Italy; valentinaiurilli@gaslini.org (V.I.); paolabarabino@gaslini.org (P.B.)
3 Stem Cell Laboratory and Cell Therapy Center, IRCCS Istituto Giannina Gaslini, via Gerolamo Gaslini 5, 16147 Genoa, Italy; alessiazorzoli@gaslini.org (A.Z.); danilomarimpietri@gaslini.org (D.M.)
* Correspondence: guendalina.zuccari@unige.it (G.Z.); eleonora.russo@unige.it (E.R.)

Abstract: Liposomal amphotericin B (Ambisome®) is the gold standard for the treatment and prevention of fungal infections both in the adult and pediatric populations. The lyophilized dosage form has to be reconstituted and diluted by hospital staff, but its management can be challenging due to the spontaneous tendency of amphotericin B to form aggregates with different biological activity. In this study, the colloidal stability of the liposomes and the chemical stability of amphotericin B were investigated over time at storage conditions. Three liposomal formulations of amphotericin B at 4.0 mg/mL, 2.0 mg/mL, and 0.2 mg/mL were prepared and assayed for changes regarding the dimensional distribution, zeta potential, drug aggregation state, and onset of by-products. Our analyses highlighted that the most diluted formulation, kept at room temperature, showed the greatest changes in the aggregation state of the drug and accordingly the highest cytotoxicity. These findings are clinically relevant since the lower dosages are addressed to the more vulnerable patients. Therefore, the centralization of the dilution of AmBisome® at the pharmacy is of fundamental importance for assuring patient safety, and at the same time for reducing medication waste, as we demonstrated using the cost-saving analysis of drug expense per therapy carried out at the G. Gaslini children hospital.

Keywords: AmBisome®; liposomes; amphotericin B; hospital pharmacy; compounding; pediatric formulations; medicines for children; heath expenditure

1. Introduction

Amphotericin B (AmB) is a macrolide polyene obtained from *Streptomyces nodosus* effective against most clinically relevant fungal species. It is one of the oldest antifungal drugs; nevertheless, up to now it remains still the gold standard of antifungal therapy thanks to its broad-spectrum activity and absence of induction of resistance [1]. Its mechanisms of action have been extensively studied, and it is acknowledged that AmB forms pores in cell membranes leading to an electrolytic imbalance and loss of essential cellular components. This efficiency in permeabilizing cell membranes is associated with a greater affinity of the drug towards ergosterol than cholesterol, leading to a high cytotoxicity towards pathogens. However, to date, all the mechanisms involved are not fully understood, and several hypotheses have been put forward [2]. Indeed, AmB can enter the cells and trigger overproduction of reactive oxygen species (ROS); thus, the increased level of these free-radicals and the imbalance of ions produce multiple detrimental effects on the cellular components (membrane, mitochondria, proteins, and DNA), resulting in fungal cell death [3]. Unfortunately, severe toxic effects are associated with AmB administration, particularly towards red blood cells and kidney cells, and the balance between toxicity/activity seems to be ascribable to the spontaneous aggregation of the drug. It has been reported that the activity of the drug is tuned by the different states of aggregation of the molecule, which spontaneously self-assembles, forming aggregates that are more water soluble [4]. As depicted in Figure 1, the chemical structure of AmB can be divided into four parts: polyene chain, polyol chain, polar tail, and polar hydrophilic zwitterionic head encompassing the mycosamine moiety and the carboxyl group.

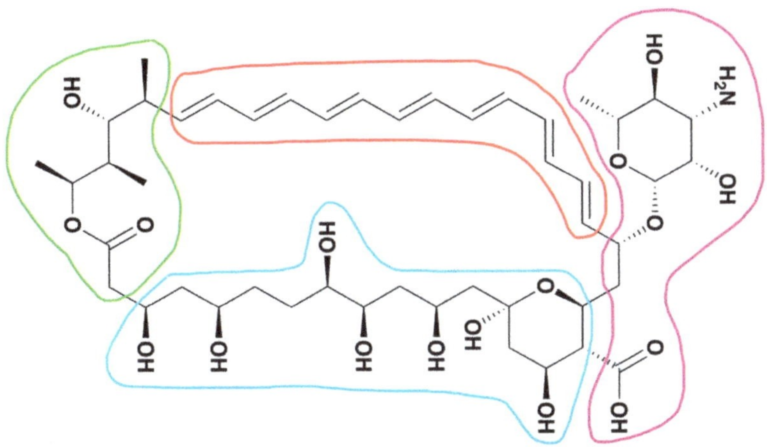

Figure 1. Chemical structure of AmB: polyene chain (red loop), polyol chain (light blue loop), polar tail (green loop), and zwitterionic head (purple loop).

Notably, at submicromolar concentrations, the monomers associate in oligomers, usually dimers, even though it is believed that they can contain between four and eight molecules of the drug [4]. Particularly, the drug's tendency for self-aggregation into dimers is driven by hydrophobic forces that lead to the formation of parallel or antiparallel dimers, while the dipole–dipole interaction between zwitterionic head groups is mostly irrelevant for the association of AmB monomers, even though it possibly modulates the parallel–antiparallel equilibrium [4]. Moreover, Zielińska et al., on the basis of previous studies [5,6], suggested that AmB monomers are capable of permeabilizing only fungal membranes, while AmB dimers are responsible for the side effects due to the interactions with cholesterol-rich membranes. Indeed, the double bond present in the lateral chain of ergosterol represents the structural element responsible for its higher affinity for AmB and consequently for its selective toxicity against fungi [6]. Particularly from studies on fungal membrane, it was found that AmB firstly binds to cell membranes and then forms complexes with ergosterol [7]. More recently, it was demonstrated that AmB–ergosterol complex spans a lipid bilayer with single-molecule length [8]. This result suggests that AmB's antifungal activity lies in its ability to form membrane pores due to aggregation of AmB–ergosterol complexes. Moreover, the effect of the aggregation state of AmB on its selectivity of interaction with ergosterol with respect to cholesterol was also demonstrated. The monomeric form (i.e., at concentrations $< 10^{-7}$ M, below the CMC) of AmB interacts selectively with ergosterol-containing and not with cholesterol-containing monolayers. On the contrary, above CMC, AmB can promote the extraction of cholesterol from the membrane and, thus, cause toxic effects. Rivnay et al. speculated that the monomeric form of AmB being present in negligible concentrations, as the drug is poorly soluble in both aqueous and highly hydrophobic media (membrane bilayers), its contribution to drug toxicity could be quite irrelevant [9].

Conversely, an increase in solubility associated with a reduction of toxicity was achieved with the transition from homo-aggregates (i.e., oligomers of pure AmB) to hetero-aggregates containing surfactants or lipids [10]. Such structures were found to be less likely to form pores in cholesterol-containing membranes, thus reducing the onset of adverse effects typically presented by the free drug. The first nano-formulation, marketed in 1958, was a combination of AmB with deoxycholate (Fungizone®); subsequently, in the 1990s, further efforts were made to ameliorate the therapeutic efficacy and lipid complex with two phospholipids (Abelcet®), liposomal AmB (AmBisome®), and colloidal dispersion with cholesteryl sodium sulphate (Amphotec®), which reached the market [10]. Simultaneously, researchers had been developing several nano-based drug-delivery systems such as polymeric nanoparticles, conjugates, lipid-based delivery systems, nano-emulsions, and nano-suspensions [11].

To date, among all the injectable formulations studied and proposed, AmBisome® is considered the gold standard for the treatment of visceral leishmaniasis and it is indicated for prophylaxis for invasive fungal infection in patients receiving immunosuppressive therapy, for empiric therapy in prolonged febrile neutropenia, invasive aspergillosis and candidiasis, and for the treatment of Cryptococcal meningitis in HIV-infected patients, both for the adult and pediatric populations [12]. In 2021, global sales of AmBisome® reached USD 540 million and are expected to amplify [13]. Although the increasing incidence of life-threatening infections and hospital-acquired infections are the major growth driver for the AmBisome®'s sales, the rising demand for targeted therapies together with the increasing number of approved indications are adjunctive factors that contribute to its high market success.

However, it should be stressed that liposomal AmB is difficult and expensive to manufacture and most of the global supply is produced by a single company. To drive down the price, bioequivalent formulations are under development, but, to date, no EMA (European Medicines Agency)-approved generic version is available on the market. As stated by the board of the European Confederation of Medical Mycology (ECMM), there is an unmet need in Europe and beyond for more affordable lipid-based AmB nano-formulations [14]. To support this requirement, EMA developed a product-specific document on the demonstration of equivalent efficacy and safety of a liposomal AmB formulation: "Liposomal amphotericin B powder for dispersion for infusion 50 mg product-specific bioequivalence guidance" [15]. Scientific experts have been questioning for a long time how to evaluate generic liposomal formulations. In this regard, in 2013, EMA released a reflection paper to support a marketing authorization of intravenous liposomal generic product [16]. In this context, several research works have been published to validate the comparability of liposomal formulations. Indeed, it has been already demonstrated that even if the qualitative and quantitative liposomal compositions are identical, the toxicity of the formulation could be higher than that of the originator if the manufacturing process is different, as seen for Anfogen® and Lambin®. The hypothetical reason for this difference probably lies in the existence of a significant difference in the drug aggregation state [9].

In recent years, despite the AmB therapeutic index having been improved by its encapsulation in the liposomal delivery system, concerns associated with the administration of this medicine still persist. The handling and managing of AmBisome® by health care staff can be challenging. One case has been reported of confusion between AmBisome® and Fungizone® which led to the rehospitalization of a 9-year-old patient [17], and the utilization of an order panel was encouraged for safe ordering and administration of AmB [18]. Although most are familiar with the high-alert and look-alike/sound-alike concerns, this medication poses other significant risks as well. Anaphylactic-like and infusion reactions have also been reported with all formulations of AmB [18]. In addition, AmB is incompatible with sodium chloride; therefore, it can be challenging to recall the appropriate sequencing of the hydration therapy. Another relevant issue is the pharmacoeconomic aspect related to the rational and cost-effective use of the liposomal formulation. On the basis of these considerations, from May 2022, the hospital pharmacy of the G. Gaslini Children Hospital (Genoa, Italy) considered restricting the preparation of AmBisome® to the pharmacy (i.e., vials unavailable in floor stock) with the aim to better preserve a check system, and to optimize dispensing and scheduling. It is well understood that the colloidal stability of nanoparticles is an important parameter that can directly affect the safety and the efficacy of the drug. For all these reasons, we evaluated the colloidal stability of AmBisome® under in-use storage times undertaken in the hospital pharmacy, thus supporting the attempt of the pharmacists to warrant clinical benefits to patients in a cost-effective manner. The aim of this research was to investigate the colloidal stability and the cytotoxic activity of AmBisome® formulations both in sterile water or in 5% glucose solution maintained at room temperature or at 4 °C up to one week from reconstitution, for better guiding the clinical use of AmBisome®. Chemical stability was also monitored by HPLC-DAD analysis to evaluate the possibility of extending the expiration date for use of AmB. Finally, we also analyzed the number of vials dispensed before and after the decision of using the pharmacist-provided medication therapy-management approach in order to establish if the procedure led to a minimization of the costs.

2. Materials and Methods

2.1. Materials

AmBisome® was purchased from Gilead Sciences Srl (Milan, Italy), sterile water was purchased from Eurospital S.p.A. (Trieste, Italy), and 5% glucose solution for infusion was from Fresenius Kabi (Isola della Scala, Verona, Italy). All solvents and reagents were of HPLC grade and purchased from Merck KGaA (Darmstadt, Germany).

2.2. Reconstitution and Dilution of Ambisome® in the Hospital Pharmacy

The reconstitution instructions and the procedures for dose adjustment are disclosed in the Summary of Product Characteristics (SmPC) agreed with Italian Medicines Agency (AIFA) [19]. Briefly, the lyophilized yellowish powder was reconstituted using 12 mL sterile water so as to have a drug concentration of 4 mg/mL AmB. Then, the liposomal suspension was vortexed for 30 s until aggregates dissolved and homogeneity was reached. The infusion to be administered in patients was obtained by transferring an aliquot of the suspension with a sterile syringe equipped with a 5 µm filter into an infusion bag containing 5% glucose whose volume had been previously adjusted so as to have a final concentration of drug ranging from 0.2 to 2 mg/mL, according to patient's weight (Figure 2).

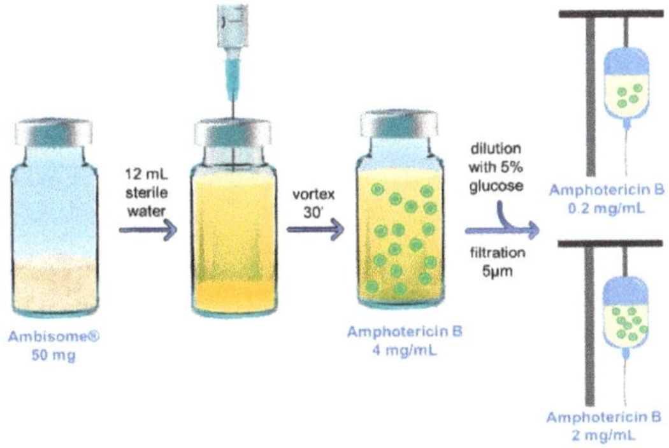

Figure 2. Sketch of reconstitution and dilution of the liposomal suspension to be infused in patients.

2.3. Sample Preparation

According to manufacturer's instructions, AmBisome® is a single-dose unpreserved sterile lyophilized powder that can be stored and administered without protection from light. Once reconstituted, the drug must be used immediately to avoid microbiological contaminations; modifications of in-use storage times and conditions are under the responsibility of the users. However, when the handling of the product is conducted under validated aseptic conditions, the manufacturer gives some indications. In Table 1, the in-use storage times after opening AmBisome® suggested by the manufacturer and those employed in the hospital pharmacy are summarized.

Table 1. In-use storage times after opening AmBisome® suggested by the manufacturer and employed in the hospital pharmacy.

Diluent	Concentration of AmB (mg/mL)	Maximum Duration of Storage at 4 °C		Maximum Duration of Storage at 25 °C	
		Manufacturer	Hospital	Manufacturer	Hospital
Water for injection	4.0	7 days	7 days	24 h	N [1]
5% glucose	2.0	7 days	24 h	48 h	N
5% glucose	0.2	4 days	4 days	24 h	N

[1] N = not in-use condition.

2.4. UV–Visible Spectrophotometry for Qualitative Analysis

The aggregation states of AmB can be identified using an UV–visible spectrophotometer (Evolution 300, ThermoFisher Scientific, Segrate, Italy), with a quartz cuvette with a path length of 1 cm. In order to determine the predominant aggregation state of Amb formulations under storage conditions, AmBisome® was reconstituted in sterile water and diluted as described above to obtain three formulations containing 4, 2, or 0.2 mg/mL AmB each. The resulting suspensions were scanned between 300 and 450 nm wavelengths at different time points (0, 1, 2, 3, and 7 days). The analysis was performed both on samples maintained at room temperature or at 4 °C. Three parameters were extracted for the characterization of the formulations: λ_{max} (main peak position, 322 nm); main peak width (at 2/3 height) reflecting heterogeneity of the species; and peak ratio. The ratio was calculated by dividing the absorbance of the first peak (322 nm), characteristic of the oligomer, by the absorbance of the fourth peak (416 nm), representative of the monomer [20]. The three liposomal formulations obtained after reconstitution and dilution with sterile water and 5% glucose (according to manufacturer's instruction) were further diluted with deionized water, prior spectrophotometric analysis, to 8.7–22.0 μM to assess the oligomer/monomer ratio. Data represent the mean ± SD of three independent experiments.

2.5. In Vitro Colloidal Stability of Liposomal AmB Formulations

Mean diameter (Z-average), polydispersity index (PDI), and zeta potential (ζ) of the liposomal formulations were recorded at 25 °C using a Malvern Nano ZS90 light scattering apparatus (Malvern Instruments Ltd., Worcestershire, UK) at a scattering angle of 90°. The apparent equivalent hydrodynamic radii of the liposomes were calculated using the Stokes–Einstein equation. For the measurements, aliquots of liposomal formulations were withdrawn and diluted when necessary to 0.2 mg/mL AmB with sterile water or 5% glucose solution according to the type of medium present in the sample. The results from these light scattering experiments were presented as the average values ± SD obtained from three different batches and carrying out three runs of ten measurements per sample. The in vitro colloidal stability of reconstituted formulations was also studied by Nanoparticle Tracking Analysis (NTA) using a Nanosight NS300 (Malvern) apparatus equipped with a 352 nm green laser, according to the manufacturer's software manual [21]. Briefly, samples were diluted in PBS to reach the ideal measurement concentration within a range of 20–100 particles per frame by preliminary tests. For this purpose, we found that samples had to be diluted 1:5 × 10^5. Camera level was increased until all particles were distinctly visible, not exceeding a particle signal saturation over 20%, and the ideal detection threshold was determined by limiting the blue crossings to 4 per frame. Each sample was measured 5 times with a syringe flow rate of 50 μL/s, at a cell temperature of 25 °C. To minimize data skewing based on single large particles, the number of completed tracks in NTA measurements was always above the minimum value of 1000. Data have been analyzed by the in-built NanoSight Software v3.4.4 and the final histogram of each sample is the result of an average of the multigraph of the five analyzes performed.

2.6. HPLC Assessment

Chromatographic experiments were performed by RP-HPLC analysis, with Hewlett-Packard HP1100 system (Palo Alto, CA, USA) consisting of a quaternary pump, continuous vacuum degasser, equipped with a Rheodyne 7125 manual sample injector and a Hewlett-Packard HP UV–vis diode array detector (DAD). A HP ChemStation data system was used for data acquisition and handling. Chromatographic separations were achieved using a LiChroCART Purospher Star RP18-e column (250 mm × 4.6 mm i.d.) (5 μm) (Merck, Darmstad, Germany) combined with a Merck LiChroCART 4-4 LiChrospher 100 RP18 (5 μm) guard column. Elution was carried out isocratically with a mobile phase acetonitrile:water (90:10, *v*/*v*) containing 0.1% trifluoroacetic acid, at a flow rate 2 mL/min, and an injection volume of 20 μL. Detection and chromatographic acquisitions were performed at 406 nm, and peak spectra were recorded by setting the diode array detector from 190 to 500 nm. Identification was carried out by comparing retention times (Rt) and UV absorbance spectra with the reference standard.

2.7. Cytotoxicity Studies

Human Embryonic Kidney (HEK) 293 were maintained in complete medium (Dulbecco's modified Eagle medium; Sigma, Livonia, MI, USA) containing 10% *v*/*v* heat-inactivated fetal bovine serum (Gibco-Invitrogen S.r.l., Carlsbad, CA, USA) and 50 IU/mL penicillin G, 50 μg/mL streptomycin sulphate, and 2 mM L-glutamine (all reagents from Euroclone S.p.A., Milan, Italy). In order to assay changes in cell viability after exposure to liposomal AmB formulations, HEK-293 cells were seeded in quadruplicate in a 96 w plate, 10,000 cells per well in 200 μL of complete medium. After 24 h, the medium was removed, and the cells were exposed for 24 h to: (i) fresh complete medium, (ii) different final drug concentrations (20, 50, 100, 150 μM) from three different stock liposomal formulations of AmB at 4.0 mg/mL (4.32 mM), 2.0 mg/mL (2.16 mM), or 0.2 mg/mL (0.22 mM), either prepared at the time (0 days) or prepared and used after 4 days and stored at two different temperatures, at 4 °C or room temperature (R.T., 25 °C), and (iii) only water for injection or 5% glucose corresponding to the volume collected from the three stock liposomal formulations (4.32, 2.16, 0.22 mM) to test the final drug concentrations of 20, 50, 100, 150, and 200 μM. The viability of HEK-293 cells was evaluated by CyQUANT® Direct Cell Proliferation Assay (Thermo Fisher Scientific, Life Technologies, Milan, Italy) in according to the manufacturer's instructions. Briefly, after 24 h of treatment, an equal volume of detection reagent was added to the cells in culture and incubated for 1 h at 37 °C. The fluorescence of the samples was measured using the monochromator-based M200 plate reader (Tecan, Männedorf, Switzerland) set at 480/535 nm.

2.8. AmBisome® Therapy Optimization: Cost-Saving Analysis

Health expenses, including costs directly related to treatments, are increasing in many countries due to the general progress in medicine that has led to an increase in the average age of populations. The optimization of medication distribution represents an opportunity to improve safety and reduce costs. Indeed, maximizing rational drug use is an important part of the drug control system. At the G. Gaslini children hospital (Genoa, Italy), until May 2022, AmBisome® was given through the nursing station and the pharmacy only supplied the drug to departments. In an attempt to minimize cost, medication floor stocks were removed, and individual prescriptions were managed only by the pharmacists. In order to quantify the amount of pharmaceutical expenditure, an analysis of the direct medical costs of administering AmBisome® was carried out before and after the establishment of the pharmacy-provided medication therapy management.

2.9. Statistical Analysis

All the experiments were performed at least three times. Concerning biological studies, each set of experimental conditions for assays was tested in 96-well plates and carried out in quadruplicate. Statistical analyses were determined by *t* test with Welch's correction two-tailed, or by two-way ANOVA with Bonferroni post hoc test, using GraphPad Prism 5 (GraphPad Software v5.0, San Diego, CA, USA). Differences were significant when p-value ranges were: * = $p < 0.05$, ** = $p < 0.01$, *** = $p < 0.001$.

3. Results and Discussion

3.1. UV–Visible Spectrophotometry

AmB possesses a very limited solubility in water at pH 7.4 (below 0.001 mg/mL), although at basic and acidic pH, its solubility is much higher (0.1 mg/mL). This is due to the ionization of the primary amine and carboxylic acid, but the consequent increase in drug degradation recommends its storage as a solid dosage form. For this poor water solubility, AmB has a high tendency to self-assemble in aqueous media by interacting with neighboring polyene chains. In this context, the monitoring and detection of an aggregation state is essential, because it is related to drug activity and toxicity [22]. As highlighted in previous studies, AmB monomers being highly unstable in aqueous medium, tend to gather quickly; it is supposed that the toxic effects (correlated to the increase in membrane permeabilization) could be affected by the presence of aggregates in solution [4], easily detectable by UV–visible spectrophotometric analysis. In this study, the monomeric state was identified by dissolving AmBisome® in methanol at an AmB concentration of 0.094 mg/mL (Figure 3 blue line), with a typical AmB UV–Vis spectrum, characterized by three main peaks at around 363, 383, and 407 nm. The methanolic spectrum mostly reflects the monomeric form of the drug, displaying two main peaks and a third peak of half intensity. Weak absorption peaks can also be observed below 350 nm. As aggregation takes place, absorption bands become prominent between 320 and 350 nm. Indeed, the spectrum of AmBisome® dissolved in water at 0.188 mg/mL showed a characteristic broad peak at 322 nm (Figure 3 red line), ascribable to the hetero-aggregates and three small peaks, typical of the monomeric state.

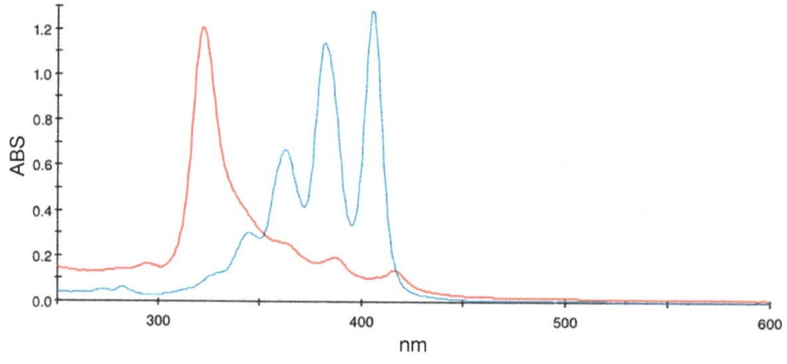

Figure 3. Representative UV–visible spectra of AmBisome® reconstituted in sterile water (0.188 mg/mL, red line) or methanol (0.094 mg/mL, blue line).

The ratio between the absorption intensity of the first peak (at 322 nm) and the fourth one (at 416 nm) can be used to monitor the aggregation state of AmB. In addition, monitoring the absorption spectra over time could be useful to reveal a drug release, as it can cause a modification of the drug aggregation forms in solution. Therefore, in order to establish if accidental leakage occurred after opening and dilution of AmBisome®, in this study, we checked the absorption ratio changing between peak 1 and peak 4. The spectral study was carried out for a week at storage conditions, in terms of temperatures, concentrations and media employed in order to monitor the aggregation state, and thus the physical stability of the formulations. According to the absorption intensity of the peaks, this ratio would be lower for a shift towards monomeric AmB forms and higher for a shift towards oligomeric AmB. Up to one week, all the liposomal formulations containing 4, 2, or 0.2 mg/mL AmB, respectively, kept at RT or 4 °C, displayed no variations in the main peak position, at λmax = 322 ± 1 nm, and the average peak width value was 10 ± 1, suggesting no differences in heterogeneity of species among all the tested formulations [9]. On the contrary, the peak intensity underwent a slight modification, as shown in Figure 4.

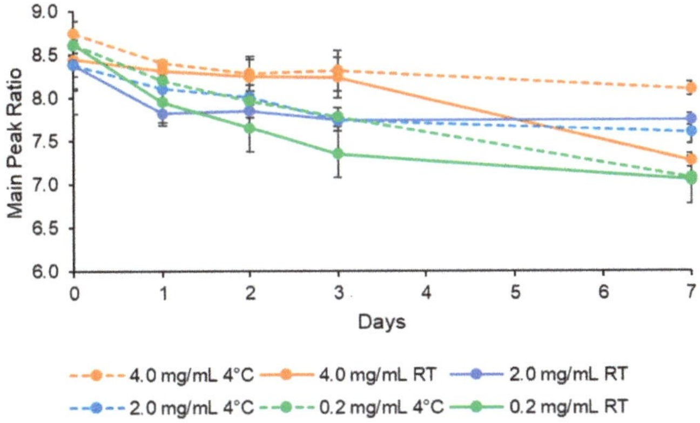

Figure 4. Changes in peak ratio over time under storage conditions. The ratio was calculated by dividing the absorbance of the first peak at 322 nm, characteristic of the oligomer, by the absorbance of the fourth peak at 416 nm, representative of the monomer. The results are reported as the mean ± SD (n = 3).

The freshly prepared liposomal formulations showed ratios ranging from 8.4 to 8.7, therefore nearly equivalent among each other. However, by increasing storage time after opening, the absorbance ratio between the first peak at 322 nm and the fourth peak at 416 nm decreases over time ranging from 8.1 to 7.1, reflecting some changes in the AmB aggregation state. The increment of the monomeric state occurred gradually and early after 24 h, more evident for the formulations kept at RT than those at 4 °C. Notably, the liposomal formulation at 0.2 mg/mL showed the highest ratio decrement, suggesting the greatest alteration in comparison to the other ones. To date, there are not comparable data in the literature, as a similar study has not been performed yet. Svirkin et al. observed a decrease in peak intensity at 415 nm after heating up to 70 °C, concluding that curing led to tighter aggregation and a decrease in drug release [23], while Liu et al. compared AmBisome® to some generical AmB formulations licensed in India and confirmed the influence of the manufacturing process on the aggregation state, drug release and toxicity [20]. However, they concluded that differences in manufacturing can induce alterations in the supramolecular structure and integrity of the liposomes, which in turn can increase the existence of free AmB, thus explaining the higher toxicity of equivalent formulations. Here, we observed a shift towards monomeric aggregates depending both on storage temperature and initial drug concentration. These changes could be related to a partial drug leakage, as corroborated by the studies of Svirkin and Liu. Indeed, in vitro release studies in clinically relevant media of AmB from AmBisome® revealed a fast drug release, characterized by a first-order kinetic model [24]. On the basis of these considerations, we hypothesized that the shift towards monomer formations followed the release of the drug from the liposome bilayer. Moreover, our samples showed neither any precipitates nor aggregation of liposomes during the period considered, as revealed by the size distribution analysis, suggesting that the arisen monomeric forms could subsequently generate the formation of new and harmful dimers in solution.

3.2. *In Vitro Colloidal Stability of Nanoformulations*

The colloidal stability of reconstituted liposomal suspensions is a prerequisite detrimental for the clinical use of AmBisome®. In this study, we assayed the size distribution, PDI, and zeta potential of nanoparticles dispersed in sterile water at 4.0 mg/mL AmB and then diluted with 5% glucose solution, reaching drug concentrations of 2.0 mg/mL and 0.2 mg/mL, according to the manufacturer's instructions. The study was performed on the three formulations at different time points: immediately after reconstitution or dilution, after 1, 2, and 4 days or 7 days under storage condition (4 °C). Notably, the solution at 4 mg/mL was kept in the fridge for up to 7 days, since the manufacturer granted for its stability for this maximum storage duration. It is important to note that the manufacturer recommends suspension filtration with a 5 µm filter, before dilution with a 5% glucose solution. The mean diameter of the freshly prepared formulations containing 0.2 mg/mL, 2.0 mg/mL, and 4.0 mg/mL AmB were 108.9 nm, 97.5 nm, and 91.9 nm for the samples, respectively (Figure 5). All liposomal formulations have mainly similar sizes around 100 nm with a polydispersity index of around 0.2.

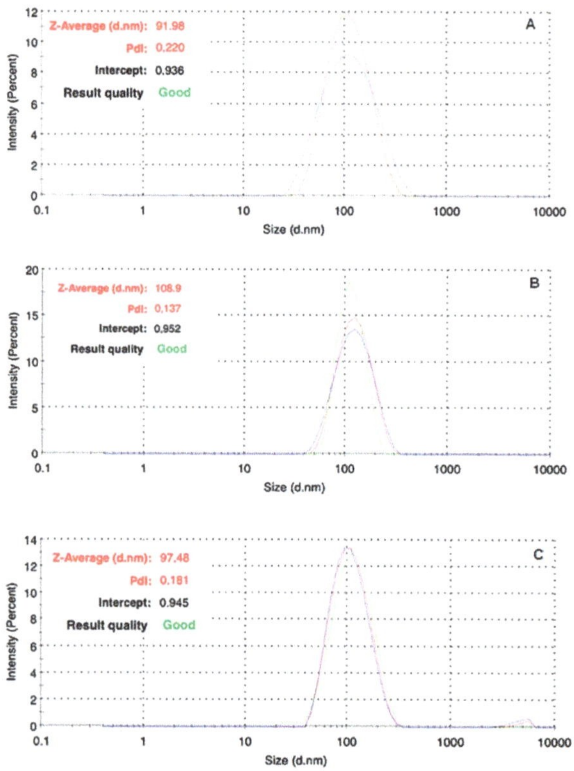

Figure 5. Representative size distributions obtained by DLS of freshly prepared liposomal formulations: (**A**) 4.0 mg/mL AmB in sterile water, (**B**) 0.2 mg/mL, and (**C**) 2.0 mg/mL AmB in 5% glucose solution.

These data are quite in agreement with those provided by Ye et al., whose findings showed an average diameter of 131 nm for a 1.0 mg/mL AmB diluted with a 5% dextrose solution [25], and more in line with the results exposed by Liu et al., which provided a value of 103 nm for the 4.0 mg/mL formulation [20]. As mentioned above, we monitored the properties of the liposomal formulations by DLS at specific time points to investigate changes occurring on the temporal scale. As reported in Table 2, the DLS technique did not evidence any significant variation within each type of sample stored at 4 °C up to 4 days or 1 week, thus confirming the high stability of the lipid bilayer of the delivery system. We furtherly prolonged the time of observation up to 14 days, but no significant changes were detected.

Table 2. Size distribution and zeta potential results of different liposomal AmB formulations detected by the DLS (dynamic light scattering) and NTA (nanoparticle tracking analysis) systems. Data represented as mean ± SD ($n = 3$).

Sample	NTA System				Dynamic Light Scattering			Storage at 4 °C
	Concentration (Particles/mL)	Mean Diameter (nm)	Mode (nm)	Percentile Values	Z-Average (nm)	PDI	Zeta Potential (mV)	Time (Days)
Liposomal AmB 4 mg/mL in sterile water	$3.94 \times 10^{13} \pm 1.43 \times 10^{12}$	87.0 ± 1.0	68.3 ± 0.7	D10 = 58.8 ± 0.2 D50 = 81.4 ± 1.1 D90 = 122.4 ± 0.8	91.9 ± 7.2	0.220	−32.6 ± 7.3	0
	$1.33 \times 10^{14} \pm 6.24 \times 10^{12}$	92.6 ± 1.1 *	75.8 ± 2.0	D10 = 64.2 ± 0.5 D50 = 84.0 ± 1.1 D90 = 135.2 ± 2.0	93.9 ± 5.2	0.189	−33.9 ± 6.7	2
	$1.28 \times 10^{14} \pm 6.81 \times 10^{12}$	104.0 ± 3.5 **	81.5 ± 2.5	D10 = 62.2 ± 2.2 D50 = 96.9 ± 3.3 D90 = 154.1 ± 3.7	92.9 ± 4.7	0.210	−32.4 ± 7.2	7
Liposomal AmB 2 mg/mL in 5% glucose	$8.47 \times 10^{13} \pm 1.80 \times 10^{12}$	89.7 ± 1.4	75.4 ± 0.8	D10 = 63.6 ± 1.9 D50 = 82.5 ± 0.8 D90 = 128.7 ± 1.7	97.5 ± 8.4	0.181	−41.4 ± 10.9	0
	$7.06 \times 10^{13} \pm 1.43 \times 10^{12}$	91.9 ± 0.3	78.9 ± 3.2	D10 = 64.0 ± 0.9 D50 = 87.3 ± 0.5 D90 = 125.3 ± 0.8	102.2 ± 4.6	0.150	−42.0 ± 11.5	1
	$8.18 \times 10^{12} \pm 2.11 \times 10^{11}$	90.9 ± 1.2	79.3 ± 0.8	D10 = 66.2 ± 2.1 D50 = 84.6 ± 0.7 D90 = 127.1 ± 3.2	99.3 ± 5.2	0.146	−42.2 ± 10.9	2
	$8.80 \times 10^{13} \pm 1.68 \times 10^{12}$	85.1 ± 0.6 *	73.6 ± 0.3	D10 = 62.2 ± 0.6 D50 = 79.5 ± 0.6 D90 = 117.0 ± 2.6	99.3 ± 6.5	0.160	−40.9 ± 10.7	4
Liposomal AmB 0.2 mg/mL in 5% glucose	$9.48 \times 10^{12} \pm 3.17 \times 10^{11}$	91.1 ± 1.1	78.8 ± 2.5	D10 = 63.5 ± 1.1 D50 = 87.0 ± 0.8 D90 = 130.0 ± 2.6	108.9 ± 7.1	0.137	−44.4 ± 15.9	0
	$9.19 \times 10^{12} \pm 1.92 \times 10^{11}$	87.6 ± 0.3	77.3 ± 2.1	D10 = 63.9 ± 0.4 D50 = 82.7 ± 0.6 D90 = 118.1 ± 1.9	112.4 ± 5.6	0.136	−45.9 ± 14.5	1
	$8.20 \times 10^{12} \pm 6.82 \times 10^{10}$	90.7 ± 0.5	77.0 ± 1.8	D10 = 64.9 ± 0.9 D50 = 83.2 ± 0.5 D90 = 131.2 ± 1.2	109.2 ± 8.2	0.133	−46.5 ± 13.9	2
	$7.47 \times 10^{12} \pm 2.62 \times 10^{11}$	88.6 ± 0.6	75.9 ± 1.4	D10 = 64.5 ± 0.7 D50 = 82.8 ± 0.9 D90 = 124.0 ± 2.7	109.0 ± 6.5	0.131	−45.7 ± 16.0	4

* $p < 0.05$, ** $p < 0.01$.

When analyzed by NTA, the same formulations always had a mean diameter slightly smaller than that determined by DLS (Table 2, Figure S1). This result is in contrast with the findings of Liu et al. [20], whose study revealed always larger values for NTA-based measurements. This slight discrepancy among the two research studies may lie in the difficulty in characterizing nano-systems like liposomes linked to the complexity of manufacturing processes and reproducibility of the scale-up, all factors that may influence the uniformity of the batches. Moreover, while the sizes remained similar over time for the two formulations diluted in 5% glucose, the liposomal AmB 4 mg/mL suspension showed an increase in the diameter from 87 nm to 104 nm. This increase in diameter could be related to the external osmotic pressure to which the liposomes are subjected, being dispersed in a hypotonic medium (sterile water) [26]. Regarding the superficial electric charge measured by DLS, we found that the zeta potential hardly changed with time within 4 days or 1 week (Table 2, Figure S2). AmBisome® consists of three lipids: hydrogenated soybean phosphatidylcholine (HSPC), distearoyl phosphatidylglycerol (DSPG), and cholesterol. DSPG is an anionic phospholipid, while HSPC and AmB are zwitterionic molecules; therefore, the surface of the liposomes became negatively charged, like most liposomal products on the market. This negative net charge assures colloidal stability and avoids flocculation processes. In fact, during the time period considered, we observed neither formation of precipitates due to drug desolvation, nor clusters of nanoparticles as confirmed by NTA. In this study, the number of particles in suspension remained almost constant or at least of the same magnitude order for each sample, highlighting the high stability of the supramolecular structure of the liposomes.

3.3. HPLC Analysis

It has been reported that AmB suffers from degradation when exposed to light, heat, radical initiators, and extreme pH conditions. The by-products have not been isolated yet, but the most probable reactions involve the highly conjugated polyene backbone, similar to a lipid oxidation [27]. Moreover, previous studies suggested that the degradation products may increase drug toxicity, such as acute hemolysis [28]. The chromatographic conditions used in this study were based on those reported by Espada et al., with some changes [29]. The detection wavelength for AmB and its related impurities, eventually present during in-use conditions storage, was set at 406 nm, as already proposed for the detection of some degradation products [27]. Linearity was maintained with stock solutions in methanol ranging from 38 to 360 μg/mL AmB. The calibration curve was generated from the average peak areas from three independent experiments, and the regression equation of the line was ($Y = 32985X + 120.07$) with a correlation coefficient of 0.9999 (Figure S3). With the chromatographic conditions adopted, the main peak of AmB appeared around 7.5632 ± 0.1782 min (Figure S4).

In order to determine if the different AmB formulations containing 4.0, 2.0, or 0.2 mg/mL AmB underwent some degradative reactions under storage conditions, HPLC-DAD analyses were performed on AmB samples after 1, 2, 3, and 7 days from the reconstitution of the lyophilized sample. Since at hospital the AmBisome® formulations, managed by the pharmacists for dose adjustments and administration to different patients, were stored in a fridge, we selected 4 °C for our stability studies. The study of recorded chromatograms, peak identity, and peak purity up to 7 days did not show any remarkable variation from the freshly prepared formulations (Figure 6), thus confirming that just storing the drug at 4 °C prevents chemical reactions and by-product formation. However, during the time period considered, the chemical stability shown by the drug in these conditions did not correspond to an unmodified aggregation state, as revealed by spectrophotometric analysis. This behavior suggests that, when the drug is kept in solution, its rearrangement (intercalated or outside the phospholipid by-layer) does not affect any chemical modifications of the molecule.

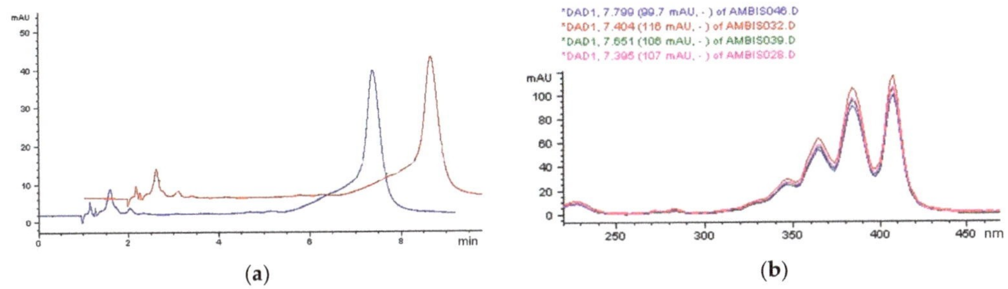

Figure 6. (**a**) Representative HPLC chromatograms of freshly prepared 4.0 mg/mL AmB in sterile water (blue line) and after 7 days (red line). (**b**) Overlaid UV–Vis spectra of AmB peak (Rt = 7.5632 min) obtained by DAD related to freshly prepared 4.0 mg/mL AmB suspension in sterile water (blue line), 0.2 mg/mL AmB in 5% glucose solution (pink line) and after 7 days at 4 °C (red line and green lines, respectively).

3.4. In Vitro Toxicity Evaluation of AmB Formulations

The in vitro toxicity of the three freshly prepared liposomal formulations, containing AmB 4.0 mg/mL (4.32 mM) in sterile water, or AmB 2.0 mg/mL (2.16 mM) in 5% glucose solution, or AmB 0.2 mg/mL (0.22 mM) in 5% glucose solution, were evaluated in HEK-293 cells due to the high incidence of nephrotoxicity exerted by AmB. We performed for the first time a time- and dose-dependent study on cell viability of the liposomal AmB formulations as they are prepared in the hospital pharmacy and then administered to patients, aiming to investigate if the handling and the storage time could exert some unexpected drug effects. Firstly, the cells were exposed for 24 h to freshly prepared formulations with or without the drug to assess if the variation in the concentration of the medium constituents could be responsible itself for some toxic effects or for a decrease in cell proliferation. Therefore, the cells were exposed to the same volume of buffer (sterile water or 5% glucose) present in the loaded formulations to evaluate possible alterations in cell viability linked to osmotic effects or lack of nutrients. As shown in Figure 7, the presence of the buffer reduces in a significative manner the cell vitality only in the case of 0.22 mM AmB formulation for a drug concentration of 200 μM. In this case, to reach that concentration of drug, the volume of the buffer added was at its highest level in comparison with the other samples. On the contrary, at all the other concentrations tested and for the other two formulations, the effects on survival rate are ascribable always to the presence of the drug. Notably, among the liposomal AmB formulations, the AmB 2.16 mM began to be toxic at 50 μM, while maintaining the same level of toxicity also at the subsequent concentrations tested, suggesting a non-dose-dependent mechanism. The formulation of AmB 4.32 mM in sterile water seems less toxic, as it exerted a slight influence on cell vitality only at 100 μM. On the contrary, the less concentrated AmB liposomal formulation (0.22 mM) showed a remarkable toxicity at the maximum concentration tested, but this effect is attributable to the excess of solvent added. Therefore, these results highlighted some differences among the formulations regarding their biological activity. It is noteworthy that the encapsulation of the drug into the liposome bilayer significantly reduces AmB cytotoxicity; indeed, the free drug is highly cytotoxic (>80% cell death) at a concentration of about 2 μM [30]. However, our study demonstrated that the liposomal formulations are not equivalent from the toxicological point of view. In fact, at the same drug concentration, the effects of the three liposomal formulations are different. If we exclude the highest drug concentration (200 μM) at which the effect of the excessive presence of solvent is not negligible, for all other concentrations the toxicity of the liposomal formulation follows the order AmB 4.32 mM < AmB 0.22 mM < AmB 2.16 mM. These results give a new insight into the safety of using nanosized drug-delivery systems, confirming the difficulties of standardization of liposomes [31].

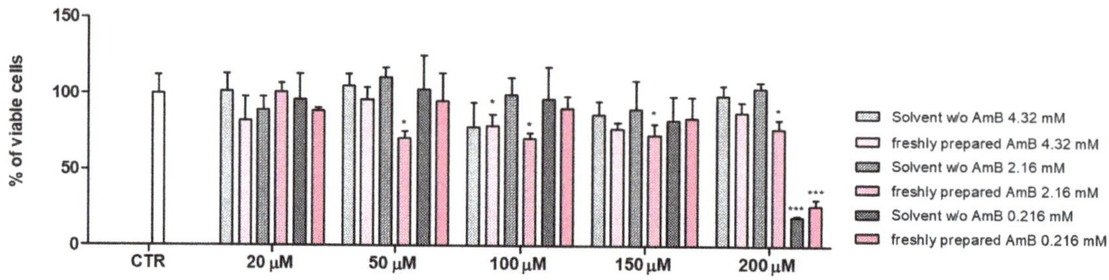

Figure 7. Three different stock concentrations of formulations containing AmB 4.32 mM, 2.16 mM, or 0.22 mM were prepared and used at different final drug concentrations 20, 50, 100, and 150 μM to treat HEK-293 cells for 24 h. Equivalent amounts of solvent without drug were used as blanks for each sample tested. Data were acquired by the use of the TECAN microplate reader, Infinite 200 (Tecan Life Sciences) set (i.e., 480/535 nm). Data are expressed as the mean ± SD of three independent experiments (* $p < 0.05$, *** $p < 0.001$ vs. CTR). CTR—control; μM—micromolar; mM—millimolar; h—hours.

In order to verify if storage conditions could further alter the biological activity of AmBisome®, we treated the cells for 24 h with the three liposomal formulations maintained for 4 days in the fridge or at RT On the basis of the results of the previous experiment, we selected only the concentrations whose blanks could not interfere with the results, therefore the 200 μM drug concentration was excluded. As shown in Figure 8, the cytotoxicity of the formulations was influenced by the storage temperature, and generally, the suspensions stored at RT were always more cytotoxic in comparison with those maintained in the fridge. Notably, the discrepancy between the storage at RT and at 4 °C was significantly more remarkable at the highest concentration (150 μM) for the formulations of AmB 4.32 mM in sterile water and for AmB 2.16 mM in 5% glucose. Probably, at the highest concentrations, the amount of free drug present in solution increases, reaching the capability of forming dimers. Indeed, when only monomers are present in solution, the drug affects only ergosterol-rich membranes, and it is less toxic. Conversely, the onset of dimerization, which is estimated to occur early at about 0.41 μM, reduces drug selectivity and increases drug toxicity towards mammalian cells [32]. Therefore, we can deduce that, at R.T., a more markedly drug leakage occurs; consequently, it is recommended not to leave the formulations outside the fridge. Curiously, the less concentrated formulation (AmB 0.22 mM) had a different behavior. In this case, the onset of a significant toxicity started at 50 μM for the sample maintained at RT and at 100 μM for the sample maintained at 4 °C. These data highlight the greater stability of the supramolecular system when stored at low temperatures, as revealed also by spectrophotometric analysis, but also show a remarkable difference among the three formulations. Particularly, it was evident that the 0.22 mM formulation after 4 days of storage was more effective in reducing cell vitality. Since the AmB toxicity is always related to its rearrangement in solution, the presence of free form of the drug outside the liposome's bilayer may be the main cause of the detrimental effect exerted on the cell viability by the drug. Our data indicate that the most diluted suspension was also the most toxic, probably due to its greater colloidal instability. These results are consistent with those obtained from the spectrophotometric analysis, which revealed that the AmBisome® dilution to the lowest concentration employed in the clinical administration was characterized by the presence of greater changes in the aggregation state. The influence of dilution on the colloidal stability of a supramolecular system is well recognized [33]. In addition, the greater instability of the most diluted formulation is consistent with the indications of storage reported in the SmPC, where it is stated that the stability at 4 °C is granted up to 7 days for AmB 4.32 mM and 2.16 mM, and only up to 4 days for AmB 0.22 mM formulation (Table 1). We confirmed that the dilution by ten times can transform the AmBisome® suspension into a less safe formulation. Consequently, pharmacists have to pay more attention to the clinical administrations involving the youngest patients, who need low dosages. In summary, it would be better to consume the more diluted formulations in a shorter period of time, considering that they are administered to the more vulnerable patients.

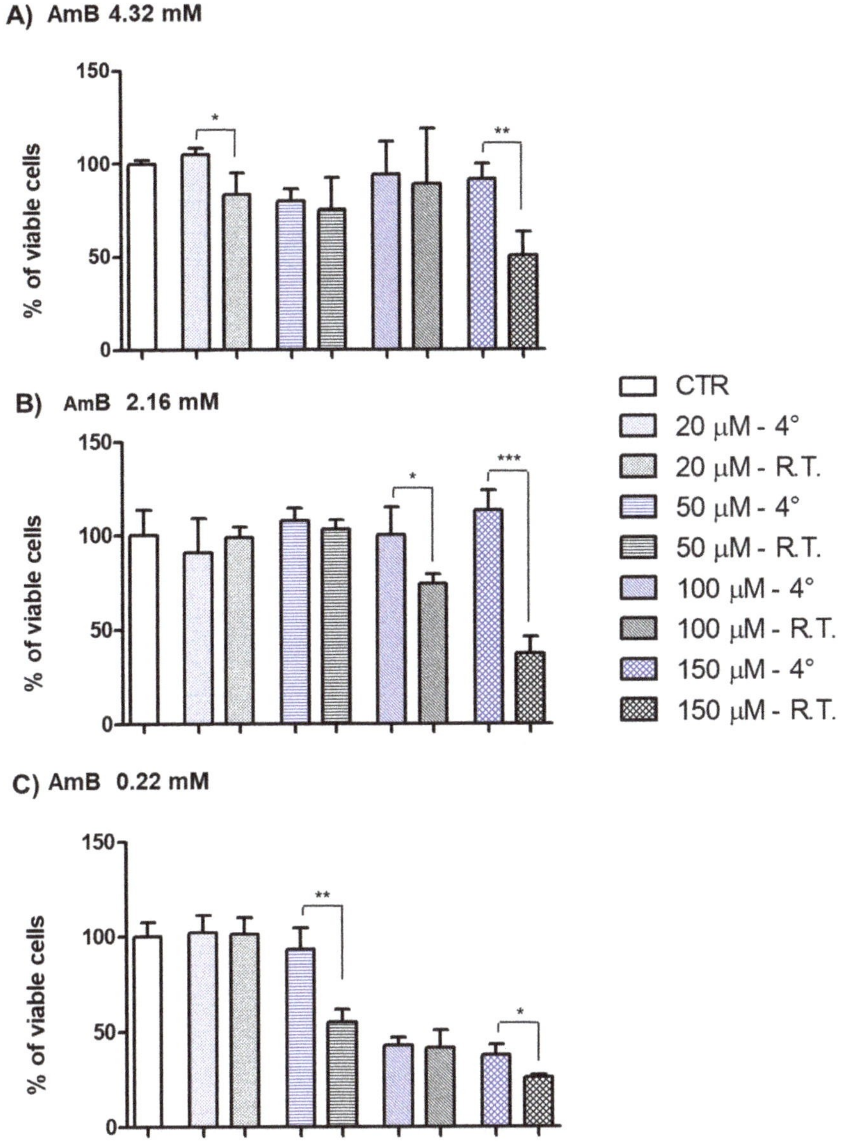

Figure 8. Three different stock concentrations of liposomal formulations containing (**A**) 4.32 mM, (**B**) 2.16 mM, or (**C**) 0.22 mM AmB were prepared and stored for 4 days at 4° (blue bars) or RT (black bars), and used at different final drug concentrations of 20, 50, 100, and 150 µM to treat HEK-293 cells for 24 h. Data were acquired using the TECAN microplate reader, Infinite 200 (Tecan Life Sciences) set (i.e., 480/535 nm). Data are expressed as the mean ± SD of three independent experiments (* $p < 0.05$, ** $p < 0.01$, *** $p < 0.001$, of 4 °C vs. RT for each final concentration). CTR—control; µM—micromolar; mM—millimolar; h—hours.

3.5. The Impact of the Centralized Compounding of AmBisome® at the G. Gaslini Children Hospital Pharmacy

The shifts towards personalized medicines on the one hand and the pressure on national health budgets and the shortage of medicines on the other have increased more and more, compounding the activity of the hospital pharmacy [34]. Among the procedures carried out by the pharmacists, the reconstitution of intravenous medicines, such as anti-infectives, analgesics, and anti-emetics represent one of the most frequent activities. Moreover, the European Association of Hospital Pharmacists (EAHP) has greatly encouraged the involvement of hospital pharmacies in reconstitution practices and in the creation of a centralized reconstitution unit, according to the Council of Europe resolution on good reconstitution practices in healthcare establishments for medicinal products for parenteral use [35]. The tasks of the hospital pharmacist in this regard include risk management, supervision of the work quality, and overall work planning.

AmBisome®'s relatively frequent use is related to its broad spectrum of activity and the limited number of alternatives, as only a few antifungal agents are licensed for use in children. Published multicenter experiences have demonstrated that liposomal AmB is the preferred antifungal choice for probable and proven invasive fungal disease in pediatric patients [36]. The safety and efficacy of AmBisome® has been established in pediatric patients aged between one month to 18 years old. Dosages can be calculated on the same per-kg body weight basis as for adults, and the maximum tolerated dose is 10 mg/kg/day, but with an increasing occurrence of hypokalemia and infusion-related vomiting with doses above 5 mg/kg/day [37].

For better monitoring of the routine drug prescriptions and to face the necessity of addressing the medication to the patient needs, the pharmacy of the G. Gaslini children hospital has opted for the centralized preparation of AmBisome® since May 2022. It has been demonstrated that the supervision of hospital pharmacists in the preparation of ready-to-administer products plays an important role in improving quality of care, patient safety, and cost saving [38]. Prior to May 2022, the reconstitution of the drug could take place on the ward. Our aim was to evaluate if the strategy of centralization would lead to a cost-effective drug, by means of waste-reduction, without any detrimental effects on patient care.

The expenditure associated with AmBisome® utilization is a direct and variable cost, depending on patient volume. For the quantification of the direct cost associated with AmBisome®, data were gathered before and after the centralization of the drug preparation. Firstly, we collected data regarding the number of vials used for all ongoing and set up therapies (Table 3). Then, we calculated the mean number of vials of AmBisome® employed per therapy, dividing the number of vials used by the number of treatments provided monthly. Then, the cost per treatment was obtained by multiplying the number of vials per treatment by the cost of 1 unit of AmBisome® at the price purchased by the hospital pharmacy (EUR 146.80). As shown in Table 3, when the medication was distributed by a ward stock system, the cost per treatment was EUR 814.74; meanwhile, when the reconstitution of the drug was carried out only at the pharmacy, the price remarkably decreased to EUR 336.17, thus leading to a cost saving of EUR 478.57 per therapy.

Table 3. Analysis of the cost per therapy associated with the administration of AmBisome® at the G. Gaslini children hospital before and after the decision of centralization of drug reconstitution.

Time Period		Vials of AmBisome® Used	Number of Therapies	Vials per Therapy	Cost per Therapy (€)
Before	January 2022	418	72	5.55 ± 0.35	814.74
	February 2022	306	58		

Table 3. *Cont.*

	Time Period	Vials of AmBisome® Used	Number of Therapies	Vials per Therapy	Cost per Therapy (€)
After	June 2022	152	83	2.29 ± 0.38	336.17
	July 2022	201	91		
	August 2022	251	99		
	September 2022	280	106		

4. Conclusions

In this study, we investigated the stability under storage conditions of three different AmBisome® formulations, corresponding to the dilutions used by the hospital staff for clinical administration: AmB 4 mg/mL (4.32 mM) in sterile water, AmB 2 mg/mL (2.16 mM), and AmB 0.2 mg/mL (0.22 mM) in 5% glucose solution. The formulations were stored at RT or at 4 °C up to 1 week and analyzed for their colloidal and chemical stabilities. The colloidal stability of the three formulations revealed a reposition of the drug during storage, starting early after 24 h and being particularly evident at RT. Indeed, we observed an increase in the monomeric drug forms, probably originating from the onset of free drug molecules released from the liposomal delivery system. The monomeric forms, having a low water solubility at submicromolar concentrations, quickly shift towards the more toxic dimeric forms. The modifications of the aggregation state were more evident for the 0.22 µM AmB formulation, highlighting a greater colloidal instability of the most diluted formulation. The biological results were in line with the changes revealed by spectrophotometric analysis, since the 0.22 µM AmB formulation was the most effective in reducing cell viability. This increased detrimental effect on cells was not ascribable to the onset of drug byproducts, as confirmed by HPLC analysis, but it probably depends on the growing presence of free drug forms of the drug in solution. Thus, our results demonstrated the difficulties related to handling nanometric supramolecular systems, since from the same batch of AmBisome®, we obtained diverse-diluted liposomal formulations highly and differently influenced by drug concentration, time, and temperature of storage. Only the colloidal stability of the liposomal suspensions remained almost constant for up to 7 days at 4 °C.

Therefore, the compounding pharmacist has to pay much attention when handling this medication. On the basis of our results, the pharmacist should avoid RT storage and consider that more diluted samples are prone to physical instability and greater toxicity. This aspect is of particular relevance, especially in a pediatric hospital, younger patients being those requiring the lowest dosages. So, in light of these considerations, the centralization of AmBisome® dilution at the pharmacy department is absolutely essential for assuring patient safety, medication quality, and cost saving, as we have demonstrated by the analysis of drug expense per therapy carried out at the G. Gaslini children hospital.

Supplementary Materials: The following supporting information can be downloaded at: https://www.mdpi.com/article/10.3390/pharmaceutics16040466/s1: Figure S1—representative size distribution obtained by NTA system of freshly prepared liposomal formulations; Figure S2—representative distribution of Zeta potentials of freshly prepared liposomal formulations; Figure S3—calibration curve of the HPLC assay method; Figure S4—chromatograms of the AmB calibration standard methanol solutions.

Author Contributions: Conceptualization, E.R., P.B. and G.Z.; methodology, D.C., E.R., G.Z., V.I., A.Z., D.M. and C.V.; validation, E.R., G.Z. and C.V.; formal analysis, D.C., C.V., E.R. and G.Z.; investigation, E.R., G.Z., V.I., A.Z., D.M., D.C. and C.V.; data curation, D.C., C.V., G.Z., E.R., A.Z. and V.I.; writing—original draft preparation, G.Z. and E.R.; writing—review and editing, G.Z., E.R., C.V., P.B., A.Z., D.C. and D.M.; supervision, E.R. and P.B.; project administration, E.R. and P.B. All authors have read and agreed to the published version of the manuscript.

Funding: This research received no external funding.

Institutional Review Board Statement: Not applicable.

Informed Consent Statement: Not applicable.

Data Availability Statement: Data are contained within the article and Supplementary Materials.

Acknowledgments: We thank the students Benedetta Senes and Gabriela Yasbek for their support during their experimental thesis period.

Conflicts of Interest: The authors declare no conflicts of interest.

References

1. Chen, L.; Zhang, L.; Xie, Y.; Wang, Y.; Tian, X.; Fang, W.; Xue, X.; Wang, L. Confronting Antifungal Resistance, Tolerance, and Persistence: Advances in Drug Target Discovery and Delivery Systems. *Adv. Drug Deliv. Rev.* **2023**, *200*, 115007. [CrossRef] [PubMed]
2. Groll, A.H.; Piscitelli, S.C.; Walsh, T.J. Clinical Pharmacology of Systemic Antifungal Agents: A Comprehensive Review of Agents in Clinical Use, Current Investigational Compounds, and Putative Targets for Antifungal Drug Development. *Adv. Pharmacol.* **1998**, *44*, 343–500. [PubMed]
3. Sangalli-Leite, F.; Scorzoni, L.; Mesa-Arango, A.C.; Casas, C.; Herrero, E.; Soares Mendes Gianinni, M.J.; Rodríguez-Tudela, J.L.; Cuenca-Estrella, M.; Zaragoza, O. Amphotericin B Mediates Killing in Cryptococcus Neoformans through the Induction of a Strong Oxidative Burst. *Microbes Infect.* **2011**, *13*, 457–467. [CrossRef] [PubMed]
4. Zielińska, J.; Wieczór, M.; Bączek, T.; Gruszecki, M.; Czub, J. Thermodynamics and kinetics of amphotericin B self-association in aqueous solution characterized in molecular detail. *Sci. Rep.* **2016**, *6*, 1910. [CrossRef] [PubMed]
5. Bolard, J.; Legrand, P.; Heitz, F.; Cybulska, B. One-Sided Action of Amphotericin B on Cholesterol-Containing Membranes Is Determined by Its Self-Association in the Medium. *Biochemistry* **1991**, *30*, 5707–5715. [CrossRef]
6. Barwicz, J.; Tancrède, P. The Effect of Aggregation State of Amphotericin-B on Its Interactions with Cholesterol- or Ergosterol-Containing Phosphatidylcholine Monolayers. *Chem. Phys. Lipids* **1997**, *85*, 145–155. [CrossRef] [PubMed]
7. Haynes, M.P.; Chong, P.L.-G.; Buckley, H.R.; Pieringer, R.A. Fluorescence Studies on the Molecular Action of Amphotericin B on Susceptible and Resistant Fungal Cells. *Biochemistry* **1996**, *35*, 7983–7992. [CrossRef]
8. Yamamoto, T.; Umegawa, Y.; Tsuchikawa, H.; Hanashima, S.; Matsumori, N.; Funahashi, K.; Seo, S.; Shinoda, W.; Murata, M. The Amphotericin B–Ergosterol Complex Spans a Lipid Bilayer as a Single-Length Assembly. *Biochemistry* **2019**, *58*, 5188–5196. [CrossRef]
9. Rivnay, B.; Wakim, J.; Avery, K.; Petrochenko, P.; Myung, J.H.; Kozak, D.; Yoon, S.; Landrau, N.; Nivorozhkin, A. Critical Process Parameters in Manufacturing of Liposomal Formulations of Amphotericin B. *Int. J. Pharm.* **2019**, *565*, 447–457. [CrossRef]
10. Hamill, R.J. Amphotericin B formulations: A comparative review of efficacy and toxicity. *Drugs* **2013**, *73*, 919–934. [CrossRef]
11. Wang, X.; Mohammad, I.S.; Fan, L.; Zhao, Z.; Nurunnabi, M.; Sallam, M.A.; Wu, J.; Chen, Z.; Yin, L.; He, W. Delivery strategies of amphotericin B for invasive fungal infections. *Acta Pharm Sin B* **2021**, *11*, 2585–2604. [CrossRef]
12. Stone, N.R.; Bicanic, T.; Salim, R.; Hope, W. Liposomal Amphotericin B (AmBisome(®)): A Review of the Pharmacokinetics, Pharmacodynamics, Clinical Experience and Future Directions. *Drugs* **2016**, *76*, 485–500. [CrossRef] [PubMed]
13. Available online: https://www.gilead.com/news-and-press/press-room/press-releases/2022/2/gilead-sciences-announces-fourth-quarter-and-full-year-2021-financial-results (accessed on 18 January 2024).
14. Available online: https://www.ema.europa.eu/en/documents/comments/overview-comments-received-liposomal-amphotericin-b-powder-dispersion-infusion-50-mg-product/chmp/559889/2021_en.pdf (accessed on 18 January 2024).
15. Available online: https://www.ema.europa.eu/en/documents/scientific-guideline/liposomal-amphotericin-b-powder-dispersion-infusion-50-mg-product-specific-bioequivalence-guidance_en.pdf (accessed on 18 January 2024).
16. Available online: https://www.ema.europa.eu/en/documents/scientific-guideline/reflection-paper-data-requirements-intravenous-liposomal-products-developed-reference-innovator_en.pdf (accessed on 18 January 2024).
17. Fleury, M.; Fonzo-Christe, C.; Normand, C.; Bonnabryet, P. Confusion between Two Amphotericin B Formulations Leading to a Paediatric Rehospitalisation. *Drug Saf. Case Rep.* **2016**, *3*, 4. [CrossRef] [PubMed]
18. Stemple, K.; Schnoor, J.; Ahern, J.; Bunnell, A. Utilization of an Order Panel to Encourage Safe Ordering and Administration of Amphotericin B. *Hosp. Pharm.* **2019**, *54*, 212–216. [CrossRef]
19. Available online: https://farmaci.agenziafarmaco.gov.it/aifa/servlet/PdfDownloadServlet?pdfFileName=footer_007212_028581_RCP.pdf&sys=m0b1l3 (accessed on 18 January 2024).
20. Liu, Y.; Mei, Z.; Mei, L.; Tang, J.; Yuan, W.; Srinivasan, S.; Ackermann, R.; Schwendeman, A.S. Analytical Method Development and Comparability Study for AmBisome® and Generic Amphotericin B Liposomal Products. *Eur. J. Pharm. Biopharm.* **2020**, *157*, 241–249. [CrossRef] [PubMed]
21. Raggi, F.; Cangelosi, D.; Consolaro, A.; Rossi, C.; Pelassa, S.; Cortese, K.; Gagliani, M.C.; Morini, M.; Segalerba, D.; Brignole, C.; et al. Extracellular Vesicle-derived microRNAs as Potential Biomarkers in Oligoarticular Juvenile Idiopathic Arthritis Patients: Methodological Challenges and New Perspectives. *Clin. Transl. Med.* **2022**, *12*, e1067. [CrossRef] [PubMed]
22. Espada, R.; Valdespina, S.; Alfonso, C.; Rivas, G.; Ballesteros, M.P.; Torrado, J.J. Effect of Aggregation State on the Toxicity of Different Amphotericin B Preparations. *Int. J. Pharm.* **2008**, *361*, 64–69. [CrossRef] [PubMed]

23. Svirkin, Y.; Lee, J.; Marx, R.; Yoon, S.; Landrau, N.; Kaisar, M.A.; Qin, B.; Park, J.H.; Alam, K.; Kozak, D.; et al. Amphotericin B Release Rate Is the Link between Drug Status in the Liposomal Bilayer and Toxicity. *Asian J. Pharm. Sci.* **2022**, *17*, 544–556. [CrossRef]
24. Díaz De León–Ortega, R.; D'Arcy, D.M.; Lamprou, D.A.; Fotaki, N. In Vitro—In Vivo Relations for the Parenteral Liposomal Formulation of Amphotericin B: A Clinically Relevant Approach with PBPK Modeling. *Eur. J. Pharm. Biopharm.* **2021**, *159*, 177–187. [CrossRef]
25. Ye, J.; Li, R.; Cheng, J.; Liu, D.; Yang, Y.; Wang, H.; Xu, X.; Li, L.; Ma, P.; Liu, Y. Comparative Colloidal Stability of Commercial Amphotericin B Nanoformulations Using Dynamic and Static Multiple Light Scattering Techniques. *Int. J. Nanomed. IJN* **2022**, *17*, 6047–6064. [CrossRef]
26. Imran, A.; Popescu, D.; Movileanu, L. Cyclic Activity of an Osmotically Stressed Liposome in a Finite Hypotonic Environment. *Langmuir* **2020**, *36*, 3659–3666. [CrossRef] [PubMed]
27. Montenegro, M.; De Souza, S.; Leão, R.; Rocha, H.; De Rezende, C.; De Souza, R. Methodology Development and Validation of Amphotericin B Stability by HPLC-DAD. *J. Braz. Chem. Soc.* **2020**, *31*, 916–926. [CrossRef]
28. Sawangchan, P.; Alexandrino, F., Jr.; Alencar, É.N.; Egito, E.S.T.; Kirsch, L.E. The Role of Aggregation and Ionization in the Chemical Instability of Amphotericin B in Aqueous Methanol. *Int. J. Pharm.* **2023**, *632*, 122586. [CrossRef] [PubMed]
29. Espada, R.; Josa, J.M.; Valdespina, S.; Dea, M.A.; Ballesteros, M.P.; Alunda, J.M.; Torrado, J.J. HPLC Assay for Determination of Amphotericin B in Biological Samples. *Biomed. Chromatogr.* **2008**, *22*, 402–407. [CrossRef] [PubMed]
30. Gurudevan, S.; Francis, A.P.; Jayakrishnan, A. Amphotericin B-Albumin Conjugates: Synthesis, Toxicity and Anti-Fungal Activity. *Eur. J. Pharm. Sci.* **2018**, *115*, 167–174. [CrossRef] [PubMed]
31. Wang, Y.; Grainger, D.W. Regulatory Considerations Specific to Liposome Drug Development as Complex Drug Products. *Front. Drug. Deliv.* **2022**, *2*, 901281. [CrossRef]
32. Fernández-García, R.; Muñoz-García, J.C.; Wallace, M.; Fabian, L.; González-Burgos, E.; Gómez-Serranillos, M.P.; Raposo, R.; Bolás-Fernández, F.; Ballesteros, M.P.; Healy, A.M.; et al. Self-Assembling, Supramolecular Chemistry and Pharmacology of Amphotericin B: Poly-Aggregates, Oligomers and Monomers. *J. Control. Release* **2022**, *341*, 716–732. [CrossRef] [PubMed]
33. Shibata, H.; Izutsu, K.; Yomota, C.; Okuda, H.; Goda, Y. Investigation of Factors Affecting in Vitro Doxorubicin Release from PEGylated Liposomal Doxorubicin for the Development of in Vitro Release Testing Conditions. *Drug Dev. Ind. Pharm.* **2015**, *41*, 1376–1386. [CrossRef]
34. Van Der Schors, T.; Amann, S.; Makridaki, D.; Kohl, S. Pharmacy Preparations and Compounding. *Eur. J. Hosp. Pharm.* **2021**, *28*, 190–192. [CrossRef]
35. Ministers' Deputies. Resolution CM/Res(2016)2 on Good Reconstitution Practices in Health Care Establishments for Medicinal Products for Parenteral Use (Adopted by the Committee of Ministers on 1 June 2016 at the 1258th Meeting of the Ministers' Deputies. Available online: https://www.edqm.eu/sites/default/files/resolution_cm_res_2016_2_good_reconstitution_practices_in_health_care_establishments_for_medicinal_products_for_parenteral_use_.pdf (accessed on 18 January 2024).
36. Seibel, N.L.; Shad, A.T.; Bekersky, I.; Groll, A.H.; Gonzalez, C.; Wood, L.V.; Jarosinski, P.; Buell, D.; Hope, W.W.; Walsh, T.J. Safety, Tolerability, and Pharmacokinetics of Liposomal Amphotericin B in Immunocompromised Pediatric Patients. *Antimicrob. Agents Chemother.* **2017**, *61*, e01477-16. [CrossRef]
37. Maertens, J.; Pagano, L.; Azoulay, E.; Warris, A. Liposomal Amphotericin B—The Present. *J. Antimicrob. Chemother.* **2022**, *77*, ii11–ii20. [CrossRef]
38. Nydert, P.; El-Edelbi, R.; Obaya, S.; Nilsson, K.M.; Lindemalm, S. 5PSQ-140 Reconstution Practice by a Paediatric and Neonatal Ward-Based Pharmacist. *Eur. J. Hosp. Pharm.* **2018**, *215*, A228–A229.

pharmaceutics

MDPI

Article

Dispensing Oral Temozolomide in Children: Precision and Stability of a Novel and Ready to Use Liquid Formulation in Comparison with Capsule Derived Mixtures

Caroline Lemarchand [1,*], Hugues Bienaymé [1], André Rieutord [2], Samuel Abbou [3], Maxime Annereau [2] and Jeremy Bastid [1,*]

1 ORPHELIA Pharma, 75005 Paris, France; hugues.bienayme@orphelia-pharma.eu
2 Clinical Pharmacy Department, Gustave Roussy Cancer Campus, 94805 Villejuif, France; andre.rieutord@gustaveroussy.fr (A.R.); maxime.annereau@gustaveroussy.fr (M.A.)
3 Children and Adolescent Oncology Department, INSERM U1015, Paris-Saclay University, 94805 Villejuif, France; samuel.abbou@gustaveroussy.fr
* Correspondence: caroline.lemarchand@orphelia-pharma.eu (C.L.); jeremy.bastid@orphelia-pharma.eu (J.B.)

Abstract: Temozolomide (TMZ) is part of the therapeutic armamentarium used in managing pediatric cancers; however, available oral forms (capsules) are not adapted for use in children. Our aim was to assess the dose accuracy and stability of TMZ using capsule contents mixed with food compared with a novel, ready-to-use liquid formulation specifically developed for children (Ped-TMZ, brand name KIZFIZO). Dose accuracy and TMZ stability testing were performed with TMZ capsule contents (90 mg) mixed with food vehicles (apple juice, apple sauce, cream, milk, and mashed potatoes) and compared to an equivalent dose of Ped-TMZ. Acceptance criteria were predefined for TMZ (95.0–105.0%) and its degradation product amino-imidazole-carboxamide (AIC; <1%) content. The delivered dose was significantly higher using Ped-TMZ (96.6 ± 1.2%) and within the predefined criteria for TMZ content, whereas it was systematically under the lower specifications of 95% using capsule-derived preparations with apple juice (91.0 ± 1.5%) and apple sauce (91.6 ± 1.4%), respectively ($p < 0.0001$). In chemical stability tests, the four food vehicles (apple sauce, cream, milk, mashed potatoes) had a significant effect on TMZ stability ($p = 0.0042$), and the AIC significantly increased with time in three of the four vehicles ($p < 0.0001$). Only 1/72 of preparations from capsules met the predefined acceptance criteria, whereas Ped-TMZ showed no TMZ loss, and the AIC remained within specifications. In conclusion, mixing TMZ capsule content with food may result in significant underexposure, possibly even greater in routine practice, as complete food intake by the child is unlikely.

Keywords: cancer; oral administration; solution; stability; temozolomide

1. Introduction

Temozolomide (TMZ) is an alkylating agent with demonstrated schedule-dependent clinical activity against malignant gliomas such as glioblastoma multiforme or anaplastic astrocytoma in patients from three years of age [1,2]. TMZ is also widely used as standard chemotherapy to treat pediatric cancers, including neuroblastoma [3–5], medulloblastoma [6], and rhabdomyosarcoma [7]. TMZ development was driven by the increasing interest in the delivery of anticancer drugs via the oral route, which is more convenient for self-administration and improves patients' quality of life. Solid dosage forms, i.e., tablets and capsules, are the most preferred pharmaceutical forms because of their advantages, such as high dosing accuracy, easy handling, long-term stability in ambient conditions, and patient compliance. As TMZ dosing is based on the body surface area (BSA), the drug is currently supplied as hard capsules of six different strengths (Temodal®: 5 mg, 20 mg, 100 mg, 140 mg, 180 mg, and 250 mg) to enable dosing flexibility [2].

Temozolomide demonstrated rapid (T_{max} ~1 h) and complete absorption (100% bioavailability) and a linear-to-dose pharmacokinetic (i.e., total body clearance) after oral administration of capsules in adult patients under fasting conditions [1,2]. However, the food effect specifically studied in a pharmacokinetic study in adult patients showed a significant impact on the pharmacokinetic profile with a T_{max} increase and C_{max} and $AUC_{0–24}$ decrease [1]. As it cannot be excluded that the change in C_{max} is clinically significant, current product guidance recommends that TMZ capsules must be swallowed whole with water on an empty stomach [2]. Nevertheless, the TMZ capsules are large (from approximately 16 mm (size 3 for TMZ 5 mg) to 22 mm (size 0 for TMZ 140 mg to 250 mg) in length), making it difficult for pediatric patients to swallow [8]. Even if the age at which children can swallow intact tablets or capsules is highly dependent on the individual and the training that they receive from healthcare professionals or caregivers, the size of tablets and capsules should be kept as small as possible [9] and less than 10 mm [10] to improve the acceptability. Furthermore, the administration of several capsules may be required to achieve the prescribed dose, which represents an additional barrier for children who are averse to swallowing the solid dosage form [11]. For TMZ treatment, according to the available dosage strengths, the common dose of 90 mg (corresponding to a child under the age of 6 exhibiting a BSA of 0.6 m^2 and treated with 150 mg/m^2 of TMZ) is achieved with four capsules of 20 mg and two capsules of 5 mg, i.e., six capsules of size 2 or 3 to be swallowed by the child. The combination of size and number of hard capsules of TMZ can affect oral acceptability and potential adherence to chemotherapy treatment.

In these cases, clinicians may often instruct caregivers to follow common administration practices in pediatrics [12,13] by opening the TMZ capsules and mixing the powder content into liquid and/or soft food before spoon-feeding or syringing the mixture to the child with the aim of improving swallowability and palatability [14,15]. Despite the lack of scientific information regarding the adverse effects associated with such drug manipulations or modifications [16], mixing medicines into foodstuffs to facilitate drug administration is frequent and occurs in one-third of medicines for oral administration to the pediatric population [11,17]. However, unless the impact of liquid or soft foods used as vehicles for drug administration on the drug product performance (i.e., drug product quality attributes) is appropriately assessed and justified [18], this approach should be avoided for several reasons. Firstly, TMZ is a cytotoxic and teratogenic alkylating agent, meaning that exposure to the powder can be harmful to caregivers and the family [8,15]. Secondly, administering the accurate dose may be inconsistent and compromised by incomplete food consumption by the child. Indeed, TMZ is a bitter substance and drug loss spilled, regurgitated, or left behind in the glass/pot is frequent. Manipulation and opening of the capsules may further increase the loss of TMZ (e.g., some powder left in the capsule shell) and thereby increase errors in accurate dosing. Third, as TMZ is unstable under light and at a pH of 7 or above, mixing the capsule contents with food may result in drug degradation and suboptimal dosing [15]. Finally, the co-administration of capsules with food may impact the bioavailability of TMZ [1] with the potential risk of subtherapeutic drug levels.

Considering these challenges, the European Medicines Agency (EMA) 'Draft Inventory of Paediatric Therapeutic Needs' highlighted the need for an age-appropriate formulation of TMZ [19].

Ped-TMZ (KIZFIZO®, temozolomide 40 mg/mL oral suspension) is a ready-to-use oral liquid pediatric formulation of TMZ that is currently in development for the treatment of relapsed or refractory neuroblastoma. This age-adapted and taste-masked formulation is designed to deliver an accurate high drug load while avoiding drug manipulation and caregiver exposure to TMZ. The objective of this study was to evaluate the impact of TMZ capsule manipulation on the main critical quality attributes, accuracy (assay), and stability of TMZ, compared with the ready-to-use Ped-TMZ suspension. Pediatric patients who require TMZ treatment typically receive doses of 80–120 mg [15]. For the purpose of this study, a dose of 90 mg was chosen corresponding to a child under the age of 6 exhibiting a BSA of 0.6 m^2 and treated with 150 mg/m^2 of TMZ. Different liquids and soft foods were selected with regard to the reported use [20] or likelihood to be used in the targeted pediatric population (children from the age of 1 year) and to cover the range of various food components (e.g., caloric content), physicochemical properties (e.g., pH, texture) and temperature administration (e.g., ambient or hot). Due to the pH-dependent hydrolysis of TMZ [21], vehicles of various pH levels were selected. Apple sauce and apple juice were selected for their acidic pH environment. The other vehicles (chocolate cream, mashed, and infant milk) were chosen for their anticipated neutral pH and their different textures, compositions, and temperature administrations. Additionally, apple sauce and apple juice (in which the chemical stability of TMZ is supposed to be favorable) were used to assess the potential impact of the vehicle texture (liquid vs. soft food) on the delivered dose, e.g., related to any potential loss of the vehicle. The holding time was assessed over one hour after the preparation of the mixture and was considered a reasonable timeframe consistent with real life.

2. Materials and Methods

2.1. Dosage Forms

In total, 20 mg capsules and 5 mg capsules of Temodal® were purchased from Merck Sharp & Dohme, Puteaux, France.

Ped-TZM (KIZFIZO®, ORPHELIA Pharma, Paris, France), a ready-to-use suspension containing 40 mg/mL of TMZ, is an investigational product comprising the following excipients: xanthan gum; citric acid, silicon dioxide, sodium benzoate, sucralose, cola flavor, and purified water. Ped-TMZ is manufactured by mixing excipients in purified water before the introduction of TMZ. After at least 30 min of stirring with TMZ, the suspension is filled into bottles [22].

2.2. Liquid and Soft Food Vehicles

Liquid and food vehicles are listed in Table 1. They were purchased from a local supermarket in France. The pH was measured at ambient temperature using the SevenGo Duo Pro pH meter (Mettler-Toledo SAS, Viroflay, France). The nutrition information of the vehicles is reported in Table 2.

Table 1. Vehicles investigated in the study.

Liquid/Soft Food	Brand Name	Packaging	pH	Texture
Apple juice	Joker	1 L bottle	3.5	Liquid
Apple sauce	Andros	100 g pot	3.8	Soft food
Chocolate cream	Danette	125 g pot	6.8	Soft food
Infant milk *	Candia baby	250 mL bottle	6.8	Liquid
Mash potatoes	Mousseline	130 g sachet	6.4	Soft food

* standard liquid infant milk formula based on cow's milk, containing mineral/vitamin supplements.

Table 2. Nutrition facts of the investigated vehicles (given for 100 mL or 100 g).

	Apple Juice	Apple Sauce	Chocolate Cream	Infant Milk	Mash Potatoes
Calories (kJ)	187	296	516	261	280
Calories (kcal)	44	70	122	62	67
Fat (g)	0	0.2	3.0	3.2	0.8
Carbohydrates (g)	10	16.0	20.0	7.0	2.5
Proteins (g)	0	0.3	3.3	1.4	2.4

2.3. Accuracy of the Delivered Dose Study (TMZ Assay)

Ninety (90) mg of TMZ powder was prepared from four Temodal® capsules of 20 mg and two capsules of 5 mg and compared to 88 mg (2.2 mL) of Ped-TMZ.

The TMZ capsules were opened, and their contents were mixed with either a soft or liquid vehicle: 100 g apple sauce or 100 mL apple juice. The apple sauce/juice preparations were mixed or agitated in the original container with a spoon for 30 s. Analytical processing was then carried out according to the sample preparation adapted from the analytical testing applied for Ped-TMZ in order to reduce the food matrix effect. The food/TMZ mixture was transferred using the same spoon as for mixing into a 2000 mL volumetric flask containing 500 mL of dilution solvent (DS) (0.5% *v*/*v* of aqueous solution of glacial acetic acid, J.T. Baker, HPLC Grade) for analytical processing. Each flask was magnetically stirred for 10 min, and the volume was increased to 2000 mL with DS. After magnetically stirring for 10 min, the solution was centrifuged for 10 min at 10,000 rpm. The supernatant was assayed by HPLC-UV to determine the percentage of TMZ recovered from the capsule-derived mixture.

The Ped-TMZ suspension was sampled using the provided co-packaged device (5 mL syringe with 0.1 mL precision) and transferred directly into a 500 mL volumetric flask containing 250 mL of DS for analytical processing. Each flask was magnetically stirred for 10 min and completed to 500 mL with DS. After an additional 10 min of stirring, 5 mL of the Ped-TMZ sample solution was diluted into 20 mL of DS and centrifuged for 10 min at 10,000 rpm. The supernatant was assayed using HPLC-UV. Temozolomide quantities in the apple sauce/juice preparations (90 mg) were compared with 2.2 mL of ready-to-use Ped-TMZ 40 mg/mL oral suspension, equivalent to 88 mg TMZ. The recovery of TMZ was calculated as the ratio of the delivered dose/theoretical dose (where the theoretical dose is 90 mg for Temodal and 88 mg for Ped-TMZ). Values were also assessed against the predefined acceptance criteria for TMZ assay (95.0–105.0%).

All experiments were replicated three times. They involved six non-analyst operators, not particularly well trained or educated in pharmaceutical practice, acting as caregivers or parents in the current study. These non-analyst operators did the mixing step, transferred the content into the flask for the Temodal manipulation, and did the sampling for Ped-TMZ. For safety reasons, analytical technicians opened and emptied the Temodal capsules into the liquid and soft food and performed the analytical sample preparation and assay.

2.4. Stability of TMZ Study

Capsule contents (90 mg of TMZ) were mixed with different children's food vehicles: in the original container for apple sauce (100 g) and chocolate cream (125 g), in 100 g of mashed potatoes, and in 100 mL of infant milk. TMZ powder was left in contact with the food vehicles for varying periods of time (0, 30, and 60 min), then transferred into a volumetric flask containing DS and centrifuged for TMZ and amino-imidazole-carboxamide (AIC) quantification according to the operating conditions previously described. All experiments were replicated three times for each tested matrix. They were performed by analytical, trained technicians.

For the Ped-TMZ, the syringes were filled with 2 mL of Ped-TMZ and stored flat for 24 h at 25 °C/60% RH and 30 °C/65% RH. The content of the syringe was then transferred into a volumetric flask containing DS and centrifuged for TMZ and amino-imidazole-carboxamide (AIC) quantification according to the operating conditions previously described. This stability study was performed on two filled syringes for each time point. It was carried out by analytical, trained technicians.

2.5. Samples Analysis

The operating conditions were similar between the TMZ assay and degradation products. TMZ and its main degradation product, AIC, were assayed using ultraviolet high-performance liquid chromatography (HPLC-UV) (Agilent HP1260, Agilent Technologies Inc., Santa Clara, CA, USA) equipped with a UV detector. A Luna C18 column

(150 × 4.6 μm, 5 μm) was utilized at the temperature of 30 °C. The injection volume of the sample was 20 μL. The mobile phase A was composed of a mixture of methanol (gradient grade) (40 mL) with a 0.5% (*v*/*v*) aqueous solution of glacial acetic acid R (HPLC grade) (960 mL) in which 0.94 g of sodium hexane sulfonate (HPLC grade) was dissolved. The mobile phase B was composed of methanol (gradient grade). The selected elution gradient started with a 100% mobile phase A, then a 45%/55% phase mobile A/phase mobile B, and again a 100% mobile phase A. TMZ and its degradation product were detected at 254 nm. The method was validated according to ICH Q2 [23]. For the TMZ assay, the method is linear over the range of 70% to 130% of the theoretical content of TMZ in the drug product (R^2 = 1.0000). The accuracy and precision were tested on the three following series: 70%, 100%, and 130% of TMZ. The mean recovery ranged from 99.8% to 99.9%, and all individual recoveries complied with the 98.0–102.0% acceptance criteria. For precision, the coefficient of variation ranged from 0.2% to 0.4% for repeatability and from 0.4% to 0.5% for intermediate precision. The specificity of the method between TMZ and its degradation products was observed. The linearity over the range of 0.05% to 8.0% of the theoretical content of TMZ in the drug product (R^2 = 1.000) was compliant with the control of TMZ degradation products. The accuracy and precision were tested on the five following series: 0.05%, 0.2%, 2.5%, 5.0%, and 8.0% of TMZ. The mean recovery ranged from 99.6% to 100.9%, and all individual recovery complied with the 75.0–125.0% and 90.0–110.0% acceptance criteria for the LOQ and 2xLOQ levels and other levels, respectively. For precision, the coefficient of variation ranged from 0.4% to 1.2% for repeatability and from 0.8% to 1.4% for intermediate precision. The stability of the solution was demonstrated for the TMZ and degradation product assays.

The method suitability was also verified in the presence of a food vehicle. Specificity was verified for TMZ and AIC in the presence of a food vehicle. Recovery ranged between 98.51% and 99.70%, whatever the vehicle. The linearity was demonstrated from 20% to 120% of the theoretical content of TMZ. Acceptance criteria were predefined according to the drug product performance of Ped-TMZ for TMZ (95.0–105.0%) and AIC (<1%) content.

2.6. Statistical Analysis

To determine the impact of the food vehicles on the amounts of TMZ and AIC in the samples, statistical analyses (JMP software used, version 16) were performed. The effect of the contact time with soft food was assessed in the stability study. The impact of the operator and repetition on TMZ content was also evaluated in both studies. One-way ANOVA or a mixed model was used to compare the dose recovery or AIC content. A Levene test was used for the comparison of variances.

3. Results

3.1. Accuracy of the Delivered Dose

Immediately after dispensing the TMZ capsules into apple juice and apple sauce, both drug manipulations presented a similar distribution of TMZ content (Figure 1). The mean ± SD TMZ recovery was 91.0 ± 1.5% and 91.6 ± 1.4%, using apple juice and apple sauce, respectively, without any significant statistical differences between both vehicles (confidence interval −1.6939/0.53059). The delivered doses consistently fell below the predefined acceptance range (95.0–105.0%). In comparison, the recovery of TMZ in the Ped-TMZ suspension was significantly higher than that observed after handling the TMZ capsules (96.6 ± 1.2%; p-value $_{ANOVA} < 0.0001$), with TMZ quantities falling within predefined specifications (Figure 1). The main degradation product (AIC) was additionally controlled, and the results were found below the limit of quantification (LOQ = 0.1%) in all samples of Temodal mixed into apple juice or apple sauce.

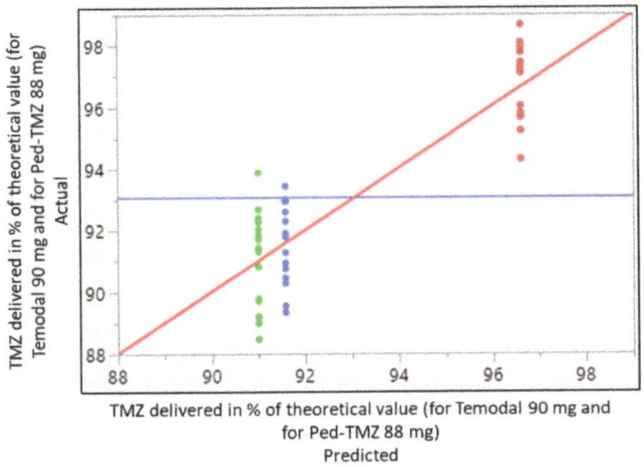

Figure 1. Whole model actual by predicted plot for the delivered dose of TMZ in % of the theoretical value (90 mg for Temodal and 88 mg for Ped-TMZ) after Temodal manipulation (● Temodal + apple juice; ● Temodal + apple sauce) or using ready-to-use Ped-TMZ (● Ped-TMZ). Predicted RMSE = 1.3778 Rsq = 0.78 p-value < 0.0001. Blue horizontal line represents the average of the delivered dose. Red diagonal line represents the line of fit for the model actual vs. predicted value. The colors are the 3 levels of the predicted delivered doses.

The ready-to-use Ped-TMZ liquid formulation was statistically different from the TMZ recovered after handling capsules with regard to the mean of the response. The liquid formulation systematically increased the percentage of the delivered dose by 3.55 points in comparison with Temodal mixed with apple sauce (estimate calculated from the linear mixed model using REML (restricted maximum likelihood) approach).

The findings were reproducible across all six operators for the three groups, as shown in the variance comparison in Table 3. The variability was equivalent regardless of the group (Ped-TMZ, Temodal + apple juice, Temodal + apple juice; Levene test p-value = 0.8648).

Table 3. Statistical analysis of the variability of the three groups: Ped-TMZ, Temodal mixed with apple juice, and Temodal mixed with apple sauce.

Group	Standard Deviation	Median Absolution Deviation (Robust Deviation Measure)
Ped-TMZ	1.246784	1.104444
Temodal + apple juice	1.488973	1.156667
Temodal + apple sauce	1.356263	1.155000

The analysis was completed with the determination of the source of variance using a linear model testing the three factors: (i) the product (Ped-TMZ, TMZ capsule mixed with apple juice, and TMZ capsule mixed with apple sauce), (ii) the operator (n = 6) and (iii) the repetition (n = 3). The product was the only source of variance in the accuracy experiments; operator or repetition did not affect the TMZ recovery (Figure 2).

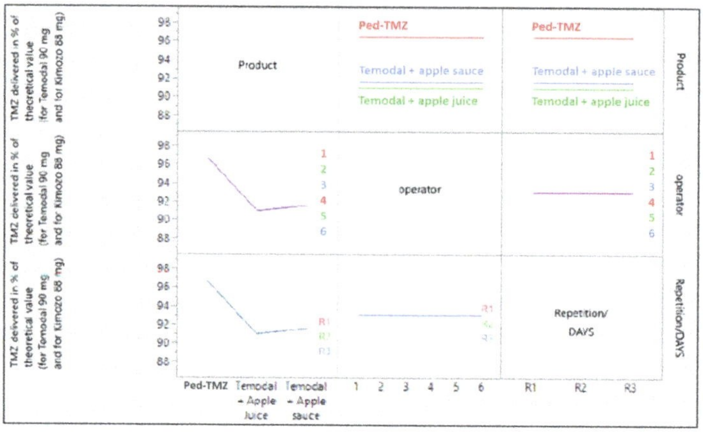

Figure 2. Effect of the three variables (product (Ped-TMZ, Temodal + Apple Juice, Temodal + Apple Sauce), operator (1 to 6), and repetition (R1, R2, R3)) on the response (TMZ delivered in % of the theoretical value).

3.2. Chemical and Physical Stability

Although the ready-to-use Ped-TMZ product is to be stored at 2–8 °C, the stability of the suspension stored in the oral syringe was investigated. The TMZ content was 100.8% or 100.4% when syringes were kept at 25 °C/60% RH or 30 °C/65% RH, respectively, for 24 h, a duration far exceeding requirements as syringes are to be prepared extemporaneously (i.e., just before administration of the drug product). This study demonstrated that the TMZ (Figure 3a) content remained within the predefined acceptance criteria (95%–105%). In addition, very limited degradation was noticed with a slight increase in the AIC from 0.05% to 0.14% or 0.2% (Figure 3b) after 24 h of storage at 25 °C/60% RH or 30 °C/65% RH, respectively. These levels are well below the predefined specification (<1% for AIC).

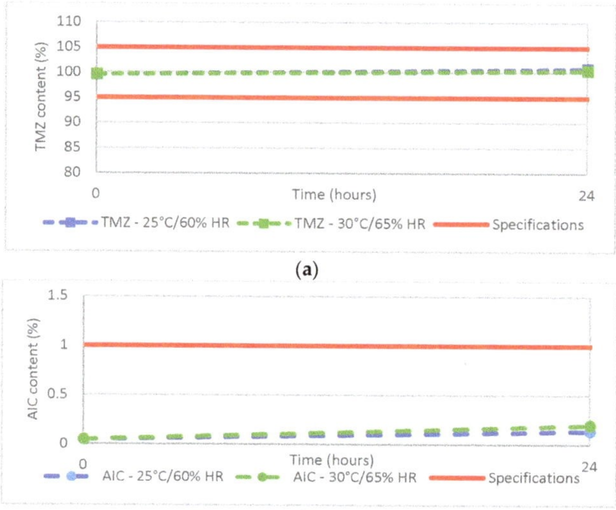

Figure 3. (**a**) TMZ and (**b**) AIC content of Ped-TMZ after 24 h storage at 25 °C or 30 °C.

Thirty-six (36) samples were prepared by mixing TMZ capsule contents with four different soft food vehicles (apple sauce, chocolate cream, infant milk, and mashed potatoes). The mean TMZ content for the 36 preparations is reported by vehicle over time in Figure 4a. The TMZ content from the mashed potatoes or apple sauce decreased from 94.2 ± 3.9% and 94.1 ± 0.4% to 89.8 ± 0.3% and 91.4 ± 0.1%, respectively, after 60 min of contact with food. TMZ from the milk mixture remained stable with content between 89.5 ± 0.2 (T0) and 91.5 ± 0.2% (60 min). TMZ content from the chocolate cream fluctuated from 88.9 ± 2.4% to 93.5 ± 0.5%. However, whatever the vehicle (apple sauce, chocolate cream, mashed potatoes, or milk) or the time point (0, 30 min, 60 min), the TMZ content was systematically below the predefined 95% lower limit except for one sample at T0. The mean AIC content over time is shown in Figure 4b, with evidence of TMZ degradation with up to 0.5%, 1.0%, and 1.3% of AIC quantified in the mixture of Temodal with chocolate cream, milk, and mashed potatoes, respectively, after 60 min of contact with food. Only the apple sauce prevented any degradation of TMZ into AIC (less than LOQ 0.1%).

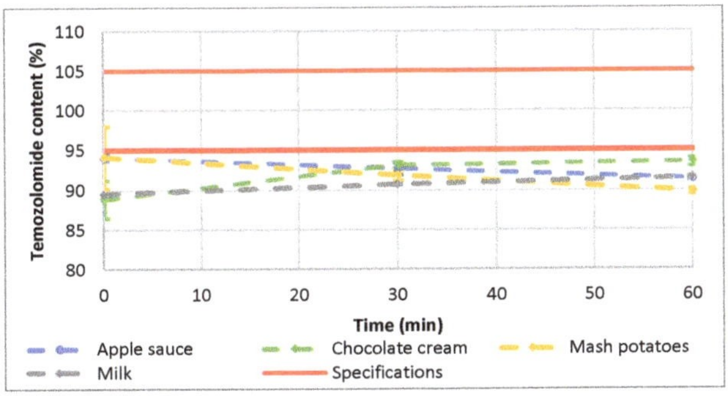

(a)

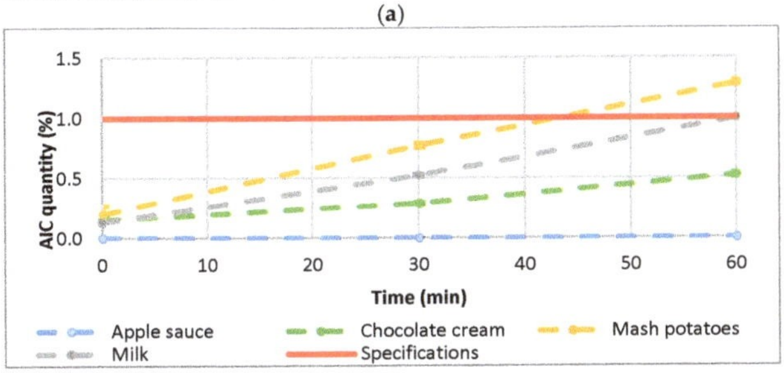

(b)

Figure 4. (**a**) mean TMZ and (**b**) mean AIC content after mixing the TMZ capsule contents with food ($n = 3$). Error bars represent SD (range for TMZ: 0.09–3.88; range for AIC: 0.01–0.07).

The impact of the different studied factors (vehicle, time, and operator) was analyzed based on a one-factor ANOVA or Kruskal–Wallis test according to normal distribution or not (test for homogeneity of variance). The four tested food vehicles (apple sauce, chocolate cream, infant milk, and mashed potatoes) had a significant impact on the TMZ delivered dose (p-value $_{\text{ANOVA}} = 0.0042$; Figure 5), whilst the vehicle factor did not have any significant effect on the degradation product AIC (p-value $_{\text{Kruskal-Wallis}} = 0.1850$). One-factor analysis has been used here for illustration purposes.

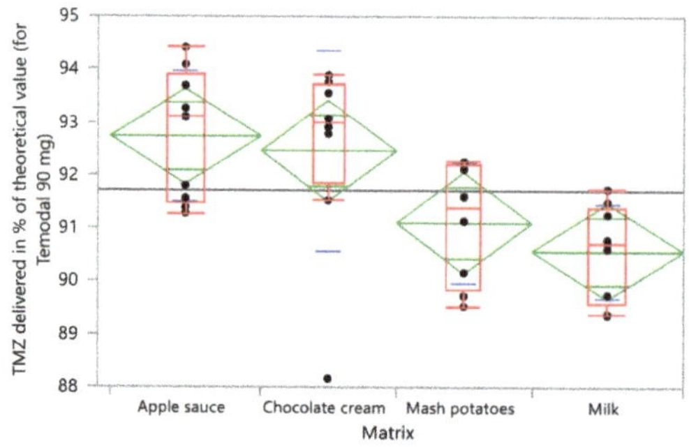

Figure 5. One-way analysis of TMZ delivered in % of the theoretical value (90 mg for Temodal) by vehicle (matrix). Box plot (median, 25th and 75th percentiles, min and max corresponding to 1.5 × IQR (Inter Quartile Range) in red, mean with confidence interval in green, and and lines that are at one standard deviation of the means in blue.

Time did not have a significant effect on the TMZ-delivered dose (p-value $_{ANOVA}$ = 0.5655). Nevertheless, one vehicle (milk) had a significant time effect on the TMZ dose, and two vehicles (milk and chocolate cream) evidenced homogeneity and physical stability issues with initial TMZ dosing below 90% and fluctuating over time (Figure 4a). The quantities of AIC, the main degradation product of TMZ, significantly increased over time when the TMZ capsules were mixed with vehicles (p-value $_{Kruskall\text{-}Wallis}$ < 0.0001) (Figure 6). In the one-way analysis, the food vehicle factor did not impact the AIC content (p-value $_{Kruskall\text{-}Wallis}$ = 0.1850). Nevertheless, the analysis of the individual food effect over time showed that AIC content increased significantly (p-value < 0.0001) when TMZ capsules were mixed with chocolate cream, milk, and mashed potatoes, the three vehicles for which pH is between 6 and 7. The AIC quantity was highest when the capsules were mixed with mashed potatoes, exceeding the predefined AIC content acceptance criteria (<1%) 60 min after mixing.

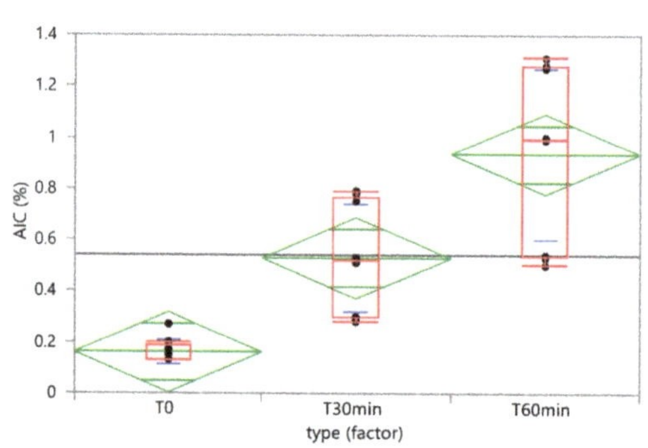

Figure 6. One-way analysis of AIC (%) by time. Box plot (median, 25th and 75th percentiles, min and max corresponding to 1.5 × IQR (Inter Quartile Range) in red, means with 95% confidence interval in green, and lines that are at one standard deviation of the means in blue.

The effect of repetition was analyzed on both the TMZ delivered and AIC results. The one-way analysis is presented in Figure 7, demonstrating the homogeneity of the variance (p = 0.8519 and p = 0.7537 for TMZ and AIC, respectively).

Combining all the assays performed, 72 samples were prepared from capsule contents mixed with 5 liquid or soft food vehicles, among which only 1 sample (1.4%) (1 out of 3 replicates using mashed potatoes at T0) delivered the right dose of TMZ (95.0%–105.0%). This means that 98.6% of samples prepared from the mixture of capsules with food would have led to underdosing of the patient.

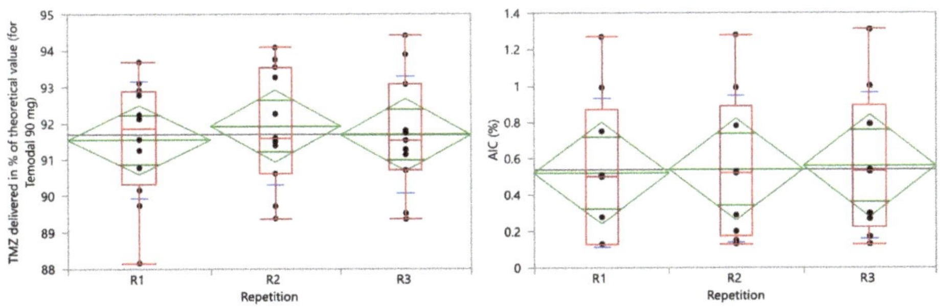

Figure 7. One-way analysis of TMZ delivered in % of the theoretical value (90 mg for Temodal) (**left**) and AIC (%) (**right**) by repetition. Box plot (median, 25th and 75th percentiles, min and max corresponding to 1.5 × IQR (Inter Quartile Range) in red, means with 95% confidence interval in green, and lines that are at one standard deviation of the means in blue.

4. Discussion

TMZ plays a crucial role in the chemotherapy treatment of pediatric oncology conditions, including recurrent or refractory gliomas [1,2], neuroblastoma [3–5], medulloblastoma [6], and rhabdomyosarcoma [7]. Despite its importance in the treatment of cancers affecting very young patients, there is currently no suitable formulation adapted for them.

When lacking appropriate pediatric forms, drug manipulations are common practices in both outpatient and inpatient settings [16]. Parents and caregivers use drug manipulation to achieve a better taste or to easily adjust the dose, whereas nurses perform it to reduce the size of the dosage forms or to facilitate administration through a feeding tube. In any case, the lack of information in SmPC or patient information leaflets or incomplete advice from their pharmacy often leads the parents, caregivers, or nurses to improvise, possibly using incompatible vehicles [24]. The impact of mixing capsules, crushed tablets, and other oral compounded formulations with foods and beverages has been evaluated in some studies [25–28]. It was highlighted that the physicochemical properties of food vehicles are an important consideration for drug exposure [29].

For TMZ administration, caregivers open capsules and mix their contents with any kind of beverage or soft foods. This practice poses multiple risks, including exposure of the caregiver to a cytotoxic drug, imprecise delivery and dosing, partial drug intake if the food or beverage is not totally ingested or consumed, and uncontrolled stability of the active compound [8,15,20]. Here, we investigated the dosing accuracy and drug stability of TMZ in various food vehicles commonly used to aid administration to pediatric patients [18,29] and whether an investigational oral suspension of TMZ could offer improved dosage accuracy and stability.

When TMZ capsules were mixed with apple sauce and apple juice, the delivered dose of TMZ consistently fell short of predefined specifications, suggesting the loss of TMZ during the preparation process, whatever the texture of the vehicle (liquid or soft food). Since the pH was acid for both vehicles (3.5–3.8), the experimental conditions were chemically favorable for TMZ stability (confirmed in the stability part of the study with apple sauce), suggesting that the loss of TMZ content may occur during the preparation. The process of twisting apart and separating the two parts of the capsule requires care and dexterity, and loss of powder onto gloves, surfaces, or utensils may occur. Some powder may also remain lodged inside the capsule, meaning that the full required dose is not dispensed into the food. This decrease in the delivered dose is likely to be underestimated in our study as the capsules were opened and emptied by skilled laboratory technicians for safety reasons. Loss may also occur after mixing the TMZ powder with the vehicle during the transfer with the spoon or syringe, mimicking administration to the child since the container was not totally emptied and/or rinsed. Interestingly, our study showed a good intra and inter-operator reproducibility. For non-analyst operators, who were not specifically well trained or educated, this minimal variability in their practice contrasts with the significant difference between nurses and hospital pharmacists in the comparative assessment highlighted by Nguyen et al. [30].

Mixing TMZ capsules with food also significantly affected the chemical stability of TMZ in a time-dependent manner. The food or drink vehicles had a significant impact on TMZ quantity, and the amount of degradation product AIC significantly increased in three out of the four food vehicles over the 60 min testing period. Mashed potato showed the most apparent degradation, while apple sauce exhibited minimal degradation. These findings are supported by a previous study involving 15 fluids, soft foods, and suspension vehicles, which indicated that drug bioavailability can be significantly influenced by various physicochemical properties of the vehicle, including pH, surface tension, and viscosity [31]. In the current study, differences in the AIC content over time may be essentially attributed to the pH of the food vehicles. Unlike apple sauce, which has an acidic pH (typically between 3.3 and 4.6) [32], the other three food vehicles had pH values ranging from 6.4 to 6.8. Since TMZ starts degrading at pH 7 and above, the increase in AIC quantity over time can be attributed to the neutral pH of the food. The fast degradation of TMZ in food presents practical challenges for parents and caregivers, as each dose needs to be freshly prepared and consumed promptly and fully to ensure proper dosage. This can be particularly challenging for children with reduced appetite or those who find the taste unpalatable, as is the case for TMZ, which exhibits a bitter taste.

Altogether, an important teaching of our study is that, despite the sample preparation being partially above the real-life standards (i.e., by skilled technicians) and assuming the complete consumption of the preparation by the child, 99% of the capsule-food/drink mixes would not have delivered the proper dose of TMZ (i.e., <95% of the targeted dose) including one sample with TMZ content as low as 86.9%, which is not acceptable for an anticancer medicine. Considering the cumulative risks associated with medicine manipulation, i.e., capsule opening and mixing by the parents, the difficulties in having a complete intake of the mixture by the child, and the time needed for this preparation that could also increase the risk of errors, the delivered dose may be dramatically reduced.

Another factor that may further contribute to TMZ underexposure is the impact of food co-administration on drug absorption. In a phase I dose-escalation and pharmacokinetic (PK) study of TMZ where 15 adult patients suffering from refractory or relapsing malignancies were enrolled, there was a 9% reduction in the $AUC_{0–24}$ and a 33% reduction in C_{max} in fed patients compared with the fasted group [1]. In the pediatric population, due to differences in physiology, anatomy, and the composition of food consumed, the food–drug interaction cannot be predicted based on adult studies [33]. That raises additional uncertainty on drug exposure when medicines are co-administered with food to children. The impact on TMZ bioavailability of co-administering 100–125 g of food, as per clinical practice or these experiments, is not known but may not be null.

Liquid formulations for oral administration are particularly crucial in pediatric patient treatment since they allow dose adjustment to weight or BSA, flexibility in administration by swallowing or feeding tube, and ease of use, and they significantly reduce the risk of manipulation [11]. Nevertheless, in the course of their development, these formulations need to address the palatability that may be an issue [11] and the patient acceptability in general [14], for which the dose volume is a major consideration [9]. The formulation of oral liquid products may also be challenging, as they generally require the use of excipients that are potentially harmful, e.g., antimicrobial preservatives for multidose containers, sweeteners, or flavoring agents [34,35]. They may also represent larger storage/transport volumes than solid dosage forms [36]. A proof-of-concept study demonstrated that preparation of a liquid formulation of TMZ from the intravenous infusion powder was feasible but it exhibited modest stability (13 weeks at 5 °C) and very low concentration (1.25 mg/mL), thereby requiring large administration volumes (e.g., 72 mL for 90 mg as in our study), not suitable for a pediatric oral formulation [8] in comparison to the recommended dose volumes for pediatric liquid products (less than 5 mL for children under 5 years and less than 10 mL for children of 5 years and older) [9]. Subsequently, the Gustave Roussy Cancer Campus developed a hospital-compounded oral suspension prepared from TMZ capsules and selected excipients, which exhibited satisfactory chemical and physical stability as well as lower distribution volumes [15]. This prototype was further developed at an industrial scale and led to the development of Ped-TMZ, with further improved long-term stability and higher TMZ concentration, allowing the administration of small volumes in line with EMA recommendations [9].

The efficacy, safety, and stability of Ped-TMZ are being tested across a range of studies. An open-label, randomized, multicenter study in patients with primary central nervous system (NCT04467346) showed the bioequivalence between Ped-TMZ and TMZ capsules [37]. An international, open-label, non-randomized, prospective, single-arm phase I study is underway to determine the PK, acceptability, and safety of Ped-TMZ in the pediatric population (NCT04610736).

5. Conclusions

TMZ dispensed with food using a spoon is systematically underdosed, as evidenced by poor recovery and instability. Our experiments suggest that mixing TMZ capsule contents with food may result in significant underexposure in pediatric patients. The ready-to-use and taste-masked oral suspension Ped-TMZ offers superior dosing accuracy and better stability than TMZ vehicle mixtures. Ped-TMZ addresses the critical and long-standing unmet medical need for young cancer patients with an age-appropriate formulation of TMZ, which was underlined by the EMA as early as 2014 [19].

Author Contributions: Conceptualization and methodology: C.L., H.B., A.R., S.A., M.A. and J.B.; validation, formal analysis, and investigation: C.L., H.B. and J.B.; writing—original draft preparation, writing—review and editing: C.L., H.B., M.A. and J.B.; supervision: C.L.; project administration and funding acquisition: H.B. All authors have read and agreed to the published version of the manuscript.

Funding: This research was funded by ORPHELIA Pharma, Paris, France.

Data Availability Statement: Due to commercial restrictions, the data is not publicly available. Data are contained within the article.

Acknowledgments: Eurofins CDMO—Amatsi group, Artigues-près-Bordeaux, France (Julien Capdeville and team) for undertaking the experimental part; Ippon Innovation, (Toulouse, France (François Bergeret and team) for statistical analyses.

Conflicts of Interest: Caroline Lemarchand, Hugues Bienaymé, and Jeremy Bastid are employees of ORPHELIA Pharma. Hugues Bienaymé, Samuel Abbou, Maxime Annereau, and Jeremy Bastid are listed as inventors in a patent or patent application related to Ped-TMZ (EP3613436). The other authors declare no conflict of interest.

References

1. Brada, M.; Judson, I.; Beale, P.; Moore, S.; Reidenberg, P.; Statkevich, P.; Dugan, M.; Batra, V.; Cutler, D. Phase I dose-escalation and pharmacokinetic study of temozolomide (SCH 52365) for refractory or relapsing malignancies. *Br. J. Cancer* **1999**, *81*, 1022–1030. [CrossRef]
2. EMA. Temodal SmPC. Available online: https://www.ema.europa.eu/en/documents/product-information/temodal-epar-product-information_en.pdf (accessed on 23 November 2023).
3. Parikh, N.S.; Howard, S.C.; Chantada, G.; Israels, T.; Khattab, M.; Alcasabas, P.; Lam, C.G.; Faulkner, L.; Park, J.R.; London, W.B.; et al. SIOP-PODC adapted risk stratification and treatment guidelines: Recommendations for neuroblastoma in low- and middle-income settings. *Pediatr. Blood Cancer* **2015**, *62*, 1305–1316. [CrossRef]
4. Moreno, L.; Rubie, H.; Varo, A.; Le Deley, M.C.; Amoroso, L.; Chevance, A.; Garaventa, A.; Gambart, M.; Bautista, F.; Valteau-Couanet, D.; et al. Outcome of children with relapsed or refractory neuroblastoma: A meta-analysis of ITCC/SIOPEN European phase II clinical trials. *Pediatr. Blood Cancer* **2017**, *64*, 25–31. [CrossRef]
5. Children's Cancer and Leukaemia Group. Options for the Treatment of Patients with Relapsed/Progressive High-Risk Neuroblastoma. 2015. Available online: https://www.cclg.org.uk/write/MediaUploads/Member%2520area/Treatment%2520guidelines/CCLG_Relapsed_Progressive_High_Risk_Neuroblastoma_Guidelines_March_2015_FINAL.pdf (accessed on 23 November 2023).

6. Hill, R.M.; Plasschaert, S.L.A.; Timmermann, B.; Dufour, C.; Aquilina, K.; Avula, S.; Donovan, L.; Lequin, M.; Pietsch, T.; Thomale, U.; et al. Relapsed Medulloblastoma in Pre-Irradiated Patients: Current Practice for Diagnostics and Treatment. *Cancers* **2022**, *14*, 126. [CrossRef]
7. Defachelles, A.S.; Bogart, E.; Casanova, M.; Merks, J.H.M.; Bisogno, G.; Calareso, G.; Gallego Melcon, S.; Gatz, S.A.; Le Deley, M.C.; McHugh, K.; et al. Randomized Phase II Trial of Vincristine-Irinotecan With or Without Temozolomide, in Children and Adults With Relapsed or Refractory Rhabdomyosarcoma: A European Paediatric Soft Tissue Sarcoma Study Group and Innovative Therapies for Children With Cancer Trial. *J. Clin. Oncol.* **2021**, *39*, 2979–2990. [CrossRef]
8. Nygren, H.; Eksborg, S. Stability of temozolomide in solutions aimed for oral treatment prepared from a commercially available powder for infusion. *Pharm. Methods* **2012**, *3*, 198–202. [CrossRef]
9. EMA. EMEA/CHMP/PEG/194810/2005, Reflection Paper: Formulations of Choice for the Paediatric Population. 2006. Available online: https://www.ema.europa.eu/en/documents/scientific-guideline/reflection-paper-formulations-choice-paediatric-population_en.pdf (accessed on 23 November 2023).
10. Bracken, L.; McDonough, E.; Ashleigh, S.; Wilson, F.; Shakeshaft, J.; Ohia, U.; Mistry, P.; Jones, H.; Kanji, N.; Liu, F.; et al. Can children swallow tablets? Outcome data from a feasibility study to assess the acceptability of different-sized placebo tablets in children (creating acceptable tablets (CAT)). *BMJ Open* **2020**, *10*, e036508. [CrossRef]
11. Venables, R.; Batchelor, H.; Hodson, J.; Stirling, H.; Marriott, J. Determination of formulation factors that affect oral medicines acceptability in a domiciliary peadiatric population. *Int. J. Pharm.* **2015**, *480*, 55–62. [CrossRef]
12. Richey, R.H.; Craig, J.V.; Shah, U.U.; Nunn, A.J.; Turner, M.A.; Barker, C.E.; Ford, J.L.; Peak, M. MODRIC–Manipulation of drugs in children. *Int. J. Pharm.* **2013**, *457*, 339–341. [CrossRef]
13. Bordes-Picard, F.; Buffangeix, C.; Celadon, M.-J.; Edeline, J.; Fayolle, N.; Gestin, P.; Lemarchand, C.; Levacher, E.; Marçon, F.; Mamecier, L.; et al. Tailor-made medication: Practices and prospects. *STP Pharma Prat.* **2020**, *6*, 2–6.
14. EMA. EMA/CHMP/QWP/805880/2012_Rev.2, Guideline on Pharmaceutical Development of Medicines for Paediatric Use. 2013. Available online: https://www.ema.europa.eu/en/documents/scientific-guideline/guideline-pharmaceutical-development-medicines-paediatric-use_en.pdf (accessed on 23 November 2023).
15. Annereau, M.; Hinterlang, M.; Bienayme, H.; Vassal, G.; Pinon, A.; Schmitt, M.; Denis, L.; Lemarchand, C.; Martin, L.; Lemare, F.; et al. Development of a Hospital Compounded, Taste-Masked, Temozolomide Oral Suspension and 5-Year Real-Life Experience in Treating Paediatric Patients. *Pharmaceuticals* **2022**, *15*, 555. [CrossRef]
16. Richey, R.H.; Shah, U.U.; Peak, M.; Craig, J.V.; Ford, J.L.; Barker, C.E.; Nunn, A.J.; Turner, M.A. Manipulation of drugs to achieve the required dose is intrinsic ot peadiatric practice but is not supported by guidelines or evidence. *BMC Pediatr.* **2013**, *13*, 81. [CrossRef]
17. Zahn, J.; Hoerning, A.; Trollmann, R.; Rascher, W.; Neubert, A. Manipulation of medicinal products for oral Adminitration to paediatric patients at a german university hospital: An observational study. *Pharmaceutics* **2020**, *12*, 583. [CrossRef]
18. FDA. Use of Liquids and/or Soft Foods as Vehicles for Drug Administration: General Considerations for Selection and In Vitro Methods for Product Quality Assessments. 2018. Available online: https://www.fda.gov/media/114872/download (accessed on 23 November 2023).
19. EMA. EMA/PDCO/381728/2014, Draft Inventory of Paediatric Therapeutic Needs–Paediatric Oncology. 2014. Available online: https://www.ema.europa.eu/en/documents/other/draft-inventory-paediatric-therapeutic-needs-paediatric-oncology_en.pdf (accessed on 23 November 2023).
20. Martir, J.; Flanagan, T.; Mann, J.; Fotaki, N. Co-administration of Paediatric Medicines with Food and Drinks in the Context of Their Physicochemical Properties—A Global Perspective on Practices and Recommendations. *AAPS J.* **2020**, *22*, 54. [CrossRef]
21. Denny, B.J.; Wheelhouse, R.T.; Stevens, M.F.; Tsang, L.L.; Slack, J.A. NMR and molecular modeling investigation of the mechanism of activation of the antitumor drug temozolomide and its interaction with DNA. *Biochemistry* **1994**, *33*, 9045–9051. [CrossRef]
22. Annereau, M.; Bastid, J.; Bienayme, H.; Lemare, F.; Schmitt, M.; Tortolano, L.; Abbou, S. Oral Suspension of Temozolomide. European Patent EP 3,613,436, 26 February 2020.
23. EMA. CPMP/ICH/381/95, ICH Topic Q 2 (R1) Validation of Analytical Procedures: Text and Methodology. 1995. Available online: https://www.ema.europa.eu/en/documents/scientific-guideline/ich-q-2-r1-validation-analytical-procedures-text-methodology-step-5_en.pdf (accessed on 23 November 2023).
24. Van der Vossen, A.; Al-Hassany, L.; Buljac, S.; Brugma, J.D.; Vulto, A.; Hanff, L. Manipulation of oral medication for children by parents and nurses occurs frequently and is often not supported by instructions. *Acta Paediatr.* **2019**, *108*, 1475–1481. [CrossRef]
25. Allen, L.V., Jr.; Stiles, M.L.; Prince, S.J.; McLaury, H.J.; Sylvestri, M.F. Stability of ramipril in water, apple juice, and applesauce. *Am. J. Health-Syst. Pharm.* **1995**, *52*, 2433–2436. [CrossRef]
26. Carrier, M.N.; Garinot, O.; Vitzling, C. Stability and compatibility of tegaserod from crushed tablets mixed in beverages and foods. *Am. J. Health-Syst. Pharm.* **2004**, *61*, 1135–1142. [CrossRef]
27. Manrique, Y.J.; Lee, D.J.; Islam, F.; Nissen, L.M.; Cichero, J.A.; Stokes, J.R.; Steadman, K.J. Crushed tablets: Does the administration of food vehicles and thickened fluids to aid medication swallowing alter drug release? *J. Pharm. Pharm. Sci.* **2014**, *17*, 207–219. [CrossRef]
28. Wu, K.W.; Zheng, K.; Tian, L.; Xia, L.; Hwang, S.Y.; Nwakama, P.E.; Sun, W.J.; Kim, M.J.; Tampal, N.; Xu, X.; et al. The effect of food vehicles on in vitro performance of pantoprazole sodium delayed release sprinkle formulation. *Int. J. Pharm.* **2023**, *635*, 122737. [CrossRef]

29. Freerks, L.; Sucher, W.; Tarnow, M.-J.; Eckert, C.; Klein, S. Vehicles for durg adminitration to children: Results and learnings form an in-depth screening of FDA-recommended liquids and soft foods for prodcut quality assessment. *Pharm. Res.* **2022**, *39*, 497–509.
30. Nguyen, D.; Secretan, P.-H.; Auvity, S.; Vidal, F.; Postaire, M.; Cisternino, S.; Schlatter, J. Assessment of practices for suspensed oral durgs by tablet crushing in pediatric units. *Eur. J. Pharm. Biopharm.* **2020**, *157*, 175–182. [CrossRef]
31. Kersten, E.; Barry, A.; Klein, S. Physicochemical characterisation of fluids and soft foods frequently mixed with oral drug formulations prior to administration to children. *Pharmazie* **2016**, *71*, 122–127.
32. Bakshi, R.A.; Aslam, A.; Khan, Z.S.; Fayaz, S.; Dar, B.N. Physiochemical, sensorial, and rheological characteristics of sauce developed from Kashmiri apples: Influence of cultivars and storage conditions. *Food Sci. Nutr.* **2022**, *10*, 1685–1693. [CrossRef]
33. Batchelor, H.; Kaukonen, A.M.; Klein, S.; Davit, B.; Ju, R.; Ternik, R.; Heimbach, T.; Lin, W.; Wnag, J.; Storey, D. Fodd effects in paediatric medicines development for products co-administered with food. *Int. J. Pharm.* **2018**, *536*, 530–535. [CrossRef]
34. Ernest, T.B.; Elder, D.P.; Martini, L.G.; Roberts, M.; Ford, J.L. Developing paediatric medicines: Identifying the needs and recognizing the challenges. *J. Pharm. Pharmacol.* **2007**, *59*, 1043–1055. [CrossRef] [PubMed]
35. Standing, J.F.; Tuleu, C. Paediatric formulations–Getting to the heart of the problem. *Int. J. Pharm.* **2005**, *300*, 56–66. [CrossRef] [PubMed]
36. WHO. Development of Paediatric Medicines: Points to Consider in Formulation. Annex 5, WHO Technical Report Series 970. 2012. Available online: https://cdn.who.int/media/docs/default-source/medicines/norms-and-standards/guidelines/trs970/annex5trs-970.pdf?sfvrsn=699cdb68_8&download=true (accessed on 23 November 2023).
37. Ducray, F.; Ramirez, C.; Robert, M.; Maxime, F.; Bronnimann, C.; Chinot, O.L.; Estrade, F.; Durando, X.; Bastid, J.; Bienaymé, H.; et al. A bioequivalence study of a novel liquid and ready-to-use temozolomide oral suspension and temozolomide capsules in patients with primary tumors central nervous system malignancies. *J. Clin. Oncol.* **2022**, *40*, e22008. [CrossRef]

pharmaceutics

MDPI

Article

A Multicenter Randomized Bioequivalence Study of a Novel Ready-to-Use Temozolomide Oral Suspension vs. Temozolomide Capsules

François Ducray [1,*], Carole Ramirez [2], Marie Robert [3], Maxime Fontanilles [4,5], Charlotte Bronnimann [6], Olivier Chinot [7], Florian Estrade [8], Xavier Durando [9,10,11,12], Stéphanie Cartalat [1], Jeremy Bastid [13], Hugues Bienayme [13] and Caroline Lemarchand [13,*]

1 Service de Neuro-Oncologie, Hôpital Neurologique, Hospices Civils de Lyon, Centre de Recherche en Cancérologie UMR INSERM 1052 CNRS 5286, Université Claude Bernard Lyon 1, 69008 Lyon, France; stephanie.cartalat01@chu-lyon.fr

2 Services de Neurologie et D'oncologie Médicale, CHU et ICHUSE de Saint-Etienne, 42055 Saint-Etienne, France; carole.ramirez@chu-st-etienne.fr

3 Institut de Cancérologie de l'Ouest, Medical Oncology, 44800 Saint Herblain, France; marie.robert@ico.unicancer.fr

4 INSERM U1245 Unit, Cancer Centre Henri Becquerel, Université Rouen Normandie, 76038 Rouen, France; maxime.fontanilles@chb.unicancer.fr

5 Le Havre Hospital Group, 76083 Le Havre, France

6 CHU de Bordeaux, Service D'oncologie Médicale, Hôpital Saint André, 33075 Bordeaux, France; charlotte.bronnimann@chu-bordeaux.fr

7 Aix-Marseille Université, Neuro-Oncology Department, APHM, CNRS, Institut de Neurophysiopathologie, CHU Timone, Service de Neuro-Oncologie, 13385 Marseille, France; olivier.chinot@ap-hm.fr

8 Centre Eugène Marquis, 35042 Rennes, France; f.estrade@rennes.unicancer.fr

9 INSERM U1240 IMoST, University of Clermont Auvergne, 63001 Clermont-Ferrand, France; xavier.durando@clermont.unicancer.fr

10 UMR 501, Clinical Investigation Centre, 63011 Clermont-Ferrand, France

11 Clinical Research and Innovation Department, Centre Jean Perrin, 63011 Clermont-Ferrand, France

12 Oncology Department, Centre Jean Perrin, 63011 Clermont-Ferrand, France

13 ORPHELIA Pharma, 75005 Paris, France; jeremy.bastid@orphelia-pharma.eu (J.B.); hugues.bienayme@orphelia-pharma.eu (H.B.)

* Correspondence: francois.ducray@chu-lyon.fr (F.D.); caroline.lemarchand@orphelia-pharma.eu (C.L.)

Abstract: Background: Temozolomide (TMZ) oral suspension (Ped-TMZ, KIZFIZO®) is being developed for the treatment of relapsed or refractory neuroblastoma, a rare cancer affecting infants and young children. The study assessed the safety and the bioequivalence of this novel pediatric formulation with existing TMZ oral capsules. Methods: In vitro dissolution profiles and the bioequivalence were evaluated following the European Medicines Agency "Guidelines on the investigation of Bioequivalence". The phase I, multicenter, randomized, open-label, crossover, single-dose bioequivalence study enrolled 36 adult patients with glioblastoma multiforme or lower-grade glioma. Each patient received 200 mg/m^2 Ped-TMZ suspension and TMZ capsules (Temodal®) on 2 consecutive days, with the order being randomly assigned. Fourteen blood samples were collected up to 10 h post-dosing. Bioequivalence was assessed by comparing the 90% confidence interval for the ratio of the geometric means of maximum TMZ plasma concentration (C_{max}) and the area under the curve (AUCt). Other endpoints included further pharmacokinetic parameters and safety. Results: Both formulations exhibited a fast in vitro dissolution profile with more than 85% of TMZ dissolved within 15 min. For the bioequivalence study, thirty patients completed the trial as per the protocol. The ratio of Ped-TMZ/TMZ capsule geometric means (90% CI) for AUCt and C_{max} were 97.18% (95.05–99.35%) and 107.62% (98.07–118.09%), respectively, i.e., within the 80–125% bioequivalence limits. No buccal toxicity was associated with Ped-TMZ liquid formulation. Conclusions: This study showed that Ped-TMZ oral suspension and TMZ oral capsule treatment are immediate release and bioequivalent medicines. There were also no unexpected safety signals or local toxicity (funded by ORPHELIA Pharma; ClinicalTrials.gov number, NCT04467346).

Keywords: temozolomide; oral suspension; bioequivalence; pediatric formulation

1. Introduction

Temozolomide (TMZ) is an alkylating agent belonging to the group of triazene compounds commonly used as chemotherapeutic drugs in cancer therapy [1]. TMZ is a second generation imidazotetrazine derivative, that does not require hepatic metabolism to form the cytotoxic methylating agent, methyl triazene imidazole-4-carboxamide (MTIC), in comparison to dimethyl triazene imidazole-4-carboxamide (DTIC) [2]. TMZ undergoes spontaneous pH-dependent hydrolysis to MTIC at a physiological pH. MTIC is then hydrolyzed to the methyldiazonium cation, which is the actual methylating agent of the DNA of tumor cells, mainly at the O^6 and N^7 positions of guanines, and the 5-aminoimidazole-4-carboxamide (AIC), which is excreted by kidney [3]. TMZ has a half-life of 1.83 h at 37 °C in phosphate buffer (0.1 M) at pH 7.4, whereas MTIC has a half-life of approximately 2 min (min) at the same pH. There is a small pH window around the physiological pH at which the propensity of TMZ to undergo ring-opening is matched by the breakdown of the MTIC in a methylating mode [2], as shown in Figure 1. The most common techniques for the determination and quantification of TMZ in human plasma are liquid chromatography coupled with mass spectrometry (in vivo investigations) [4–6] and the UV spectroscopic method for analytical samples (in vitro studies) [7].

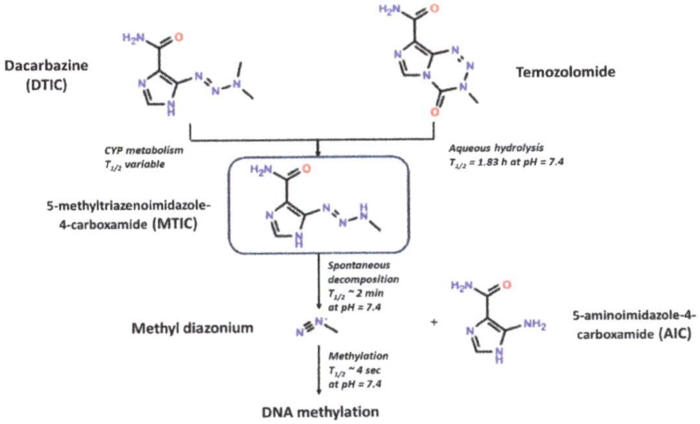

Figure 1. TMZ mechanism of action.

TMZ has been commercialized since 1999 under the tradename Temodal® in Europe and Temodar® in the US, with several oral-dose presentations: hard gel capsules 5 mg, 20 mg, 100 mg, 140 mg, 180 mg and 250 mg. TMZ is indicated for the treatment of adult patients with newly diagnosed glioblastoma multiforme and children from the age of three years, adolescents, and adult patients with recurrent malignant glioma [8]. As recommended by the International Pediatric Medical Associations, TMZ is also used off-label as a standard backbone chemotherapy for the treatment of various pediatric malignancies, notably relapsed or refractory neuroblastoma, a solid tumor affecting very young children, [9–11] as well as relapsed medulloblastoma [12] and rhabdomyosarcoma [13].

TMZ hard-gel capsules are not adapted for use in the pediatric population [14]. Although the intravenous (IV) dosage form was approved in 2009 with the same indications [8], the IV route increases toxicity (e.g., pain, irritation, pruritus, warmth, swelling and erythema at infusion site, petechia and hematoma) [15] and patients prefer oral chemotherapies, which are more convenient, administered at home with a good perception of efficacy [16]. As highlighted in the draft inventory of peadiatric therapeutic needs [14], an age-adapted oral TMZ formulation is of paramount importance for children suffering from neuroblastoma to ensure a good quality of life for these young patients treated in an outpatient setting and usually attending school. Facing the lack of age-adapted formulations, caregivers are instructed to open TMZ capsules and mix the contents with soft food to overcome swallowing difficulties. As TMZ is a bitter, highly toxic and unstable substance, this practice poses significant challenges to caregivers and the pediatric population. These include dose inaccuracy and drug instability [17], poor compliance, exposure to a cytotoxic drug, and environmental waste. To overcome this situation, the TMZ oral suspension (Ped-TMZ; KIZFIZO®) was developed as a novel pediatric oral liquid formulation that is taste-masked and ready to use. Ped-TMZ aims to prevent the inappropriate handling and exposure to toxic ingredients for parents and caregivers and is being developed for children with relapsed or refractory neuroblastoma to allow for a more precise dosage and a better compliance with treatment.

The present study aimed to evaluate the bioequivalence between Ped-TMZ and Temodal in order to assess if Ped-TMZ can be considered therapeutically equivalent to the reference oral capsule formulation. According to the EMA and FDA guidelines [18,19], with TMZ being a Biopharmaceutical Classification System (BCS) class I drug [20], a comparison of in vitro dissolution profiles can be used as a surrogate evaluation of bioequivalence. The in vitro dissolution method strategy comparing the two formulations was based on the recommendation described in the Draft Guidance on Temozolomide [21] and the FDA Guidance applied on dissolution testing [22].

As TMZ is sparingly soluble in water [23], a proportion of TMZ is already in solution in the Ped-TMZ suspension, which could potentially impact the absorption rate of TMZ (e.g., absorption from the buccal cavity) or exert formulation-specific local toxicity (e.g., mucositis). As these potential formulation-specific effects cannot be assessed in vitro, a formal bioequivalence study between Ped-TMZ and the reference product Temodal was conducted. First-in-human phase I or bioequivalence clinical studies are traditionally conducted in healthy volunteers, except for oncology drugs such as TMZ that are evaluated in cancer patients. Although the Ped-TMZ oral suspension is developed for pediatrics, the bioequivalence study was conducted in adult patients (18 years or older) with newly diagnosed glioblastoma multiforme or lower-grade glioma for ethical reasons, considering the number of blood sampling required for the pharmacokinetic (PK) analysis.

Here, we report the in vitro dissolution profiles of Ped-TMZ and Temodal capsules and the results of the formal bioequivalence study undertaken in adult patients comparing the PK parameters of both formulations after a single-dose administration. We describe the general and local safety of Ped-TMZ.

2. Materials and Methods

2.1. Products

The commercially available Temodal capsules, 100 mg, were purchased from Merck Sharp & Dohme, Puteaux, France. The investigational product Ped-TMZ, TMZ oral suspension, 40 mg/mL (brand name: KIZFIZO) was provided by ORPHELIA Pharma, Paris, France.

2.2. Reagents and Chemicals

For dissolution testing, analytical reagents were purified water (Milli-Q Elix Essential 5, Merck Chimie SAS, Fontenay-Sous-Bois, France) and hydrochloric acid R (37%) grade for analysis (J.T. Baker). For the bioanalytical assays, TMZ and the internal standard temozolomide-d3 (TMZ-d3) were purchased from TRC (North York, ON, Canada). The reagent-grade acetonitrile, isopropanol and methanol of gradient grade purity were purchased from Carlo Erba, trichloroacetic acid (TCA), ammonium acetate 7.5 M solution and formic acid were purchased from Sigma (St Louis, MO, USA), glacial acetic acid was from Honeywell (Charlotte, NC, USA) and dimethyl sulfoxide (DMSO) was from ACROS. Acetic acid used to prepare acetic acid 10% solution was purchased from Thermo Fisher

Scientific (Waltham, MA, USA), and purified water (Milli-Q direct 8, Merck Chimie SAS, Fontenay-Sous-Bois, France) was used. Human plasma from healthy donors was provided by BioIVT (UK). Microtubes in polypropylene were purchased from Sarstedt (Nümbrecht, Germany) and Nunc™ 96 DeepWell™ Polystyrene Plates (DWP) were purchased from Thermo Fisher Scientific (Waltham, MA, USA).

2.3. In Vitro Dissolution Testing

The in vitro dissolution testing was performed using the basket (USP 1) apparatus (Dissolutest apparatus, Sotax, Aesch, Switzerland) described in the 10th Edition of European Pharmacopoeia 2.9.3 monograph [24] or US Pharmacopeia <711> [25] at 37 °C ± 0.5 °C and setting the agitation speed at 100 rpm. One hundred milligrams was used for the dissolution test by introducing one 100 mg TMZ capsule or 2.5 mL of Ped-TMZ (40 mg/mL) into 500 mL of dissolution medium (0.1 N HCl prepared via dilution of 8.5 mL of hydrochloric acid R (37%) to 1000.0 mL with purified water). Samples were collected using peristaltic pump (Sotax, Aesch, Swizerland) at 5, 10, 15, 20, 30 and 45 min and analyzed online by direct UV-reading after filtration on 1 µm glass filter (Macherey-Nagel, Düren, Germany). Dissolved TMZ is quantified by UV spectrophotometry (Lambda 75 UV/visible spectrophotometer Perkin Elmer, Shelton, CT, USA) at 328 nm. The evaluation is based on absorbance measurement and external standardization with relative response. The dissolution medium was used as blank solution. The assay of TMZ was validated for linearity, accuracy and precision according to the guideline ICH Q2 (R1) [26]. The method is linear over the range 20% to 100% (R = 1.0000). The accuracy and precision were tested on the three following series: 20%, 100% and 120% of TMZ. The mean recovery ranged from 99.78% to 101.4%, and all individual recovery complied with the 95.0–105.0% acceptance criteria. Regarding the precision, the coefficient of variation ranged from 0.4% to 0.7% for repeatability and from 0.7% to 1.8% for intermediate precision. The dissolution profile of TMZ was determined for both pharmaceutical forms (n = 12).

2.4. Bioequivalence Study Design and Oversight

We conducted a phase I, multicenter, randomized, open-label, crossover, single-dose bioequivalence study in seven centers in France (Hôpital Neurologique and Neurobiotec, Hospices Civils de Lyon, Lyon, France; Centre Hospitalier Universitaire de Saint-Etienne, Saint-Etienne, France; Institut de Cancérologie de l'Ouest, Medical Oncology, Saint Herblain, France; Cancer Centre Henri Becquerel, Rouen, France; Hôpital St André, Bordeaux, France; CHU Hôpital de La Timone, Marseille, France; Centre Eugène Marquis, Rennes, France; and Oncology Department, Centre Jean Perrin, Clermont-Ferrand, France).

Patient medical history was assessed and a physical examination, including buccal examination, was conducted, as detailed in the clinical study protocol (CSP). The CSP was approved by an independent ethics committee in France. The sponsor (ORPHELIA Pharma) designed the study and oversaw its conduct in collaboration with the contracted research organization, Eurofins Optimed. The study was conducted in accordance with the principles of the Declaration of Helsinki, Good Clinical Practice guidelines (ICHE6) and any relevant local regulatory requirements. Investigators were responsible for data collection and analysis.

2.5. Participants

Adult patients (18 years or older) with newly diagnosed glioblastoma multiforme or lower-grade glioma (grade 2 or grade 3) treated with exactly 200 mg/m^2 TMZ as monotherapy participated in the bioequivalence study. Eligible patients had a body mass index (BMI) in the range of 18.5 to 30 kg/m^2 and were non-pregnant and non-breast feeding. All participants provided written informed consent prior to the screening visit. Key exclusion criteria were the co-administration of sodium valproate or valproic acid (which may reduce TMZ clearance [8]) and the use of nasogastric tubes. A full list of the eligibility criteria is provided in Supplementary S1.

Patients were able to withdraw or discontinue the study if they decided to do so at any time, irrespective of the reason. A follow-up visit was planned by the investigator to conduct end-of-study visit examinations. Further criteria for withdrawal or premature discontinuation were adverse events (AEs). According to the investigator's decision, participants experiencing AEs were monitored until conditions were resolved, or the patient was lost to follow-up.

2.6. Interventions

Participants were randomly assigned in a 1:1 ratio, using an interactive web-based response system, to receive a single oral administration of 200 mg/m^2 of each formulation (Ped-TMZ suspension [test product] or TMZ capsule, Temodal [reference product]) on D1 or D2 of a five-day cycle (Figure 2). No wash-out period was required between administrations, owing to the short half-life of TMZ (approximately 1.8 h [8]). Hospitalization was planned for 10 h (from 8:00 a.m. to 6:00 p.m.) for D1 and D2 or for the 48 h (h). During this period, TMZ was administered as a daily dose rounded to 300 mg or 400 mg. Prior to TMZ administration, participants were asked to maintain fasting conditions for 8 h. All patients were pre-medicated with 8 mg ondansetron (orodispersible tablet or tablet) 30 min prior to TMZ administration to prevent the nausea and vomiting associated with chemotherapy. TMZ administration took place around 8:00 a.m., after which 240 mL of tap water was used for study standardization and mouth rinsing, in a sitting position. Fasting conditions continued for 4 h post-dose, after which a standardized lunch was served. Additionally, any concomitant medications, except corticosteroid and anti-epileptic treatment, were delayed for 4 h post-dose. Concomitant treatments with valproate or valproic acid were excluded; other antiepileptic drugs were permitted.

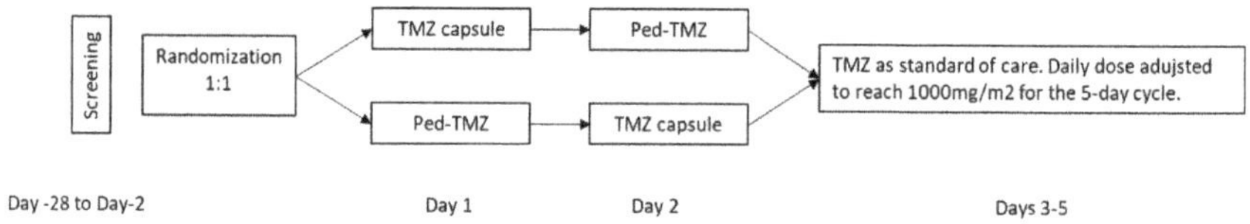

Figure 2. Bioequivalence study design. Screening procedures were conducted from Day 28 to Day 2 before starting study medication. Patients were treated on Day 1 and Day 2 of a treatment cycle. Patients received, under fasting conditions, 200 mg/m^2 Ped-TMZ oral suspension on one day and 200 mg/m^2 TMZ capsule treatment on the other day, with the order being randomly assigned in a 1:1 ratio. From D3 to D5 (outside the scope of the trial), patients received TMZ as standard of care.

From D3 to D5 of the treatment cycle, TMZ was administered outside of the scope of the trial as the standard of care, with the daily dose adjusted to reach a total of 1000 mg/m^2 for the five-day treatment cycle.

2.7. Blood Sample Collection

Visit-specific blood handling procedures, along with clinical and biological examinations at baseline, D1, D2 and end-of study visit are detailed in the Supplementary S2. In brief, for TMZ concentration measurements, a total of 28 $\times$ 6 mL blood samples were drawn per patient (14 blood samples of 6 mL per study day). Blood samples were collected pre-dose (T0), at 10 min, 20 min, 30 min, 45 min, 1 h (h), 1.5 h, 2 h, 2.5 h, 3 h, 4 h, 6 h, 8 h and 10 h post-dose in each period (Supplementary S3). The 6 mL of venous blood was collected using a pre-chilled vacuum tube with K_2EDTA. The blood samples were cooled in an ice-water bath immediately after sampling and centrifuged (4 °C, 2500$\times$ g, 5 min) to separate plasma within 30 min of blood collection.

For the determination of TMZ plasma concentrations, plasma samples were prepared in duplicate. Two aliquots of 1.0 mL of plasma sample were placed in a polypropylene tube containing 50 µL of 10% acetic acid solution (stabilizer) within 5 min after centrifugation.

The acidified plasma was vortexed, and the tube was then sealed and stored frozen at −80 ± 10 °C until bioanalysis.

2.8. TMZ Bioanalysis

All plasma samples were prepared by protein precipitation and TMZ in human plasma extracts was assayed according to a liquid chromatography-tandem mass spectrometry (LC-MS/MS) validated analytical method.

2.8.1. Sample Preparation

Plasma samples were thawed at room temperature in water batch and vortexed. Twenty (20) µL of the samples were spiked with 20 µL of Internal Standard (IS) (TMZ-d3) solution prepared in DMSO, and then, 70 µL of TCA 10% were added. The samples were vortexed for approximately 30 s and centrifuged at 20,000× *g* and 4 °C for 5 min. Twenty-five µL of supernatant were transferred into 96 DWP plates. Following addition of 400 µL of solvent A (see below the composition), plates were mixed and centrifuged at 2500× *g* and 4 °C for 5 min. The rinsing solvent consisted of a mix of acetonitrile, methanol, isopropanol and water (1/1/1/1; *v*/*v*/*v*/*v*) with 0.1% of formic acid. Then, injection of samples in LC-MS/MS was performed.

The solution of TMZ and IS (TMZ-d3) used for calibration standard and quality control (QC) are prepared in DMSO. As TMZ is unstable at physiological pH, blank matrix is prepared by acidification of plasma with acetic acid 10%. The calibration standard and QC are prepared by addition of solution of TMZ and IS to blank matrix previously centrifugated at 2500× *g* and 4 °C for 5 min.

2.8.2. Chromatographic Conditions

A LC-MS API4000 (Applied Biosystems/Sciex LLC, Framingham, MA, USA) equipped with HPLC pumps LC-20AD or LC-20-ADXR (Shimadzu Corp, Japan) and an automatic temperature-controlled sampler SIL-10AC or SIL-20ACXR (Shimadzu Corp., Kyoto, Japan) was used to chromatographically separate TMZ and its Internal Standard (IS) from the plasma matrix obtained after protein precipitation. Chromatographic analysis was achieved using a Synergi Hydro-RP 2 × 100 mm, 2.5 µm column (Phenomenex, Torrance, CA, USA). The mobile phases consisted of ammonium acetate 10 mM solution containing 0.20% of formic acid (solvent A) and methanol containing 0.10% of formic acid (solvent B). The gradient elution was started with 30% of solvent B, then increased up to 95% for 0.5 min, maintained for 1.0 min, and then decreased to 30% of phase B for 0.01 min. The final composition was maintained until the end of the run (4 min). The column temperature was maintained at 40 °C throughout all measurements, whereas the sample temperature was kept at 4 °C. A volume of 5 µL sample was injected at the flow rate of 0.3 $mL{\cdot}min^{-1}$. The column eluent was directed into a triple quadrupole mass spectrometer API4000 (Applied Biosystems/Sciex LLC, Framingham, MA, USA) with an electrospray ionization source (ESI). The TMZ and TMZ-d3 were detected by monitoring mass transition using Multiple Reaction Monitoring (MRM) scan mode. The mass transitions were 198.2 > 138.3 for TMZ and 195.1 > 138.0 for TMZ-d3 with Dwell of 200 ms, the declustering potential of 60 v, the collision energy of 14 eV and a collision cell exit potential of 15 v for each transition. The data were acquired using the Analyst® software (version 1.6.3, Applied Biosystems/Sciex LLC, Framingham, MA, USA).

The method was validated according to the bioanalytical method validation guidelines of the US FDA [27] and EMA [28]. The specificity of the method was demonstrated towards TMZ in presence of AIC and MTIC. The TMZ plasma assay was linear over the range of 0.1 to 25 µg/mL weighting with quadratic regression ($1/x^2$). The deviation ranged from −5.88 to 10.17%. Intra-run and inter-run precision ranged from 1.01 to 9.76% and from 1.10 to 6.82%, respectively, for the 4 tested concentrations (0.1, 0.3, 12.5 and 20 µg/mL). No carry over was observed. The absence of TMZ contribution on IS and vice versa was verified. A

10-fold dilution process was validated. Bench-top and long-term stabilities at -80 ± 10 °C were validated to cover the handling and the storage of plasma samples before bioanalysis.

Finally, the robustness of the analytical method was demonstrated by sample reanalysis, with 90.15% of incurred sample reanalysis results meeting the acceptance criteria.

2.9. Calculation of Pharmacokinetic Parameters

The co-primary endpoints were two pharmacokinetic parameters determined from TMZ plasma concentrations obtained on D1 and D2: the observed maximum plasma concentration (C_{max}) and the area under the plasma concentration curve from administration to the last quantifiable concentration at time t (AUC_t). Secondary endpoints were the area under the plasma concentration curve extrapolated to infinity (AUC_{inf}), the first time to reach C_{max} (T_{max}), elimination rate constant (λ) and the plasma elimination half-life ($t_{1/2}$). Additionally, the residual area of TMZ ($\%AUC_{extra}$) was determined from TMZ plasma concentrations obtained on D1 and D2. Safety was assessed throughout the study, including physical and buccal examination, vital signs, adverse events, concomitant treatments, electrocardiogram and laboratory examinations.

2.10. Statistical Analyses

Sample size calculations were based on previous TMZ bioequivalence studies [29–31]. It was estimated that 30 patients were required to achieve the lower limit of the 90% confidence interval (CI) and the upper limit of the 90% CI for the primary endpoints.

All randomized patients were included in the intention-to-treat set (ITTS), which provided the basis for descriptive statistics regarding quantitative and qualitative parameters. Quantitative parameters were provided using mean, standard deviation (SD), standard error of the mean (SEM), minimum, median, maximum, and number of observations, whereas qualitative parameters were provided using frequencies (n) and percent frequencies (%). Patient medical history was listed and summarized by system organ class and preferred term (Medical Dictionary for Regulatory Activity; MedDRA), if relevant. Abnormal physical findings at baseline were listed. Concomitant treatments were listed (coding performed according to the World Health Organization drug dictionary) by treatment group and patient.

Patients from the ITTS that completed the study without protocol deviations or violations thought to significantly affect the pharmacokinetic analysis (e.g., observed AEs such as vomiting and diarrhea) were included in the PK set. The pharmacokinetic and statistical analyses were carried out using Phoenix WinNonlin™ software (Version 8.1; Certara, Princeton, NJ, USA) based on an independent model method (non-compartmental analysis). The primary endpoints C_{max} and AUC_t were analyzed using an analysis of variance (ANOVA) of two treatments, two periods and two-way crossover general linear model with the fixed effects of sequence, subject tested within sequence, period and treatment to determine error variance of ANOVA. Each ANOVA included the calculation of least-square means, adjusted differences between treatment means and the standard error associated with these differences. The level of significance for period and sequence was 0.05. However, since the difference between treatments is being tested with 90% CI, the treatment effect from ANOVA for any pharmacokinetic parameter was not considered. For the pharmacokinetic parameters C_{max} and AUC_t, the CI for test and reference product averages were calculated using the ANOVA output from the analysis of the ln-transformed data. Inter-patient variability (%CV) was calculated for plasma concentration vs. time data and all pharmacokinetic parameters (T_{max}, C_{max}, AUC_t, AUC_{inf}, elimination rate constant [K_{el}], $t_{1/2}$ and $\%AUC_{extra}$). Intra-patient variability (%CV) was calculated for pharmacokinetic parameters C_{max} and AUC_t based on ln-transformed data. The ratio of geometric mean for C_{max} and AUC_t are reported as point estimates. The bioequivalence between the test and reference products was assessed if the 90% CI fell within the [80–125%] bioequivalence limits for C_{max} and AUC_t [18,32]. The assessment of bioequivalence was based on 90% CIs for the ratio of the population geometric means (test/reference) for the parameters under consideration. This method is equivalent to two one-sided tests with the null hypothesis of bio-inequivalence at the 5% significance level.

Patients from the ITTS who received at least one study treatment dose were included in the safety set for reporting safety parameters. AEs were coded according to the MedDRA. They were classified into pre-defined standard categories according to chronological criteria. Treatment-emergent AEs (TEAEs) were defined as AEs that occurred for the first time or, if present before, worsened during exposure to the drug(s). TEAEs were summarized by primary System Organ Class (SOC), Preferred Term (PT) and treatment group, with evaluations of the number of AEs and the number of patients reporting these AEs. Non-TEAEs were defined as AEs that occurred prior to study drug administration (also called "pre-dose event") and summarized by SOC, PT, and sequence. Any potential local toxicity reaction in the mouth relating to Ped-TMZ oral suspension intake, such as but not limited to intensive local pain or ulcerative lesion of the mucosa, were categorized as AEs of special interest (AESI). The statistical analysis for safety parameters consisted of individual data listings and descriptive/inferential statistics using the SAS® computer program (release 9.4, SAS Institute, Cary, NC, USA).

3. Results

3.1. *In Vitro Dissolution Testing*

Prior to the initiation of the bioequivalence study, an in vitro dissolution study was conducted on Ped-TMZ 40 mg/mL oral suspension compared to TMZ 100 mg capsules following the EMA and FDA Guidelines [18,19]. The in vitro dissolution testing was carried out using the basket method according to a strategy based on the recommendation for the TMZ capsule described in the Draft Guidance on Temozolomide [21] and the FDA Guidance on Dissolution Testing [22]. As shown in Figure 3, 94.5% and 88.9% of TMZ is released at 15 min for Ped-TMZ and TMZ 100 mg capsules, respectively. According to the guideline, as more than 85% of TMZ is dissolved within 15 min for both products, they can be considered as immediate-release medicines and no statistical calculation is required for the demonstration of similarity according to the EMA guideline [18]. Of note, the difference between the dissolution profiles at 5 min (33.9% for Temodal compared to 98.1% for Ped-TMZ) is expected and reflects the progressive solubilization of the hard gel capsule (gelatin) of Temodal. From the 10 min dissolution timepoint, both profiles have a similar shape.

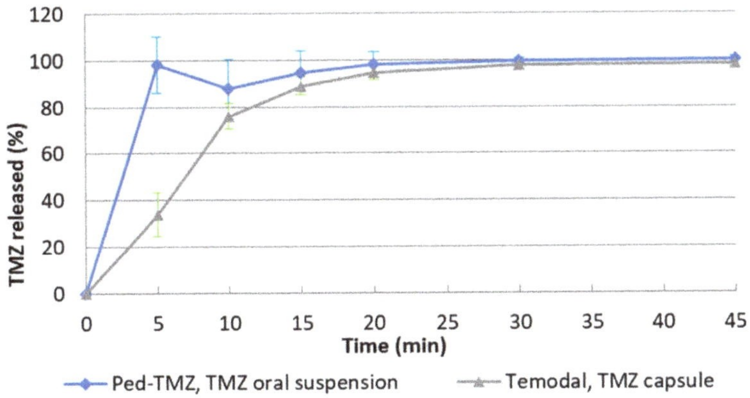

Figure 3. In vitro dissolution rates of Ped-TMZ oral suspension and TMZ capsules in HCl 0.1 N ($n = 12$). Error bars represent SD.

3.2. *Pharmacokinetic Bioequivalence Study*

3.2.1. Baseline Demographics

From September 2020 through to December 2021, 36 patients were enrolled in the study and comprised the ITTS. Three patients were withdrawn, two upon the investigator's decision and one due to a treatment administration error (for TMZ capsule treatment, a dose of 500 mg was administered instead of 300 mg). Four major deviations involving three additional patients were detected during the study and led to the exclusion and replacement of these patients (two missing pharmacokinetic samplings in one patient and two patients did not follow the fasting protocol). Thirty (30) patients completed the study without protocol deviations or violations (PK set). Patient disposition and details regarding the different population sets are presented in Figure 4.

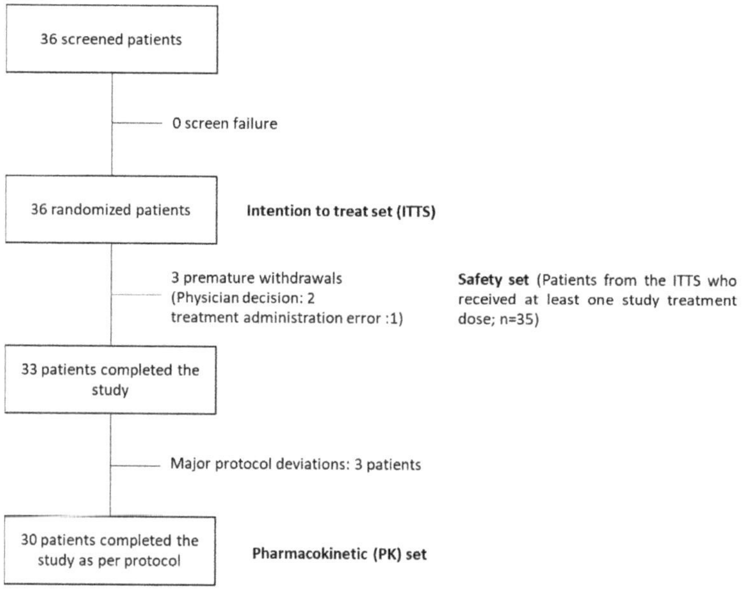

Figure 4. Patient disposition according to CONSORT and details of the different population sets.

Patient demographics and baseline characteristics are summarized in Table 1 and further described in Supplementary Table S1. Most participants were male (27/36, 75%), with a mean age of 52 years. Their BMIs ranged from 19.8 to 30.6 kg/m^2. Most patients (30/36) had a Karnofsky index equal to or higher than 80. In the ITTS, the Karnofsky performance score ranged from 60 to 100%, with a mean of 85.3 $\pm$ 11.3%. Most patients (30/36, 83.3%) had at least a medical or surgical history, but this was not considered to have an impact on safety and pharmacokinetic assessment criteria. Concomitant treatments, including anti-epileptics and steroids, are described in Supplementary Table S2.

Table 1. Baseline demographics from the ITT (n = 36), Safety (n = 35) and PK (n = 30) sets. BMI, body mass index; BSA, body surface area; ITT, intention-to-treat set; Max, maximum; Min, minimum; PK, pharmacokinetic set; SD, standard derivation.

	ITTS (n = 36)	**Safety Set (n = 35)**	**PK Set (n = 30)**
Age (years)			
Mean $\pm$ SD	52.3 $\pm$ 14.8	52.0 $\pm$ 14.9	52.8 $\pm$ 14.6
Min/Max	20/79	20/79	20/79

Table 1. *Cont.*

	ITTS (*n* = 36)	**Safety Set** (*n* = 35)	**PK Set** (*n* = 30)
Sex, n (%)			
Female	9 (25.0)	9 (25.7)	8 (26.7)
Male	27 (75.0)	26 (74.3)	22 (73.3)
Height (cm)			
Mean ± SD	173.22 ± 8.00	173.11 ± 8.09	172.93 ± 7.97
Min/Max	157/188	157/188	157/188
Weight (kg)			
Mean ± SD	74.45 ± 10.96	74.38 ± 11.11	74.40 ± 11.79
Min/Max	58.0/102.0	58.0/102.0	58.0/102.0
BMI (kg/m^2)			
Mean ± SD	24.79 ± 2.91	24.79 ± 2.95	24.82 ± 2.93
Min/Max	19.8/30.6	19.8/30.6	19.8/30.6
BSA (m^2)			
Mean ± SD	1.89 ± 0.17	1.89 ± 0.17	1.89 ± 0.18
Min/Max	1.6/2.3	1.6/2.3	1.6/2.3

3.2.2. Pharmacokinetic Parameters and Plasma Concentrations

For the 30 patients of the pharmacokinetic (PK) set, 28 × 6 mL blood samples were drawn per patient (14 blood samples per day) from T0 (pre-dose) to 10 h post-dose. The mean plasma concentration–time curves are shown in Figure 5.

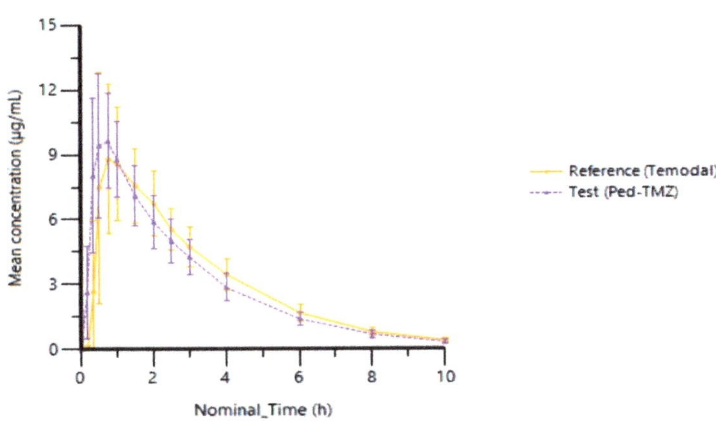

Figure 5. Plasma TMZ concentration after a single administration of 200 mg/m^2 Ped-TMZ oral suspension (test) and TMZ capsule (Temodal, reference) (mean ± SD, *n* = 30 patients).

The PK parameters calculated following the oral administration of the TMZ capsule (reference) or Ped-TMZ oral suspension (test) are presented in Table 2. The co-primary endpoints C_{max} and AUC_t were similar after oral administration of the two formulations and even showed less variability after administration of the Ped-TMZ oral suspension (%CV = 23.2% and 16.2%) than after administration of the TMZ capsule treatment (%CV = 37.1% and 18.2%). The mean C_{max} (±SD) was 10.94 ± 2.54 µg/mL for Ped-TMZ and 10.51 ± 3.89 µg/mL for TMZ capsule. The mean AUC_t (±SD) was 30.47 ± 4.94 h·µg/mL for Ped-TMZ and 31.47 ± 5.73 h·µg/mL for the TMZ capsule treatment. Secondary endpoints (mean ± SD) for Ped-TMZ vs. TMZ capsule treatment included AUC_{inf} (31.38 ± 5.06 vs. 32.58 ± 5.84), T_{max} (0.65 ± 0.30 vs. 0.91 ± 0.41 h), K_{el} (0.37 ± 0.04 vs. 0.36 (0.03) 1/h) and $t_{1/2}$ (1.91 ± 0.21 vs. 1.93 ± 0.16 h).

Table 2. Pharmacokinetic data of the pharmacokinetic set (n = 30 patients). Results are displayed as arithmetic mean. $\%AUC_{extra}$, percentage of extrapolated AUC; AUC_{inf}, area under the plasma concentration curve extrapolated to infinity; AUC_t, area under the plasma concentration curve from administration to the last quantifiable concentration at time t; C_{max}, observed maximum plasma concentration of TMZ; CV, subject variability; K_{el}, estimated by the linear regression of the logarithm of the terminal concentration as a function of time; Max, maximum; Min, minimum; n, number of patients; SD, standard derivation; $t_{1/2}$, plasma elimination half-life, calculated as $t_{1/2} = \ln_2/K_{el}$; T_{max}, first time to reach C_{max}.

Parameter (Unit)	Statistic	TMZ Capsule (Reference) (n = 30)	Ped-TMZ Oral Suspension (Test) (n = 30)
T_{max} (h)	Mean	0.909	0.649
	SD	0.405	0.302
	Median	0.77	0.63
	Min-max	0.33–2.00	0.33–1.53
C_{max} (μg/mL)	Mean	10.506	10.939
	SD	3.894	2.540
	% CV	37.1	23.2
AUC_t (h·μg/mL)	Mean	31.471	30.467
	SD	5.727	4.939
	% CV	18.2	16.2
AUC_{inf} (h·μg/mL)	Mean	32.584	31.376
	SD	5.840	5.062
	% CV	17.9	16.1
K_{el} (1/h)	Mean	0.362	0.367
	SD	0.031	0.035
	% CV	9.5	9.5
$t_{1/2}$ (h)	Mean	1.928	1.909
	SD	0.163	0.205
	% CV	8.4	10.7
$\%AUC_{extra}$ (%)	Mean	3.454	2.901
	SD	0.954	0.895
	% CV	27.6	30.8

3.2.3. Bioequivalence of Ped-TMZ Oral Suspension vs. TMZ Capsules

Assessment of bioequivalence was based upon the 90% two-sided CI of the geometric means ratio for the AUC_t and C_{max} parameters. Two products are deemed bioequivalent if the 90% two-sided CIs are within the acceptance interval (80% to 125%). The geometric means for Ped-TMZ vs. TMZ capsule treatment were 30.09 h·μg/mL vs. 30.96 h·μg/mL for AUC_t and 10.67 μg/mL vs. 9.92 μg/mL for C_{max}, respectively (Table 3). The ratios of geometric means (Ped-TMZ/TMZ capsule) for AUC_t and C_{max} were 97.18% and 107.62%, respectively, and the 90% CIs for AUC_t (95.05–99.35%) and C_{max} (98.07–118.09%) were within the 80% to 125% limits for bioequivalence. Intra-patient variability for AUC_t and C_{max} were 2.53% and 4.47%, respectively. The results satisfied the bioequivalence criteria of the Bioequivalence Guidelines (90% CIs between 80% and 125%). The two examined medications Ped-TMZ oral suspension and TMZ capsules are bioequivalent.

Table 3. Summary of pharmacokinetic parameters from the PK set (n = 30) treated with Ped-TMZ oral suspension and TMZ oral capsule. Results are displayed as geometric mean.; AUC_t, area under the plasma concentration curve from administration to the last quantifiable concentration at time t; CI, confidence interval; C_{max}, observed maximum plasma concentration of TMZ.

	TMZ Oral Capsule (Reference) (n = 30)		Ped-TMZ Oral Suspension (Test) (n = 30)
C_{max} (μg/mL)	9.92		10.67
C_{max} ratio (%) (90% CI)		107.62 (98.07;118.09)	
C_{max} % CV		4.47	
AUC_t (h·μg/mL)	30.96		30.09
AUC_t ratio (%) (90% CI)		97.18 (95.05;99.35)	
AUC_t % CV		2.53	

3.2.4. Safety Assessment

Among the 35 patients included in the safety set, 34 patients received at least one study treatment dose, as scheduled in the protocol. No serious adverse events (SAEs) were reported during this study. During the overall study period, five patients (14.3%) reported the occurrence of six treatment-emergent AEs (TEAEs), i.e., AEs that occurred after treatment initiation. Of these, four TEAEs were experienced by four patients after Ped-TMZ oral suspension administration. These included two episodes of headache of mild intensity, judged by the investigators to be unrelated or unlikely to be related to the study treatment; one episode of mild nausea, judged to be related to the treatment; and one episode of mild diarrhea, judged by the investigators to be unrelated to the treatment. Two TEAEs (one episode of moderate lymphopenia and one episode of headache of mild intensity) were experienced by two patients after TMZ capsule administration and were all judged to be unrelated to the treatment. Three pre-dose events, that were not TEAEs, were also reported. All the TEAEs were resolved before the end of the study. There was no evidence of clinically relevant treatment-related abnormalities for laboratory parameters, vital signs, physical findings or electrocardiogram recordings.

As Ped-TMZ is the first oral liquid dosage form of TMZ, buccal adverse events of special interest (AESIs), defined as any potential local toxicity reaction in the mouth, such as intensive local pain or ulcerative lesion of the mucosa, were carefully monitored. Importantly, no such buccal toxicity associated with the use of Ped-TMZ was detected during this study.

4. Discussion

TMZ is widely used as standard chemotherapy to treat a broad range of pediatric malignancies, including relapsed or refractory neuroblastoma [9–11], which affects very young children. However, the currently available oral dosing forms are not adapted to the pediatric population, and an age-appropriate TMZ formulation is on the priority list established by the EMA [14]. Ped-TMZ, an oral suspension of TMZ (KIZFIZO), has been developed with the aim of providing an age-appropriate formulation to the pediatric population, with accuracy, flexibility of dose adjustment according to the BSA, ease of use and taste masking.

Here, we investigated the in vitro dissolution profile as well as the pharmacokinetic properties and safety of the TMZ oral suspension (Ped-TMZ) developed to address the needs of pediatric patients. This open-label and randomized clinical study was conducted, in adult patients with gliomas for ethical reasons, to assess the bioequivalence of a single dose of 200 mg/m^2 of TMZ administered as an oral suspension (Ped-TMZ) or capsule (Temodal) under fasting conditions. The plasma concentration–time profile and PK parameters were similar for both treatments. The 90% CIs of the geometric means of the exposure

PK parameters, C_{max} and AUC_t, were contained within the bioequivalence limits of 80% to 125%, demonstrating the bioequivalence between Ped-TMZ, TMZ oral suspension and TMZ capsules.

Our PK findings (mean PK parameters) are in-line with previous PK analyses from 359 adult patients collected in three phase I studies (patients with advanced cancer without bone marrow involvement) and three phase II studies (patients with glioblastoma multiforme or anaplastic astrocytoma) as described in the Temodal European public assessment report (EPAR) [33]. Since Temodal approval, many PK clinical investigations of TMZ have been conducted, currently offering a bigger set of patients. Thirty-one (31) PK studies of TMZ in adult patients [3,6,34–62] and 12 PK studies conducted in children [58,63–73], where the AUC and C_{max} mean value are reported with or without CV, were selected for the determination of PK parameters in these two populations. Despite the limitations of pooling the data (e.g., quality not necessarily the same across all studies), the mean value of the AUC and C_{max} calculated from the pooled data of these studies were reported in the Figures 6 and 7, as a function of the administrated dose in mg/m^2. The linear regression was also calculated without intercept (i.e., the parameter is predicted to be 0 when the dose is 0).

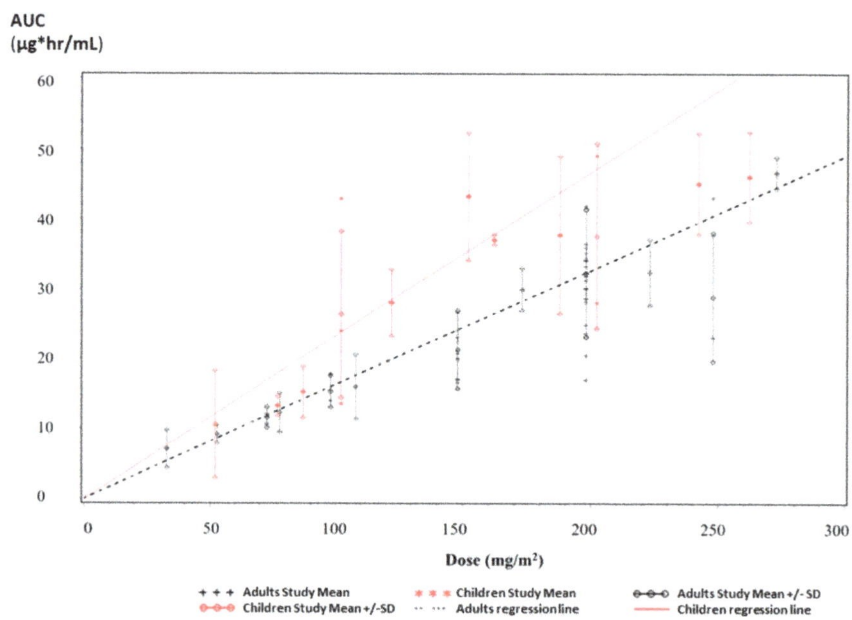

Figure 6. AUC from TMZ PK studies in adults and children.

The mean AUC value of Ped-TMZ after a dose of 200 mg/m^2 (30.47 µg·hr/mL), which is close to the one of Temodal in our study (31.47 µg·hr/mL), is very consistent with the published data (Figure 6). For the dose of 200 mg/m^2, AUC values collected from the literature ranged from 17.00 to 41.80 µg·hr/mL [3,44], with a mean of 32.03 µg·hr/mL from the pooled data set. Similarly, C_{max} determined for Ped-TMZ (10.94 µg/mL) and Temodal (10.51 µg/mL) are consistent with the data collected from the literature (Figure 7). C_{max} ranged from 5.20 to 15.3 µg/mL [3,35], with a mean value from the pooled data of 9.98 µg/mL for the dose of 200 mg/m^2.

In the perspective of pediatric use of Ped-TMZ, the PK data (AUC and C_{max}) from clinical studies conducted in adults was compared to those coming from clinical studies conducted in the pediatric population. This descriptive analysis interestingly highlights some differences and similarities of the main PK parameters (AUC and C_{max}) when comparing the data in adults and in children. The AUC values observed in children are higher than in adults (Figure 6), which is consistent with the EPAR of Temodal [33] and the current EMA summary of product characteristics (SmPC) [8], and which is expected when dosing is carried out by BSA in children. There was no difference in C_{max} between children and adults (Figure 7), which is not in agreement with the EPAR of Temodal reporting higher C_{max} in children [33]. The ongoing TEMOkids pediatric PK population study will help to better characterize the exposure of children to Ped-TMZ.

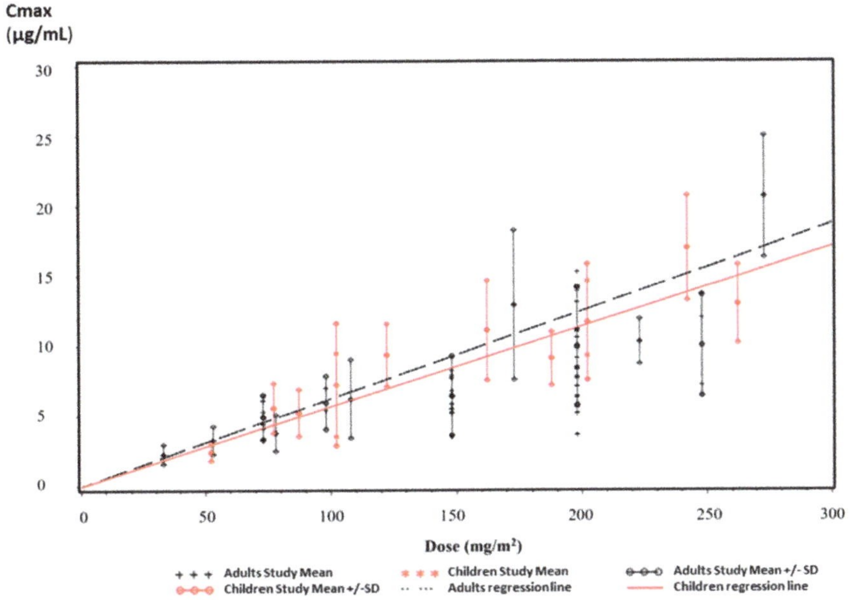

Figure 7. C_{max} from TMZ PK studies in adults and children.

Our investigations showed that Ped-TMZ reached T_{max} after 0.6 h, whereas the mean $t_{1/2}$ was 1.91 h, values which are congruent with known T_{max} between 0.5 and 1.5 h and $t_{1/2}$ of approximately 1.8 h for TMZ capsules [2,8,15].

Despite the water-soluble and immediately bioavailable fraction of TMZ (approximately 8%, data not shown) in the Ped-TMZ suspension, the C_{max} and T_{max} did not differ to the reference product Temodal. No rapid oromucosal absorption of TMZ can be suspected from the buccal cavity: the total dose of TMZ in Ped-TMZ is swallowed and absorbed from the gastrointestinal tract. The absorption PK profile is consistent with an in vitro, dissolution profile, showing the fast release of TMZ (more than 85% dissolved within 15 min). The slight difference of the TMZ release observed at the very early timepoint of the dissolution profile (close to 100% for Ped-TMZ vs. 30% for Temodal) reflects the solubilization of the hard gel capsule of Temodal and is confirmed as insignificant regarding the in vivo bioequivalence.

As a first in human trial, this study aimed to report the short-term safety profile of the Ped-TMZ oral suspension, which is in accordance with that expected for the TMZ capsule treatment [8,74]. No serious AEs were reported. A total of six TEAEs were reported including gastrointestinal disorders, blood and lymphatic system disorders or nervous system disorders. All were mild to moderate in severity and only 1/6 was considered to be related to the study drug (Ped TMZ) by the investigator. They were resolved before the end of the study. One limitation of the present study is that it assessed the safety of Ped-TMZ for a short treatment period (only 2 days). The full safety profile of Ped-TMZ, including the evaluation of any potential oral complications following administration of Ped-TMZ in the longer term and in the targeted population (pediatrics), is being investigated in the TEMOkids trial (NCT04610736).

This study aimed at collecting any potential signal of buccal toxicity specifically related to a liquid formulation of a chemotherapeutic drug. The lack of selectivity of antineoplastic oral chemotherapy may result in direct toxicity, upon action of the drug on the oral mucosa, or indirect toxicity, as a consequence of chemotherapeutic drug-induced bone-marrow suppression or myelosuppression. Local adverse events such as oropharyngeal mucositis are not mentioned in the Temodal SmPC [8]. Areview of the literature led us to identify one study evaluating alisertib in combination with irinotecan and oral TMZ in pediatric and young adult neuroblastoma patients, in which mucositis was reported in 9% of the 244 courses [75], although most likely attributable to alisertib. Nevertheless, a liquid formulation of a cytotoxic drug such as Ped-TMZ may potentially irritate the mucosa when administered orally. Some precautions were taken with administration of 240 mL of water immediately after the treatment with Ped-TMZ. Buccal toxicity was specifically monitored during the study with buccal examination before and after administration of Ped-TMZ and at the end of the study. The first signs of oral complications (inflammatory/vascular phase) generally occur shortly after the administration of chemotherapy, with the release of epithelial cytokines producing local tissue damage that leads to early stage of mucositis [76]. In this clinical study, no acute buccal toxicity (i.e., early stage of mucositis) occurring after the administration of Ped-TMZ was detected, which is in line with the safety profile of a hospital compounded liquid formulation [77]. Further potential oral complications are being specifically monitored in the pediatric TEMOkids study, in which patients receive up to six cycles of treatment.

5. Conclusions

Ped-TMZ oral suspension (KIZFIZO) is the first drinkable form of TMZ specifically developed to address the needs of pediatric cancer patients or patients presenting swallowing difficulties. This study demonstrated the bioequivalence of the Ped-TMZ oral suspension vs. TMZ oral hard-gel capsules (Temodal), meaning that the two formulations are therapeutically equivalent. The safety profile of Ped-TMZ in this first in human study is similar to the one of the TMZ capsules, without any acute buccal complication occurring after the administration of Ped-TMZ; although, the short treatment duration is a limitation of the present study. The PK and safety profile of Ped-TMZ in childhood populations is currently being further evaluated in the TEMOkids trial (NCT04610736).

Supplementary Materials: The following supporting information can be downloaded at: https://www.mdpi.com/article/10.3390/pharmaceutics15122664/s1, Table S1: Medical and surgical history from the ITTS (>10%); Table S2: Concomitant medications starting before/after TMZ administration from the ITTS (>10%) by treatment sequence and totalled over all patients; Supplementary S1: Full list of eligibility criteria; Supplementary S2. Study period flow chart; Supplementary S3. Collection of blood samples.

Author Contributions: Conceptualization, J.B., H.B. and C.L.; Methodology, H.B., C.L. and F.D; Validation, C.L.; Formal Analysis, C.L.; Investigation, F.D., C.R., M.R., M.F., C.B., O.C., F.E., X.D. and S.C.; Resources, F.D., C.R., M.R., M.F., C.B., O.C., F.E., X.D. and S.C.; Data Curation, C.L.; Writing—Original Draft Preparation, J.B., H.B. and C.L.; Writing—Review and Editing, J.B., H.B., C.L., F.D., C.R., M.R., M.F., C.B., O.C., F.E., X.D. and S.C.; Visualization, J.B., H.B. and C.L.; Supervision, J.B., H.B. and C.L.; Project Administration, C.L.; Funding Acquisition, H.B. All authors had full access to study data, participated in drafting the manuscript (assisted by a sponsor-funded medical writer) and approved its submission for publication. All authors have read and agreed to the published version of the manuscript.

Funding: This research was funded by ORPHELIA Pharma.

Institutional Review Board Statement: The study was conducted in accordance with the Declaration of Helsinki and was approved by the Ethics Committee of Comité de Protection des Personnes Sud-Méditerranée I, France (protocol ORP-TMZ-1—EudraCT 2020-000293-23 on 11 March 2020).

Informed Consent Statement: Informed consent was obtained from all patients involved in the study.

Data Availability Statement: Due to commercial restrictions, the data is not publicly available.

Acknowledgments: We would like to thank the patients who participated in the trial and their families. We would like to acknowledge the institutions (Hôpital Neurologique and Neurobiotec, Hospices Civils de Lyon, Lyon, France; Centre Hospitalier Universitaire de Saint-Etienne, Saint-Etienne, France; Institut de Cancérologie de l'Ouest, Medical Oncology, Saint Herblain, France; Cancer Centre Henri Becquerel, Rouen, France; Hôpital St André, Bordeaux, France; CHU Hôpital de La Timone, Marseille, France; Centre Eugène Marquis, Rennes, France; Oncology Department, Centre Jean Perrin, Clermont-Ferrand, France) and their teams (research assistants, nurses, laboratory assistants, pharmacists) who participated in the current study. We would also like to thank Hospital Gustave Roussy, Villejuif, France; Eurofins ADME (Julien Fernandez as Study Director and team); and Eurofins Optimed for bioanalysis and pharmacokinetic assessments and clinical operations; Eurofins CDMO for dissolution testing; and Effi-stat (Jean-Christophe Lemarié) for statistical support. Medical writing support to draft the outline of the article was provided by Health Unlimited.

Conflicts of Interest: C.B., F.E., S.C. and X.D. have no conflicts of interest. C.R. has received honoraria from Novocure and Leo Pharma. F.D. has received honoraria and meeting support from Novocure. M.F. has received honoraria from Novocure and meeting support from Gilead and Pfizer. M.R. has received honoraria from Lilly and Novartis and meeting support from AstraZeneca and Creafirst. O.C. has received consulting fees from Ipsen and AbbVie, honoraria from Bristol-Meyer Squib, meeting support from Kyowa Kirin Pharma, leadership role at Beta Innov and received materials and other services from Novocure. C.L., H.B. and J.B. are employees of ORPHELIA Pharma.

References

1. Strobel, H.; Baisch, T.; Fitzel, R.; Schilberg, K.; Siegelin, M.D.; Karpel-Massler, G.; Debatin, K.M.; Westhoff, M.A. Temozolomide and Other Alkylating Agents in Glioblastoma Therapy. *Biomedicines* **2019**, *7*, 69. [CrossRef]
2. Denny, B.J.; Wheelhouse, R.T.; Stevens, M.F.; Tsang, L.L.; Slack, J.A. NMR and molecular modeling investigation of the mechanism of activation of the antitumor drug temozolomide and its interaction with DNA. *Biochemistry* **1994**, *33*, 9045–9051. [CrossRef]
3. Baker, S.D.; Wirth, M.; Statkevich, P.; Reidenberg, P.; Alton, K.; Sartorius, S.E.; Dugan, M.; Cutler, D.; Batra, V.; Grochow, L.B.; et al. Absorption, metabolism, and excretion of 14C-temozolomide following oral administration to patients with advanced cancer. *Clin. Cancer Res.* **1999**, *5*, 309–317.
4. El Mubarak, M.A.; Stylos, E.K.; Chatziathanasiadou, M.V.; Danika, C.; Alexiou, G.A.; Tsekeris, P.; Renziehausen, A.; Crook, T.; Syed, N.; Sivolapenko, G.B.; et al. Development and validation of simple step protein precipitation UHPLC-MS/MS methods for quantitation of temozolomide in cancer patient plasma samples. *J. Pharm. Biomed. Anal.* **2019**, *162*, 164–170. [CrossRef]
5. Peer, C.J.; Ronner, L.; Rodgers, L.; Lester McCully, C.M.; Warren, K.E.; Figg, W.D. Quantification of Temozolomide in Nonhuman Primate Fluids by Isocratic Ultra-High Performance Liquid Chromatography-Tandem Mass Spectrometry to Study Brain Tissue Penetration Following Intranasal or Intravenous Delivery. *Separations* **2016**, *3*, 4. [CrossRef] [PubMed]
6. Muggeri, A.; Vago, M.; Perez, S.; Rubio, M.; Gonzalez, C.; Magarinos, C.; Rosenberg, M.; Costa, F.; Perez-Lloret, S. A Randomized, Open-Label, Two-Way Crossover, Single-Dose Bioequivalence Study of Temozolomide 200 mg/m^2 (Dralitem® vs. Temoda® Capsules) in Patients with Primary Tumors of the Central Nervous System Under Fasting Conditions. *Drugs R D* **2017**, *17*, 427–434. [CrossRef] [PubMed]
7. Waghule, T.; Narayan Saha, R.; Singhvi, G. UV spectroscopic method for estimation of temozolomide: Application in stability studies in simulated plasma pH, degradation rate kinetics, formulation design, and selection of dissolution media. *Spectrochim. Acta A Mol. Biomol. Spectrosc.* **2021**, *258*, 119848. [CrossRef]
8. EMA. Temodal SmPC. Available online: https://www.ema.europa.eu/en/documents/product-information/temodal-epar-product-information_en.pdf (accessed on 13 September 2023).
9. Children's Cancer and Leukaemia Group. Options for the Treatment of Patients with Relapsed/Progressive High-Risk Neuroblastoma. 2015. Available online: https://www.cclg.org.uk/write/MediaUploads/Member%20area/Treatment%20guidelines/CCLG_Relapsed_Progressive_High_Risk_Neuroblastoma_Guidelines_March_2015_FINAL.pdf (accessed on 13 September 2023).
10. Moreno, L.; Rubie, H.; Varo, A.; Le Deley, M.C.; Amoroso, L.; Chevance, A.; Garaventa, A.; Gambart, M.; Bautista, F.; Valteau-Couanet, D.; et al. Outcome of children with relapsed or refractory neuroblastoma: A meta-analysis of ITCC/SIOPEN European phase II clinical trials. *Pediatr. Blood Cancer* **2017**, *64*, 25–31. [CrossRef]
11. Parikh, N.S.; Howard, S.C.; Chantada, G.; Israels, T.; Khattab, M.; Alcasabas, P.; Lam, C.G.; Faulkner, L.; Park, J.R.; London, W.B.; et al. SIOP-PODC adapted risk stratification and treatment guidelines: Recommendations for neuroblastoma in low- and middle-income settings. *Pediatr. Blood Cancer* **2015**, *62*, 1305–1316. [CrossRef] [PubMed]
12. Hill, R.M.; Plasschaert, S.L.A.; Timmermann, B.; Dufour, C.; Aquilina, K.; Avula, S.; Donovan, L.; Lequin, M.; Pietsch, T.; Thomale, U.; et al. Relapsed Medulloblastoma in Pre-Irradiated Patients: Current Practice for Diagnostics and Treatment. *Cancers* **2022**, *14*, 126. [CrossRef] [PubMed]

13. Defachelles, A.S.; Bogart, E.; Casanova, M.; Merks, J.H.M.; Bisogno, G.; Calareso, G.; Gallego Melcon, S.; Gatz, S.A.; Le Deley, M.C.; McHugh, K.; et al. Randomized Phase II Trial of Vincristine-Irinotecan with or without Temozolomide, in Children and Adults with Relapsed or Refractory Rhabdomyosarcoma: A European Paediatric Soft Tissue Sarcoma Study Group and Innovative Therapies for Children with Cancer Trial. *J. Clin. Oncol.* **2021**, *39*, 2979–2990. [CrossRef]
14. EMA. EMA/PDCO/381728/2014, Draft Inventory of Paediatric Therapeutic Needs—Paediatric Oncology. 2014. Available online: https://www.ema.europa.eu/en/documents/other/draft-inventory-paediatric-therapeutic-needs-paediatric-oncology_en.pdf (accessed on 13 September 2023).
15. Garcia, M.; Clopès, A.; Bruna, J.; Martinez, M.; Fort, E.; Gil, M. Critical appraisal of temozolomide formulations in the treatment of primary brain tumors: Patient considerations. *Cancer Manag. Res.* **2009**, *1*, 137–150. [CrossRef]
16. Eek, D.; Krohe, M.; Mazar, I.; Horsfield, A.; Pompilus, F.; Friebe, R.; Shields, A.L. Patient-reported preferences for oral versus intravenous administration for the treatment of cancer: A review of the literature. *Patient Prefer. Adherence* **2016**, *10*, 1609–1621.
17. Lemarchand, C.; Bienaymé, H.; Rieutord, A.; Tortolano, L.; Annereau, M.; Bastid, J. Dispensing oral temozolomide in children: Precision and stability of a novel ready-to-use liquid formulation in comparison with capsule derived mixtures. In *Supplement: Abstracts from the 54th Congress of the International Society of Paediatric Oncology (SIOP) September 28–October 1, 2022*; Wiley: New York, NY, USA, 2022; Volume 69. [CrossRef]
18. EMA. EMA/CPMP/EWP/QWP/1401/98, Guideline on the Investigation of Bioequivalence. 2010. Available online: https://www.ema.europa.eu/en/documents/scientific-guideline/guideline-investigation-bioequivalence-rev1_en.pdf (accessed on 13 September 2023).
19. FDA. Bioavailability and Bioequivalence Studies Submitted in NDAs or INDs—General Considerations. 2014. Available online: https://www.fda.gov/regulatory-information/search-fda-guidance-documents/bioavailability-and-bioequivalence-studies-submitted-ndas-or-inds-general-considerations (accessed on 13 September 2023).
20. EMA. Temozolomide Teva EPAR. 2010. Available online: https://www.ema.europa.eu/en/documents/assessment-report/temozolomide-teva-epar-public-assessment-report_en.pdf (accessed on 13 September 2023).
21. FDA. Draft Guidance on Temozolomide. 2008. Available online: https://www.accessdata.fda.gov/drugsatfda_docs/psg/Temozolomide_cap_21029_RC12-08.pdf (accessed on 13 September 2023).
22. FDA. Dissolution Testing and Acceptance Criteria for Immediate-Release Solid Oral Dosage form Drug Products Containing High Solubility Drug Substances. 2018. Available online: https://www.fda.gov/files/drugs/published/Dissolution-Testing-and-Acceptance-Criteria-for-Immediate-Release-Solid-Oral-Dosage-Form-Drug-Products-Containing-High-Solubility-Drug-Substances-Guidance-for-Industry.pdf (accessed on 13 September 2023).
23. European Pharmacopoeia 11.0. Temozolomide Monograph, 04/2019:2780. 3973-3974. Available online: https://pheur.edqm.eu/app/11-0/content/11-0/2780E.htm (accessed on 15 November 2023).
24. European Pharmacopoeia 11.0. 2.9.3. Dissolution Test for Solid Dosage Forms, 01/2023:20903. 2023, pp. 348–355. Available online: https://pheur.edqm.eu/app/11-0/content/11-0/20903E.htm?highlight=on&terms=dissolution (accessed on 15 November 2023).
25. United States Pharmacopeial. *General Chapter, <711> Dissolution*; USP-NF; United States Pharmacopeia: Rockville, MD, USA, 2023. [CrossRef]
26. EMA. CPMP/ICH/381/95, ICH Topic Q 2 (R1) Validation of Analytical Procedures: Text and Methodology. 1995. Available online: https://www.ema.europa.eu/en/documents/scientific-guideline/ich-q-2-r1-validation-analytical-procedures-text-methodology-step-5_en.pdf (accessed on 13 September 2023).
27. FDA. Bioanalytical Method Validation—Guidance for Industry. 2018. Available online: https://www.fda.gov/files/drugs/published/Bioanalytical-Method-Validation-Guidance-for-Industry.pdf (accessed on 13 September 2023).
28. EMA. CHMP/EWP/192217/2009 Rev. 1 Corr. 2**, Guideline on Bioanalytical Method Validation. 2011. Available online: https://www.ema.europa.eu/en/documents/scientific-guideline/guideline-bioanalytical-method-validation_en.pdf (accessed on 13 September 2023).
29. FDA. NDA# 22-277, Schering-Plough, Pivotal Bioequivalence Study P02467. 2008. Available online: https://www.accessdata.fda.gov/drugsatfda_docs/nda/2009/022277s000_ClinPharmR.pdf (accessed on 15 November 2023).
30. EMA. Temozolomide Sandoz SmPC. Available online: https://www.ema.europa.eu/en/documents/product-information/temozolomide-sandoz-epar-product-information_en.pdf (accessed on 13 September 2023).
31. EMA. Temozolomide TEVA SmPC. Available online: https://www.ema.europa.eu/en/documents/product-information/temozolomide-teva-epar-product-information_en.pdf (accessed on 13 September 2023).
32. FDA. DRAFT Guidance for Industry. Bioequivalence Studies with Pharmacokinetic Endpoints for Drugs Submitted Under an ANDA. 2021. Available online: https://www.fda.gov/regulatory-information/search-fda-guidance-documents/bioequivalence-studies-pharmacokinetic-endpoints-drugs-submitted-under-abbreviated-new-drug (accessed on 13 September 2023).
33. EMA. Temodal EPAR. 2005. Available online: https://www.ema.europa.eu/en/documents/scientific-discussion/temodal-epar-scientific-discussion_en.pdf (accessed on 13 September 2023).
34. Agarwala, S.S.; Kirkwood, J.M. Temozolomide in combination with interferon alpha-2b in patients with metastatic melanoma: A phase I dose-escalation study. *Cancer* **2003**, *97*, 121–127. [CrossRef]
35. Aoki, T.; Nishikawa, R.; Mizutani, T.; Nojima, K.; Mishima, K.; Adachi, J.; Matsutani, M. Pharmacokinetic study of temozolomide on a daily-for-5-days schedule in Japanese patients with relapsed malignant gliomas: First study in Asians. *Int. J. Clin. Oncol.* **2007**, *12*, 341–349. [CrossRef]

36. Azzabi, A.; Hughes, A.N.; Calvert, P.M.; Plummer, E.R.; Todd, R.; Griffin, M.J.; Lind, M.J.; Maraveyas, A.; Kelly, C.; Fishwick, K.; et al. Phase I study of temozolomide plus paclitaxel in patients with advanced malignant melanoma and associated in vitro investigations. *Br. J. Cancer* **2005**, *92*, 1006–1012. [CrossRef]
37. Beale, P.; Judson, I.; Moore, S.; Statkevich, P.; Marco, A.; Cutler, D.L.; Reidenberg, P.; Brada, M. Effect of gastric pH on the relative oral bioavailability and pharmacokinetics of temozolomide. *Cancer Chemother. Pharmacol.* **1999**, *44*, 389–394. [CrossRef]
38. Brada, M.; Judson, I.; Beale, P.; Moore, S.; Reidenberg, P.; Statkevich, P.; Dugan, M.; Batra, V.; Cutler, D. Phase I dose-escalation and pharmacokinetic study of temozolomide (SCH 52365) for refractory or relapsing malignancies. *Br. J. Cancer* **1999**, *81*, 1022–1030.
39. Britten, C.; Rowinsky, E.; Baker, S.; Agarwala, S.; Eckardt, J.; Barrington, R.; Diab, S.; Hammond, L.; Johnson, T.; Villalona-Calero, M.; et al. A Phase I and Pharmacokinetic Study of Temozolomide and Cisplatin in Patients with Advanced Solid Malignancies. *Clin. Cancer Res.* **1999**, *5*, 1629–1637.
40. Brock, C.S.; Newlands, E.S.; Wedge, S.R.; Bower, M.; Evans, H.; Colquhoun, I.; Roddie, M.; Glaser, M.; Brampton, M.H.; Rustin, G.J. Phase I Trial of Temozolomide Using an Extended Continuous Oral Schedule. *Cancer Res.* **1998**, *58*, 4363–4367.
41. Dhodapkar, M.; Rubin, J.; Reid, J.M.; Burch, P.A.; Pitot, H.C.; Buckner, J.C.; Ames, M.M.; Suman, V.J. Phase I trial of temozolomide in patients with advanced cancer. *Clin. Cancer Res.* **1997**, *3*, 1093–1100. [PubMed]
42. Diez, B.D.; Statkevich, P.; Zhu, Y.; Abutarif, M.A.; Xuan, F.; Kantesaria, B.; Cutler, D.; Cantillon, M.; Schwarz, M.; Pallotta, M.G.; et al. Evaluation of the exposure equivalence of oral versus intravenous temozolomide. *Cancer Chemother. Pharmacol.* **2010**, *65*, 727–734. [CrossRef] [PubMed]
43. Gander, M.; Leyvraz, S.; Decosterd, L.; Bonfanti, M.; Marzolini, C.; Shen, F.; Lienard, D.; Perey, L.; Colella, G.; Biollaz, J.; et al. Sequential administration of temozolomide and fotemustine: Depletion of O6-alkyl guanine-DNA transferase in blood lymphocytes and in tumours. *Ann. Oncol.* **1999**, *10*, 831–838. [CrossRef]
44. Gojo, I.; Beumer, J.H.; Pratz, K.W.; McDevitt, M.A.; Baer, M.R.; Blackford, A.L.; Smith, B.D.; Gore, S.D.; Carraway, H.E.; Showel, M.M.; et al. A Phase 1 Study of the PARP Inhibitor Veliparib in Combination with Temozolomide in Acute Myeloid Leukemia. *Clin. Cancer Res.* **2017**, *23*, 697–706. [CrossRef]
45. Hammond, L.A.; Eckardt, J.R.; Baker, S.D.; Eckhardt, S.G.; Dugan, M.; Forral, K.; Reidenberg, P.; Statkevich, P.; Weiss, G.R.; Rinaldi, D.A.; et al. Phase I and pharmacokinetic study of temozolomide on a daily-for-5-days schedule in patients with advanced solid malignancies. *J. Clin. Oncol.* **1999**, *17*, 2604–2613. [CrossRef] [PubMed]
46. Hammond, L.A.; Eckardt, J.R.; Kuhn, J.G.; Gerson, S.L.; Johnson, T.; Smith, L.; Drengler, R.L.; Campbell, E.; Weiss, G.R.; Von Hoff, D.D.; et al. A randomized phase I and pharmacological trial of sequences of 1,3-bis(2-chloroethyl)-1-nitrosourea and temozolomide in patients with advanced solid neoplasms. *Clin. Cancer Res.* **2004**, *10*, 1645–1656. [CrossRef] [PubMed]
47. Hottinger, A.F.; Aissa, A.B.; Espeli, V.; Squiban, D.; Dunkel, N.; Vargas, M.I.; Hundsberger, T.; Mach, N.; Schaller, K.; Weber, D.C.; et al. Phase I study of sorafenib combined with radiation therapy and temozolomide as first-line treatment of high-grade glioma. *Br. J. Cancer* **2014**, *110*, 2655–2661. [CrossRef]
48. Jackson, S.; Weingart, J.; Nduom, E.K.; Harfi, T.T.; George, R.T.; McAreavey, D.; Ye, X.; Anders, N.M.; Peer, C.; Figg, W.D.; et al. The effect of an adenosine A2A agonist on intra-tumoral concentrations of temozolomide in patients with recurrent glioblastoma. *Fluids Barriers CNS* **2018**, *15*, 2. [CrossRef]
49. Jen, J.F.; Cutler, D.L.; Pai, S.M.; Batra, V.K.; Affrime, M.B.; Zambas, D.N.; Heft, S.; Hajian, G. Population Pharmacokinetics of Temozolomide in Cancer Patients. *Pharm. Res.* **2000**, *17*, 1284–1289. [CrossRef]
50. Lassman, A.B.; Van Den Bent, M.J.; Gan, H.K.; Reardon, D.A.; Kumthekar, P.; Butowski, N.; Lwin, Z.; Mikkelsen, T.; Nabors, L.B.; Papadopoulos, K.P.; et al. Safety and efficacy of depatuxizumab mafodotin + temozolomide in patients with EGFR-amplified, recurrent glioblastoma: Results from an international phase I multicenter trial. *Neuro Oncol.* **2019**, *21*, 106–114. [CrossRef]
51. Lee, E.Q.; Puduvalli, V.K.; Reid, J.M.; Kuhn, J.G.; Lamborn, K.R.; Cloughesy, T.F.; Chang, S.M.; Drappatz, J.; Yung, W.K.; Gilbert, M.R.; et al. Phase I study of vorinostat in combination with temozolomide in patients with high-grade gliomas: North American Brain Tumor Consortium Study 04-03. *Clin. Cancer Res.* **2012**, *18*, 6032–6039. [CrossRef]
52. Marzolini, C.; Decosterd, L.A.; Shen, F.; Gander, M.; Leyvraz, S.; Bauer, J.; Buclin, T.; Biollaz, J.; Lejeune, F. Pharmacokinetics of temozolomide in association with fotemustine in malignant melanoma and malignant glioma patients: Comparison of oral, intravenous, and hepatic intra-arterial administration. *Cancer Chemother. Pharmacol.* **1998**, *42*, 433–440. [CrossRef] [PubMed]
53. Middleton, M.R.; Grob, J.J.; Aaronson, N.; Fierlbeck, G.; Tilgen, W.; Seiter, S.; Gore, M.; Aamdal, S.; Cebon, J.; Coates, A.; et al. Randomized phase III study of temozolomide versus dacarbazine in the treatment of patients with advanced metastatic malignant melanoma. *J. Clin. Oncol.* **2000**, *18*, 158–166. [CrossRef]
54. Newlands, E.S.; Blackledge, G.R.P.; Slack, J.A.; Rustin, G.J.; Smith, D.B.; Stuart, N.S.; Quarterman, C.P.; Hoffman, R.; Stevens, M.F.G.; Brampton, M.H.; et al. Phase I trial of temozolomide. *Br. J. Cancer* **1992**, *65*, 287–291. [CrossRef] [PubMed]
55. Ostermann, S.; Csajka, C.; Buclin, T.; Leyvraz, S.; Lejeune, F.; Decosterd, L.A.; Stupp, R. Plasma and cerebrospinal fluid population pharmacokinetics of temozolomide in malignant glioma patients. *Clin. Cancer Res.* **2004**, *10*, 3728–3736. [CrossRef] [PubMed]
56. Portnow, J.; Badie, B.; Chen, M.; Liu, A.; Blanchard, S.; Synold, T.W. The neuropharmacokinetics of temozolomide in patients with resectable brain tumors: Potential implications for the current approach to chemoradiation. *Clin. Cancer Res.* **2009**, *15*, 7092–7098. [CrossRef] [PubMed]

57. Reardon, D.A.; Nabors, L.B.; Mason, W.P.; Perry, J.R.; Shapiro, W.; Kavan, P.; Mathieu, D.; Phuphanich, S.; Cseh, A.; Fu, Y.; et al. Phase I/randomized phase II study of afatinib, an irreversible ErbB family blocker, with or without protracted temozolomide in adults with recurrent glioblastoma. *Neuro Oncol.* **2015**, *17*, 430–439. [CrossRef]
58. Riccardi, A.; Mazzarella, G.; Cefalo, G.; Garre, M.L.; Massimino, M.; Barone, C.; Sandri, A.; Ridola, V.; Ruggiero, A.; Mastrangelo, S.; et al. Pharmacokinetics of temozolomide given three times a day in pediatric and adult patients. *Cancer Chemother. Pharmacol.* **2003**, *52*, 459–464. [CrossRef]
59. Rudek, M.A.; Donehower, R.C.; Statkevich, P.; Batra, V.K.; Cutler, D.L.; Baker, S.D. Temozolomide in patients with advanced cancer: Phase I and pharmacokinetic study. *Pharmacotherapy* **2004**, *24*, 16–25. [CrossRef]
60. Schold, S.C., Jr.; Kuhn, J.G.; Chang, S.M.; Bosik, M.E.; Robins, H.I.; Mehta, M.P.; Spence, A.M.; Fulton, D.; Fink, K.L.; Prados, M.D. A phase I trial of 1,3-bis(2-chloroethyl)-1-nitrosourea plus temozolomide: A North American Brain Tumor Consortium study. *Neuro Oncol.* **2000**, *2*, 34–39. [CrossRef]
61. Tawbi, H.A.; Beumer, J.H.; Tarhini, A.A.; Moschos, S.; Buch, S.C.; Egorin, M.J.; Lin, Y.; Christner, S.; Kirkwood, J.M. Safety and efficacy of decitabine in combination with temozolomide in metastatic melanoma: A phase I/II study and pharmacokinetic analysis. *Ann. Oncol.* **2013**, *24*, 1112–1119. [CrossRef]
62. Wen, P.Y.; Omuro, A.; Ahluwalia, M.S.; Fathallah-Shaykh, H.M.; Mohile, N.; Lager, J.J.; Laird, A.D.; Tang, J.; Jiang, J.; Egile, C.; et al. Phase I dose-escalation study of the PI3K/mTOR inhibitor voxtalisib (SAR245409, XL765) plus temozolomide with or without radiotherapy in patients with high-grade glioma. *Neuro Oncol.* **2015**, *17*, 1275–1283. [CrossRef]
63. Baruchel, S.; Diezi, M.; Hargrave, D.; Stempak, D.; Gammon, J.; Moghrabi, A.; Coppes, M.J.; Fernandez, C.V.; Bouffet, E. Safety and pharmacokinetics of temozolomide using a dose-escalation, metronomic schedule in recurrent paediatric brain tumours. *Eur. J. Cancer* **2006**, *42*, 2335–2342. [CrossRef]
64. Broniscer, A.; Chintagumpala, M.; Fouladi, M.; Krasin, M.J.; Kocak, M.; Bowers, D.C.; Iacono, L.C.; Merchant, T.E.; Stewart, C.F.; Houghton, P.J.; et al. Temozolomide after radiotherapy for newly diagnosed high-grade glioma and unfavorable low-grade glioma in children. *J. Neurooncol.* **2006**, *76*, 313–319. [CrossRef]
65. Broniscer, A.; Gururangan, S.; MacDonald, T.J.; Goldman, S.; Packer, R.J.; Stewart, C.F.; Wallace, D.; Danks, M.K.; Friedman, H.S.; Poussaint, T.Y.; et al. Phase I trial of single-dose temozolomide and continuous administration of o6-benzylguanine in children with brain tumors: A pediatric brain tumor consortium report. *Clin. Cancer Res.* **2007**, *13*, 6712–6718. [CrossRef] [PubMed]
66. Broniscer, A.; Iacono, L.; Chintagumpala, M.; Fouladi, M.; Wallace, D.; Bowers, D.C.; Stewart, C.; Krasin, M.J.; Gajjar, A. Role of temozolomide after radiotherapy for newly diagnosed diffuse brainstem glioma in children: Results of a multiinstitutional study (SJHG-98). *Cancer* **2005**, *103*, 133–139. [CrossRef] [PubMed]
67. Estlin, E.; Lashford, L.; Ablett, S.; Price, L.; Gowing, R.; Gholkar, A.; Kohler, J.; Lewis, I.; Morland, B.; Pinkerton, C.R.; et al. Phase I study of temozolomide in paediatric patients with advanced cancer. *Br. J. Cancer* **1998**, *78*, 652–661. [CrossRef] [PubMed]
68. Horton, T.M.; Thompson, P.A.; Berg, S.L.; Adamson, P.C.; Ingle, A.M.; Dolan, M.E.; Delaney, S.M.; Hedge, M.; Weiss, H.L.; Wu, M.F.; et al. Phase I pharmacokinetic and pharmacodynamic study of temozolomide in pediatric patients with refractory or recurrent leukemia: A Children's Oncology Group Study. *J. Clin. Oncol.* **2007**, *25*, 4922–4928. [CrossRef] [PubMed]
69. Meany, H.J.; Warren, K.E.; Fox, E.; Cole, D.E.; Aikin, A.A.; Balis, F.M. Pharmacokinetics of temozolomide administered in combination with O6-benzylguanine in children and adolescents with refractory solid tumors. *Cancer Chemother. Pharmacol.* **2009**, *65*, 137–142. [CrossRef]
70. Panetta, J.C.; Kirstein, M.N.; Gajjar, A.; Nair, G.; Fouladi, M.; Heideman, R.L.; Wilkinson, M.; Stewart, C.F. Population pharmacokinetics of temozolomide and metabolites in infants and children with primary central nervous system tumors. *Cancer Chemother. Pharmacol.* **2003**, *52*, 435–441. [CrossRef]
71. Rubie, H.; Geoerger, B.; Frappaz, D.; Schmitt, A.; Leblond, P.; Ndiaye, A.; Aerts, I.; Le Deley, M.C.; Gentet, J.C.; Paci, A.; et al. Phase I study of topotecan in combination with temozolomide (TOTEM) in relapsed or refractory paediatric solid tumours. *Eur. J. Cancer* **2010**, *46*, 2763–2770. [CrossRef]
72. Wagner, L.M.; Crews, K.R.; Iacono, L.C.; Houghton, P.J.; Fuller, C.E.; McCarville, M.B.; Goldsby, R.E.; Albritton, K.; Stewart, C.F.; Santana, V.M. Phase I trial of temozolomide and protracted irinotecan in pediatric patients with refractory solid tumors. *Clin. Cancer Res.* **2004**, *10*, 840–848. [CrossRef]
73. Wagner, L.M.; Villablanca, J.G.; Stewart, C.F.; Crews, K.R.; Groshen, S.; Reynolds, C.P.; Park, J.R.; Maris, J.M.; Hawkins, R.A.; Daldrup-Link, H.E.; et al. Phase I trial of oral irinotecan and temozolomide for children with relapsed high-risk neuroblastoma: A new approach to neuroblastoma therapy consortium study. *J. Clin. Oncol.* **2009**, *27*, 1290–1296. [CrossRef]
74. Stupp, R.; Hegi, M.E.; Mason, W.P.; van den Bent, M.J.; Taphoorn, M.J.; Janzer, R.C.; Ludwin, S.K.; Allgeier, A.; Fisher, B.; Belanger, K.; et al. Effects of radiotherapy with concomitant and adjuvant temozolomide versus radiotherapy alone on survival in glioblastoma in a randomised phase III study: 5-year analysis of the EORTC-NCIC trial. *Lancet Oncol.* **2009**, *10*, 459–466. [CrossRef]
75. DuBois, S.G.; Marachelian, A.; Fox, E.; Kudgus, R.A.; Reid, J.M.; Groshen, S.; Malvar, J.; Bagatell, R.; Wagner, L.; Maris, J.M.; et al. Phase I Study of the Aurora A Kinase Inhibitor Alisertib in Combination with Irinotecan and Temozolomide for Patients with Relapsed or Refractory Neuroblastoma: A NANT (New Approaches to Neuroblastoma Therapy) Trial. *J. Clin. Oncol.* **2016**, *34*, 1368–1375. [CrossRef]

76. Chavelli-Lopez, B. Oral toxicity produced by chemotherapy: A systematic review. *J. Clin. Exp. Dent.* **2014**, *6*, 81–90. [CrossRef]
77. Annereau, M.; Hinterlang, M.; Bienayme, H.; Vassal, G.; Pinon, A.; Schmitt, M.; Denis, L.; Lemarchand, C.; Martin, L.; Lemare, F.; et al. Development of a Hospital Compounded, Taste-Masked, Temozolomide Oral Suspension and 5-Year Real-Life Experience in Treating Paediatric Patients. *Pharmaceuticals* **2022**, *15*, 555. [CrossRef]

pharmaceutics

MDPI

Review

Circulating Biomarkers for Monitoring Chemotherapy-Induced Cardiotoxicity in Children

Luigia Meo [1], Maria Savarese [2], Carmen Munno [2], Peppino Mirabelli [3], Pia Ragno [1], Ornella Leone [2] and Mariaevelina Alfieri [2,*]

[1] Department of Chemistry and Biology, University of Salerno, Via Giovanni Paolo II, 132, 84084 Salerno, Italy; lmeo@unisa.it (L.M.); pragno@unisa.it (P.R.)
[2] Clinical Pathology, Santobono-Pausilipon Children's Hospital, 80123 Naples, Italy; m.savarese@santobonopausilipon.it (M.S.); c.munno@santobonopausilipon.it (C.M.); o.leone@santobonopausilipon.it (O.L.)
[3] Clinical and Translational Research Unit, Santobono-Pausilipon Children's Hospital, 80123 Naples, Italy; p.mirabelli@santobonopausilipon.it
* Correspondence: m.alfieri@santobonopausilipon.it

Abstract: Most commonly diagnosed cancer pathologies in the pediatric population comprise leukemias and cancers of the nervous system. The percentage of cancer survivors increased from approximatively 50% to 80% thanks to improvements in medical treatments and the introduction of new chemotherapies. However, as a consequence, heart disease has become the main cause of death in the children due to the cardiotoxicity induced by chemotherapy treatments. The use of different cardiovascular biomarkers, complementing data obtained from electrocardiogram, echocardiography cardiac imaging, and evaluation of clinical symptoms, is considered a routine in clinical diagnosis, prognosis, risk stratification, and differential diagnosis. Cardiac troponin and natriuretic peptides are the best-validated biomarkers broadly accepted in clinical practice for the diagnosis of acute coronary syndrome and heart failure, although many other biomarkers are used and several potential markers are currently under study and possibly will play a more prominent role in the future. Several studies have shown how the measurement of cardiac troponin (cTn) can be used for the early detection of heart damage in oncological patients treated with potentially cardiotoxic chemotherapeutic drugs. The advent of high sensitive methods (hs-cTnI or hs-cTnT) further improved the effectiveness of risk stratification and monitoring during treatment cycles.

Keywords: pediatric cancer; children; chemotherapy; cardiotoxicity; troponin; high-sensitivity-troponin; cardiac biomarkers; heart failure

1. Introduction

Cancer is the top disease-related cause of death for children and teens, although most cancers (99%) develop in adults. However, increasing research aims to discover new treatments for childhood cancers, greatly improving the overall survival rate, which has reached more than 80% for children. In the pre-chemotherapy era, the cure rate of childhood cancer was <25%, and most cancers were treated with surgery and radiation. With the advent of chemotherapy in the 1960s, and the development of novel therapies, a crescent increase in survival was observed. In the last years the development of next-generation sequencing technologies (NGS) and the advent of -omic sciences have shed light on molecular and genomic mechanisms underlying pediatric cancer disease, demonstrating that the genomic landscape is very various and, frequently, the etiology and tumorigenic mechanisms are quite different from that of common adult cancers [1–3].

Every year there are about 1400 diagnoses of cancer in pediatric population (Available online: https://apps.who.int/iris/handle/10665/347370, accessed on 29 July 2022; Available online: https://seer.cancer.gov, accessed on 29 July 2022) (Figure 1). However, despite the progress in the treatment of pediatric cancers based on the use of radiotherapy and poly-chemotherapy, several challenges remain, such as the management of severe acute and chronic toxicities caused by chemotherapies. More effective and less toxic treatments for pediatric cancers could be obtained by therapies that specifically target tumor cells, or inhibit oncogenic molecular aberrations as well as personalized chemotherapies through pharmacogenetics and precision medicin. Chemotherapy targets cells that are growing and dividing actively through cell cycle and especially cancer cells that grow faster than healthy cells. However, normal cells can be damaged by the chemotherapy as well, giving rise to several side effects. Although different for each person, side effects associated with chemotherapy administration comprise secondary malignancies, neurocognitive dysfunction, cardiopulmonary toxicity, impairment of kidney function, endocrinopathy, whose frequency and severity depend on several variables such as sex, age at diagnosis, and exposures to cumulative doses of specific treatment modalities [4]

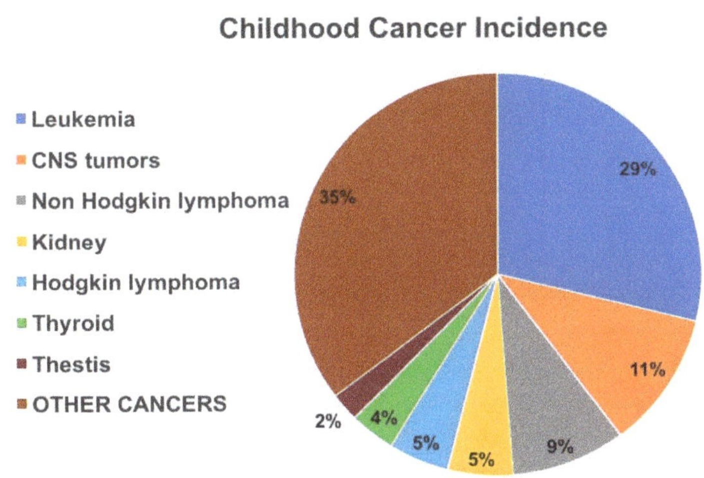

Figure 1. Frequency of pediatric cancers in pediatric population (0–19 years), calculated from Global Cancer observatory, accessed on 1 September 2023 (https://gco.iarc.fr/today/home).

Exposure to alkylating agents, anthracyclines, and epipodophyllotoxins, for treating hematologic malignancies, solid tumors and preconditioning regiments for hematopoietic stem cell transplantation (HSCT), has been associated with increased risk of developing secondary malignant neoplasms (SMN), histologically distinct malignancies, that may develop after completion of therapies for the primary tumor and remain the main cause of morbidity for pediatric patients [5]. Neurologic complications were observed in 33% of children with non-Central Nervous System (CNS) solid tumors. In fact, side effects of chemotherapy on central and peripheral nervous system are well-known and widely described and represent a significant source of morbidity in the treatment of cancer patients. CNS side effects are also found in patients subjected to new therapies, such as biologic therapy and immunotherapy; they occur during treatments or months/years later. Several symptoms and complications have been reported such as edema, seizures, fatigue, psychiatric disorders, and venous thromboembolism, that can earnestly impact the quality of life. Oxidative injuries from oxygen radicals generated by chemotherapy agents often result in acute or chronic cardiovascular complications. The cardiotoxicity of anthracyclines is widely known, but also alkylating agents (cyclophosphamide, ifosfamide, cisplatin, busulfan, mitomycin), vinca alkaloids, fluorouracil, cytarabine, amsacrine, asparaginase and the more recent agents as paclitaxel, trastuzumab, etoposideand teniposide, have also been associated with cardiotoxicity. Cardiac effects may occur during or immediately after treatment or months or years later after treatments including a wide spectrum of manifestations such as asymptomatic electrocardiographic abnormalities, blood pressure changes, arrhythmias, myocarditis, pericarditis, cardiac tamponade, acute myocardial infarction, cardiac failure, shock, and long-term cardiomyopathy. The assumption of anthracyclines (Doxorubicin and Daunorubicin) at doses higher than 300 mg/m^2 results in symptomatic cardiotoxicity and is associated with high morbidity and mortality in children [6,7].

Cancer-therapy-related cardiac dysfunction (CTRCD) includes a spectrum of cardiac dysfunctions ranging from asymptomatic cardiac injury characterized only increased levels of cardiac biomarkers to clinical signs of heart failure. CTRD is less studied than in adults, although the toxic limited doses of chemotherapy agents are well known in children. In fact, doses of most chemotherapy agents in pediatric (but also in adult) population are established considering toxicity. The Children's Oncology Group Chemotherapy Standardization Task force developed a method of dosing anticancer drugs in infants based on body surface area (BSA) dose banding incorporated in dosing tables for infants and children. These tables start from doses for children and infant with a BSA < 0.6 m^2 and gradually switch from body weight based to BSA-based dosing [8,9]. Due to the increasing number of surviving children, CTRCD will continue to increase in the future flanked by the rapid evolution of the "cardio-oncology" aiming to detecting, monitoring, and treating cardiotoxic side effects of cancer therapy [10]. The National Comprehensive Cancer Network's "Adolescents and Young Adults with Cancer" and The Children's Oncology Group's "Long-Term Follow-Up Guidelines for Survivors of Childhood, Adolescent, and Young", have established guidelines containing detailed informations to establish programs for childhood cancer survivors (Available online: https://cancerprogressreport.aacr.org/wp-content/uploads/sites/2/2022/09/AACR_CPR_2022.pdf, accessed on 26 August 2023; Available online: http://survivorshipguidelines.org, accessed on 26 August 2023). Prevention of cardiotoxicity may be achieved by screening for risk factors, monitoring for symptoms and events during treatments, electrocardiographic and echocardiographic studies, angiography, measurements of biochemical markers of myocardial injury. A second level of prevention aims to minimize progression of heart dysfunction by monitoring cardiac function during and after cancer therapy, using cardioprotectants reducing oxidative stress during chemotherapy, using analogs or formulations having milder cardiotoxicity, altering the dose, schedule or approach to drug delivery.

In this review, we recapitulate the effects of different chemotherapy drugs on heart function and of main biomarkers used to detect and follow cardiotoxicity underlining the key role of the high-sensitivity troponin as a biomarker for monitoring chemotherapy-induced cardiotoxicity in pediatric patients.

2. Chemotherapy-Induced Cardiotoxicity in Children

Knowledge of the pediatric heart, compared to the adult heart, is essential to address the issue of chemotherapy-related cardiotoxicity. Long term cardiotoxicity is observed especially in pediatric patients who experiences relapses and second line treatments [11]. The fetal and neonatal heart express high levels of cyclin-dependent kinases and cyclins, positive cell cycle regulators, not expressed in the adult heart [12]. Moreover, in neonatal cardiomyocytes, the telomerase activity promotes S-phase entry and suppresses cyclin-dependent kinase inhibitors thus inducing cell proliferation [13].

Anthracyclines are the chemotherapy drugs mostly associated with cardiotoxicity. However, cardiac complications could be associated also with other chemotherapy agents under trial or commonly used for the treatment of pediatric cancers, such as paclitaxel, tyrosine kinase inhibitors and alkylating agents [14].

2.1. Anthracyclines

Anthracyclines are chemotherapeutic drugs acting by targeting both the isoenzymes of topoisomerase II (TOP2) (TOP2A and TOP2B) and stabilizing the TOP2 DNA complex. Disruption of the TOP2B on mice and human embryonic stem cells prevents the cardiotoxicity associated with anthracyclines demonstrating that TOP2B is responsible for the cardiotoxicity associated with anthracyclines [15,16]. Doxorubicin, the most commonly used anthracycline, act inducing lipid peroxidation at the cell and mitochondrial membranes by forming complexes with Fe^{2+}, thus resulting in apoptosis, mitochondrial DNA damage producing reactive oxygen species (ROS) [17,18] whose persistence could lead to late CTRCD. Specifically, anthracycline is a lipophilic molecule that easily diffuses through the cell membrane, reaching the inner mitochondrial membrane. It acts by binding cardiolipin and converting its quinone into semiquinone thus realizing free radicals. This mechanism induces the production of ROS that contribute to lipid peroxidation, cell membrane damage and the release of intracellular proteins such as lactate dehydrogenase (LDH) and cardiac troponins [19,20]. The use of the iron chelator Dexrazoxane, in a preclinical study in mice with upregulated mitochondrial iron exporters, reduces the generation of ROS in mitochondria providing cardioprotection from anthracycline treatment without reducing its anticancer efficacy, thus mitigating CTRCD [21,22]. Dexrazoxane has been approved by FDA as a cardioprotective agent and has been employed to improve cardiac toxicity observed in anthracycline-treated oncologic patients, such as breast cancer patients or small-cell lung cancer and adult patients with soft tissue sarcomas [23]. This drug is administered intravenously in combination with the anthracycline to reduce the incidence of cardiac complications. Dexrazoxane can also be used to treat tissue damage caused by extravasation of anthracyclines during their administration [24]. However, since Dexrazoxane does not wholly eliminate the risk of anthracycline- induced cardiotoxicity, it is critical to verify cardiac function before and during therapy to monitor the left ventricular ejection fraction (LVEF) [23].

Genetic Variants Associated with Anthracycline Sensitivity

Several studies identified genetic variants associated with Anthracycline sensitivity in pediatric oncologic patients. A number of single nucleotide polymorphism (SNP) variations in specific genes, resulting in changes in signal transduction, cell cycle regulation, mitochondrial function and cellular transport, were identified (Table 1). These variants are responsible for the anthracycline-associated cardiotoxicity (ACT). The polymorphism rs1056892 in carbonyl reductase (CBR3) is related to a tripled risk of ACT [21]. The polymorphism rs3743527 within the 3′ Untranslated Region (3′ UTR) of the ATP binding cassette subfamily C member 1 (ABCC1) gene in children affected by Acute Lymphoblastic Leukemia (ALL) decreased the ABCC1 expression, through a posttranscriptional mechanism, promoting ACT [25]. The SNP rs10426377 of sulfotransferase family cytosolic member 2B1 (SULT2B1), which increases the solubility of drugs in water and promotes renal excretion, is also associated with ACT in men, probably decreasing the excretion of anthracycline through kidneys [26,27]. The SNP rs13058338 in the RAC2 subunit of NADPH oxidase is strongly related with ACT susceptibility. Indeed, NADPH oxidase knockout mice were protected from heart failure induced by doxorubicin; further NADPH oxidase inhibitors showed a reduction in the damaged cardiomyocytes after anthracycline exposure. Altogether, these studies confirm that the NADPH oxidase, and thus SNP rs13058338, plays a key role in the ACT [28]. The SNP rs10836235 in catalase (CAT), that converts hydrogen peroxide into water preventing the conversion to hydroxyl free radical, increases expression of CAT and is associated with ACT resistance [29]. The glutathione S transferase (GSTP1) conjugates free glutathione to free radical chemotherapeutic drug metabolites, thus preventing damaging interactions with molecules like DNA, protein and lipids. The SNP rs1695 of GSTP1 leads to a reduced activity of GSTP1 and, consequently, to ACT susceptibility [30]. Increased risk and severity of ACT was also associated to the missense mutation rs12468485 in the G protein-coupled receptor 35 (GPCR35) [31]. Hyaluronan synthase-3 (HAS3) is responsible of the synthesis of the glycosaminoglycan Hyaluronan, that serves as scaffolds during tissue remodeling. The SNP rs2232228 in HAS3 was reported to influence the risk of ACT [32]. The SNP rs1786814 in the CUGBP Elav-like family member 4 (CELF4) is associated to the propensity to develop cardiomyopathy post-anthracyclines in childhood cancer survivors [33]. CELF4 is an RNA binding protein that regulates the alternative splicing of the transcript of the TNNT2 gene encoding for cardiac troponin T, a component of the thin filaments of sarcomeres [33]. The embryonic heart predominantly expresses the variants of cardiac troponin T with an alternative exon 5, which, by contrast, is strongly down-regulated in adults. The CELF4 variant shows a lower affinity to the TNNT2 in the adult heart, impairing the contractility and in some cases LV ejection fraction [34]. Magdy and colleagues demonstrated that primary cardiomyocytes recapitulated the cardio-protective effect of the SLC28A3 locus and that SLC28A3 expression modulated the severity of anthracycline-induced cardiotoxicity [35]. A novel cardio-protective SNP, rs11140490, identified in the SLC28A3 locus, exerted its effect modulating the expression of the antisense long noncoding RNA SLC28A3-AS1 overlapping SLC28A3 locus, thus impairing the expression of doxorubicin–related genes like *SLC28A3*, and eventually protecting patients from ACT [35]. The SNP rs2229774, identified in retinoic acid receptor-γ (RARG) that binds the TOP2B promoter, was associated with an increased risk of anthracycline-induced cardiotoxicity. This nucleotide variation induces a decreased repression of the TOP2B, thus resulting in increased cardiomyocyte death [17]. In fact, human induced pluripotent stem cell-derived cardiomyocytes (hiPSC-CMs) derived from patients with rs2229774 were more sensitive to doxorubicin. This variant acts through the suppression of TOP2B expression and the activation of the cardio-protective extracellular regulated kinase (ERK) pathway [36]. The Canadian Pharmacogenomics Network for Drug Safety (CPNDS) identified, several genetic variants playing a significant role in the risk of developing ACT. In particular, three variants emerged as consistently associated with ACT, including the previously cited variant RARG (rs2229774, G>A), the variant UGT1A6 (rs17863783, G>T) and the protective variant in SLC28A3 (rs7853758, G>A). The UGT1A6 (rs17863783, G>T) variant reduces the UGT1A6 glucuronidation activity, that causes the accumulation of cardiotoxic metabolites resulting in an increased risk of developing ACT. The SLC28A3 (rs7853758, G>A) reduces the expression of the SLC28A3 gene encoding for a drug transporter of anthracyclines thus impairing the influx of anthracyclines in cardiac cells, producing a protective effect [37]. A missense variant (p.Thr253Met, c.758C>T variant) of the gene GPR35, identified using exome array data, was associated with an higher risk of chronic anthracycline-induced cardiotoxicity and more severe cardiac manifestations at low anthracycline doses [38]. A summary of identified genetic variants associated with Antracycline-related ACT is presented in Table 1.

Table 1. Genetic variants associated with Anthracycline sensitivity in pediatric oncologic patients.

SNP	Locus	Effects	Reference
rs2229774	RARG	increased cardiomyocyte death	Aminkeng et al., 2015 [17]
rs1056892	CBR3	tripled risk of ACT	Blanco et al., 2012 [21]
rs3743527	3′ UTR of ABCC1	ACT	Semsei et al., 2012 [25]
rs10426377	SULT2B1	ACT	Visscher et al., 2012 [26] Visscher et al., 2013 [27]
rs13058338	RAC2 subunit of NADPH	ACT susceptibility	Zhao et al., 2010 [28]
rs10836235	CAT	ACT resistance	Rajić et al., 2009 [29]
rs1695	GSTP1	susceptibility to ACT	Windsor et al., 2012 [30]
rs12468485	GPCR35	increased risk and severity of ACT	Min et al., 2010 [31]
rs2232228	HAS3	manipulate the risk of ACT	Wang et al., 2014 [32]
rs1786814	CELF4	increased cardiomyopathy	Wang et al., 2016 [33]
rs11140490	SLC28A3 locus	cardio-protective effect	Magdy et al., 2022 [35]
rs2229774	RARG	increased risk of ACT	Magdy et al., 2022 [35]
rs17863783	UGT1A6	increased risk of ACT	Loucks et al., 2022 [37]
rs7853758	SLC28A3	cardio-protective effect	Loucks et al., 2022 [37]
p.Thr253Met, c.758C>T variant	GPR35	increased risk of ACT	Ruiz-Pinto et al., 2017 [38]

2.2. Taxanes

Taxanes, diterpenes originally isolated from TAXUS, induce cardiotoxic events in 3–20% of patients [39]. Among taxanes, paclitaxel exacerbates anthracycline-induced toxicity increasing heart failure (HF) events [40] and histo-pathological alterations of cardiac tissue, with extensive necrosis [41]. Paclitaxel is an alkaloid extracted from vinca, acts by interrupting microtubule formation. It targets tubulin and stabilizes the microtubule polymer, protecting it from disassembly, thus impairing the metaphase spindle configuration and the progression of mitosis. Paclitaxel is highly effective in the treatment of recurrent childhood brain tumors and is becoming a prospective management option for pediatric tumors [42]. Another study demonstrated the effectiveness of paclitaxel treatment on children affected by Kaposi sarcoma [43]. Perez-Somarriba and colleagues observed a strong response with normalization of tumor markers in three patients showing relapsed intracranial NGGCT, after treatment with gemcitabine, paclitaxel, and oxaliplatin [44]. However, although taxanes have demonstrated high efficacy in adults affected by solid tumors and in pediatric solid tumor in vitro models, their use in children has been restricted by dose-limiting toxicity especially due to the solvent formulation of these drugs [45,46], so these drugs are not yet introduced in clinical practice for pediatric patients.

However, it has a cardiotoxic effect in the adult population such as bradycardia, cardiac ischemia, atrioventricular block, ventricular arrhythmias, probably due to the fact that the disruption of microtubular functions can definitely impact on subcellular organelle, indirectly interfering with myocardial functioning [47]. However, the cellular and molecular mechanisms underlying taxane-induced cardiotoxicity have not been fully elucidated.

2.3. Tyrosine Kinase Inhibitors

Tyrosine kinase inhibitors (TKIs) block the enzymes tyrosine kinases. Tyrosine kinases mediate the activation of growth signals in cells, thus impairing cell proliferation.

In particular, TKIs act by interfering with the ATP binding site of the tyrosine kinase or blocking the ligand-binding site impairing its function. Examples of TKIs include axitinib, dasatinib, erlotinib, imatinib, nilotinib, pazopanib, sunitinib. Used to treat cancers in children such as chronic myeloid leukemia (CML), acute myeloid leukemia (AML), acute lynphoblastic leukemia (ALL), gastrointestinal stromal tumor (GIST), neuroblastoma, renal cell carcinoma, etc. [48]. These drugs activate the endoplasmic reticulum (ER) stress response; the prolonged activation can promote cell death pathways that finally lead to apoptotic and necrotic death of the cardiac tissue.

2.4. Alkylating Agents

Alkylating agents, such as Cisplatin and Carboplatin, commonly used during bone marrow transplantation in children, can induce late-onset CTRCD [49]. These drugs cause an increased ROS production and direct injury to the endothelium causing extravasation of blood in the myocardium, deposition of fibrin in the interstitium, and capillary microthrombi [50]. Cardiomyocyte apoptosis, inflammation, endothelial dysfunction, calcium dysregulation, and mitochondrial damage, promoting hypertension, cardiomyopathy, myocardial infarction, arrhythmias, and heart failure (HF) have been observed in patients treated with Cyclophosphamide [51]. 5-Fluorouracil (5-FU) has been associated with the acute coronary syndrome, probably due to a decrease in nitric oxide locally, causing coronary artery spasm and vasoconstriction, microvascular thrombus, and finally myocardial ischemia [52].

2.5. Radiation Therapy

The 10–30% of patients receiving radiation therapy (RT) develop cardiac complications [53]. The effect of radiation onto water molecules in the cell produces ROS thus damaging mitochondria and DNA in myocytes thus promoting myocardial fibrosis. Cardiotoxicity severity depends on the total radiation dose and the volume of the heart exposed and its incidence increases by 60% for every 1-Gy increase in mediastinal radiation dose [54]. Further, cardiotoxicity is more commonly observed in patients who previously received anthracycline-based chemotherapy or showing cardiac risk factors. Radiation also causes endothelial dysfunction, resulting in intravascular thrombosis, myocardial ischemia, and interstitial fibrosis [55].

3. Cardiac Biomarkers

As stated by the American College of Cardiology and the European society of Cardiology, cardiac biomarkers are central in the diagnosis of major cardiovascular diseases. A good cardiac biomarker should be highly expressed in the cardiac tissue, show sensitivity and specificity and early detectable in the blood after the onset of clinical symptoms, such as chest pain [56–58]. There are many cardiac biomarkers, classified into different patho-physiologic groups, including myocardial ischemia or necrosis, inflammation, hemodynamics, angiogenesis, atherosclerosis, or plaque instability [59].

Aspartate transaminase, a not cardio-specific enzyme, was the first biomarker used for the diagnosis of Acute Myocardial Infarction (AMI) in the 1960s [60]. For this reason, later different other enzymes with increased sensitivity and specificity, such as LDH, creatine kinase (CK), CK isoenzyme MB (CK-MB), and myoglobin, were employed in the diagnostic algorithm, thus improving the diagnosis accuracy [61,62]. In the 1990s, a sensitive radioimmunoassay was developed to detect circulating troponin, for the biochemical diagnosis of AMI, with a sensitivity near to 100% in detection of AMI at 6–12 h after the onset of chest pain. Cardiac troponins T and I levels increase early after the onset of AMI, reaching a peak in the serum after 12–48 h and remaining elevated for 4–10 days [63]. In 2007–2010, a high-sensitivity assay (hs-cTn) became the gold standard in the diagnostic algorithm in the last universal definition of MI. The most largely employed cardiac biomarkers are troponins in the diagnosis of AMI and the natriuretic peptides in the diagnosis and prognosis of heart failure. Elevated cardiac troponin is the main criterion with high sensitivity and specificity, for the diagnosis of AMI in the presence of ischaemia signs while BNP and its N-terminal fragment proBNP (NT-proBNP) are considered markers with high sensitivity but low specificity for HF [64].

Cardiac troponin (cTn) is a component of the thin filament playing a key role in the muscle contraction by mediating the interaction between actin and myosin.

Three similar isoforms have been identified: the isoform C (cTnC) binds Calcium ions; the isoform I (cTnI) inhibits the ATPase activity of actomyosin; and isoform T (cTnT), interacts with actomyosin. Plasmatic levels of cTn are elevated also in acute or chronic heart failure, myocarditis, Takotsubo cardiomyopathy, atrial fibrillation, aortic dissection and stroke. cTn is released in the blood consequently to cell turnover, myocyte apoptosis or necrosis. It has been demonstrated that in response to ischemia without necrosis, membranous blebs release cTn. Isoforms cTnI and cTnT, expressed only in the cardiac muscle (contrary, the isoform C is expressed also in the skeletal muscle), are the most specific markers for acute coronary syndromes among the isoforms, and their plasmatic increase are considered the "gold standard" in AMI diagnosis [65].

In various studies, the diagnostic value of cTn after the treatment with cardiotoxic chemotherapy was investigated. Lipshultz and colleagues investigated cTnT blood levels in 51 sampled patients (median = 5.7 years) subjected to surgical cardiovascular (n = 19) or non-cardiovascular (n = 17) treatment or who took doxorubicin for acute lymphoblastic leukemia (ALL) (n = 15). They demonstrated that increased levels of cTnT in the serum of children corresponded to a more severe myocardial damage and predicted consequent subclinical and clinical cardiac morbidity and mortality [66].

However, another study showed that measurement of cTnT within 24 h after assumption of chemotherapy drug did not show high sensitivity to identify patients with following subclinical cardiotoxicity. cTnT levels were measured at three time points in 163 samples from 38 children, 24 h after chemotherapy cycles. In this study, increased levels of cTnT (>0.010 ng/mL) was observed in 6 samples from 3 patients. Finally, at the end of chemotherapy cycles, 7 out of the 38 patients showed LV dysfunction and only 1 of these 7 showed increased cTnT levels, while 2 children with higher cTnT levels did not show LV dysfunction up to 7 months after the cTnT measurement [67].

From the advent of high-sensitivity cardiac troponin (hs-cTn) assays, attention was more focused on the predictive value of cTn for cardiovascular disease beside its diagnostic use for acute coronary syndrome [68]. Actually, in most of worldwide laboratories the hs-cTn assays have been recognized and recommended by European Society of Cardiology Guidelines for rapid rule-in/rule-out of myocardial infarctions. These assays are used in the early evaluation of the typical chest pain and also for prognosis, to predict the risk of long-term events and mortality, not only in cardiovascular diseases but also in different pathologies. Compared to classical assays, hsTn assays are able to detect troponins at a much lower concentration, with high precision, with small coefficient of variation even at the 99th percentile, in the reference population, thus allowing a faster recognition of AMI (rule-in/rule-out) [69]. It is important to underline that there is a variability of troponin levels also in healthy patients, for example men show higher levels than women, there is a circadian variability (lightly higher in the morning). In addition, there is also a correlation with age and a variability in patients affected by diseases such as chronic kidney disease and diabetes [70].

The methods for the detection of hsTn are mainly immunochemical methods, such as enzyme linked immunoassay (ELISA), immunofluorescence assay, radioimmunoassay (RIA), and immune-chemiluminescence assay that share similar bases: an immunological phase, in which there is a specific interaction between an anti-cTn antibody and a cTn N-terminal amino acid antigen; a second phase characterized by either an enzymatic reaction or another antibody-antigen reaction, based on the method chosen; the final phase varies depending on the detection method employed: a spectrophotometer measuring color intensity for ELISA a radiometer detecting radionuclides emissions for RIA and, a fluorometer detecting fluorophores for immunofluorescence. The intensity of the signal is directly proportional to the amount of troponin molecules, allowing their quantification.

A comprehensive reference table of hsTn methods available either on automated laboratory platforms or as point of care (POC) systems is regularly updated by the IFCC Committee on Clinical Applications of Cardiac Bio Markers (C-CB) and it is publicly accessible on the IFCC website [71]. For the purpose of this review, we focused on POC hsTn methods, which are amenable to bedside testing and are suitable for pediatric patients as they require small volume whole blood samples. As reported by the IFCC Committee on Clinical Applications of Cardiac Bio-Markers (C-CB), only three analytical systems for the measurement of cardiac troponin respond to both the definition of high sensitivity assays [72] and the most recent definition given by IFCC of point of care devices [73]: PATHFAST hs-cTnI (LSI Medience, Tokio, Japan), Quidel TriageTrue High Sensitivity Troponin I Test (Quidel, CA, USA) and Siemens Atellica VTLi hs-cTnI (Siemens Healthcare Diagnostics Inc., Erlangen, Germany). Their analytical and instrument characteristics are summarized in the Table 2.

BNPs belongs to the group of Natriuretic peptides (NPs), composed of three peptides with similar structures: the atrial natriuretic peptide (ANP), the B-type (or brain) natriuretic peptide (BNP), and the C-type natriuretic peptide (CNP). BNPs play a key role in the maintenance of the cardiovascular homeostasis, regulating volume and pressure overload. Circulating BNP and the N-terminal pro-B-type natriuretic peptide (NT-proBNP) increase their levels consequently to increased wall stretching due to volume or load stress in HF caused by systolic and/or diastolic dysfunction, valvular heart disease, left ventricular hypertrophy, ischemia, or a combination of these factors.

Table 2. Analytical and instrument characteristics of high-sensitivity cTn assay.

Characteristic	PATHFAST hs-cTnI	Quidel TriageTrue hs-cTnI	Siemens Atellica VTLi hs-cTnI
LoB	1.23 ng/L	0.4 ng/L (plasma) 0.5–0.8 ng/L (whole blood)	0.55 ng/L
LoD	2.33 ng/L	0.7–1.6 ng/L (plasma) 1.5–1.9 ng/L (whole blood)	1.2 ng/L (plasma) 1.6 ng/L (whole blood)
% CV at 99th Percentile	6.1%	5.0–5.9% at 21 ng/L (plasma) 5.9–6.5% at 22 ng/L (whole blood)	6.5% (plasma) 6.1% at 22.9 ng/L (whole blood)
Concentration at 20% CV	4 ng/L	2.1–3.6 ng/L (plasma) 2.8 ng/L (whole blood)	2.1 ng/L (plasma) 3.7 ng/L (whole blood)
Concentration at 10% CV	15 ng/L	4.4–8.4 ng/L (plasma) 5.8–6.2 ng/L (whole blood)	6.7 ng/L (plasma) 8.9 ng/L (whole blood)
99th Percentile	Overall: 27.9 ng/L F: 20.3 ng/L M: 29.7 ng/L	Overall: 20.5 ng/L F: 14.4 ng/L M: 25.7 ng/L	Overall: 22.9 ng/L F: 18.5 ng/L M: 27.1 ng/L
Reference population	Overall n = 734 F: 352 M: 382	Overall n = 789 F: 391 M: 398	Overall n = 694 F: 331 M: 363
Specimen type	Heparin-Na, heparin-Li or EDTA whole blood or plasma	EDTA whole blood or plasma	Li Hep whole blood and plasma, capillary blood
POCT definition (according to Collinson 2023)	Desktop	Portable	Portable
Instrument size	475 × 343 × 569 mm	190 × 70 × 225 mm	250 × 52 × 85 mm (analyzer) 290 × 60 × 100 mm (docking station)
Instrument weight	28 kg	0.7 kg	780 g (analyzer) 460 g (docking station)
Single-test technology	No	Yes	Yes
Other markers available on the same analyzer	NT-proBNP, myoglobin, CK-MB, D-dimer, presepsin, CRP, PCT	BNP, NT-proBNP, myoglobin, CK-MB, D-dimer, drugs of abuse, PLGF	No
Included in ESC 2023 guidelines for ACS [74]	Yes	Yes	No

BNP and inactive NT-proBNP derive from the cleavage of the precursor proBNP and are then secreted in equal concentrations in the blood, where the BNP can bind to NP receptors (NPRs) thus activating the intracellular cGMP signaling pathways to decrease the volume or the pressure overload. BNP is mainly eliminated by degradation mediated by endopeptidases and in part through and renal excretion and the uptake by NPR [75].

Further, the levels of BNP or NT-proBNP are definitely helpful for risk stratification and management of patients with suspected heart failure. In fact, their decreasing levels indicates effective management strategies [76].

A study conducted on samples of 2525 patients three days after the onset of ischemic symptoms showed that measurement of the BNP could provide predictive information on the risk of new or recurrent MI episodes [77].

For an appropriate diagnosis, risk stratification, and management of patients affected by cardiovascular diseases, other biomarkers can be evaluated in routine clinical practice. Among these, C-Reactive Protein (CRP) and Interleukin-6 (IL-6) are both significantly up-regulated in acute coronary syndrome [78]. CRP, most widely used as inflammatory marker in routine clinical practice, whose levels have been observed to significantly increase in ACS patients as compared to the patients without a story of ischemic cardiomyopathy [79].

Copeptin, is a peptide deriving from the C-terminus of the vasopressin prohormone. It is released with arginine vasopressin (AVP) within 0–4 h after the onset of cardiac symptoms [80] improving efficacy in combination with troponin levels measurement for early rule-out of AMI [81–84]. However, it is as a nonspecific prognostic marker, since its level is also influenced by other pathologic conditions also such as renal disease and lower respiratory tract infections [85].

Among emerging biomarkers still under study there are some cytokines such as Interleukin 6 (IL-6) and Interleukin 37 (IL-37) and a member of lectin family, Galectin-3 (Gal-3).

IL-6, as well as CRP, is an inflammatory biomarker showing high expression levels in MI induced by trans-coronary ablation of septal hypertrophy [86,87]. IL-6 is also related to adverse cardiac events [88]. These observations suggest the diagnostic value and the potential use as therapeutic target in unstable ischemic heart disease [89]

IL-37 is an anti-inflammatory cytokine belonging to the IL-1 ligand family [90] that plays a crucial role in innate immunity and adaptive immunity. It inhibits the secretion of cytokines IL-1β, IL-6, and TNF-α in monocytes, macrophages, dendritic cells, and epithelial cells [91] a is involved in the onset and development of chronic inflammation and autoimmune diseases such as systemic lupus erythematosus, diabetes and rheumatoid arthritis [92,93]. As demonstrated by clinical and and pre-clinical studies in animal models, IL-37 participates in atherosclerotic disease and its levels are highly upregulated in acute coronary syndrome in which increased IL-37 levels are correlated with poor outcomes [94,95].

Gal-3 is involved in inflammation processes and its levels increase in cardiac injury [96]. It is a member of the lectin family; it is related to left ventricular dilation and contributes in the prediction of the outcome and the follow up of patients with both acute or chronic HF [97,98].

In the last decade, potential prognostic value of lnRNA and miRNA emerged as new and sensitive biomarkers of myocardial infarction probably acting as molecular sponge [99–105].

Adachi and colleagues demonstrated that significant increased levels of circulating miRNA-208b and miRNA-499, specifically expressed in cardiomyocytes, have been detected in AMI patients compared with the health control group [106]. Serum levels of miRNA-1 and miRNA-133a, muscle-specific microRNAs, are involved in the regulation of cardiac hypertrophy; their serum levels resulted increased in a group of patients with unselected AMI. In particular, it has been shown that miRNA-133a detected in the serum can be emplyed as a marker for cardiomyocyte death [107]. The long noncoding RNA LIPCAR is considered a marker in patients with ST-segment elevation MI and can contribute to predict survival in patients with heart failure [108,109]. lnRNA HOTAIR is an essential mediator of acute myocardial infarction [110].

4. Role of hs-cTn in the Diagnosis and Monitoring of Chemotherapy-Induced Cardiotoxicity in Pediatric Population

The European Society of Cardiology (ESC) position paper on cancer therapy and cardiovascular toxicity (2016) recommends the use of high-sensitivity troponins to predict left ventricular (LV) dysfunction in patients undergoing chemotherapy [111]. The 2020 European Society for Medical Oncology (ESMO) consensus cites the importance of the measurement of hs-cTn in detecting or predicting cardiovascular toxicity, during oncologic therapy [112]. In addition, Recent Clinical Practice Guidelines in Cardio-Oncology suggested that myocardial biomarkers, are considered diagnostic indicators of CTRCD [113]. A number of studies demonstrated that hs-cTn could be used as a marker for early monitoring of CTRCD in chemo-radiotherapy-treated patients [114–121]. In general, an increase in Tn concentration by 3–5 ng/L, measured by the hs-cTn corresponds to 10–20 mg of myocardial tissue necrosis, which could not be detected by cardiac imaging techniques [122].

However, so far, reference values for pediatric population have not been established thus limiting the use of hs-cTn dosage for the diagnosis and managements of cardiac diseases in children. As demonstrated by some studies hs-cTnI and hs-cTnT values are generally more elevated in infants and children if compared to those observed in adults [123–127]; moreover, boys have usually higher values than girls confirming the trend already reported for the conventional methods [128–130]. In particular, values of hsTn are highest in the first month of life, then rapidly decline in the next six months and finally continue to decline slower to reach a plateau during adolescence. Some studies demonstrated the increase of hsTn values in healthy adolescents after athletic training, returning to baseline values in 24–48 h [131–136]. Although based on few studies, increased levels of hsTn are considered a marker of myocardial injury also in pediatric population [137]. The incidence of myocardial infarction is much lower than in adults but myocardial injury can be found in neonates, infants and children affected by bronchiolitis, sepsis, and has recently been observed in pediatric patients with SARS-CoV-2 [138–140].

In order to shed light on the relevance in using hsTnI method to detect TnI in children patients, we report here some data that we obtained in our hospital, presented in the 27° Annual Symposium ELAS-Italia, Ligand Assay (November 2022, Bologna, Italy). 46 plasma EDTA samples coming from 15 patients undergoing chemotherapy (age: 7 months–16 years) were analyzed retrospectively, with the high-sensitive hsTnI method following manufacturer instructions (Triage MeterPro/TriageTrue hs-cTnI Assay). Samples were selected as their cTn values were below the lower measuring limit of the cTnI method (0.05–30 ng/mL). Results were interpreted based on the overall 99th percentile URL reported for the high-sensitive method (20.5 ng/L). Out of the 49 samples resulting in values <0.05 ng/mL (<50 ng/L) with the cTnI method, 28 were below the overall 99th percentile URL of the high-sensitive method (<20.5 ng/L), 18 were above it (≥20.5 ng/L). Out of these 18 samples, 9 resulted in hs-cTnI values above 50 ng/L. These results suggest that the measurement of hs-cTnI granted us a higher level of analytical detail during the monitoring of chemotherapy-induced cardiotoxicity. Not only it was possible to observe values below the threshold of the cTnI traditional method, but in some cases hs-cTnI levels were found to be above it (up to 154 ng/L), due to the considerably higher precision of the new method. Moreover, in some patients, sequential hs-cTnI measurement revealed troponin oscillations following treatment, opening for its routine use in monitoring potential cardiac damage by chemotherapy agents (Figure 2) [141].

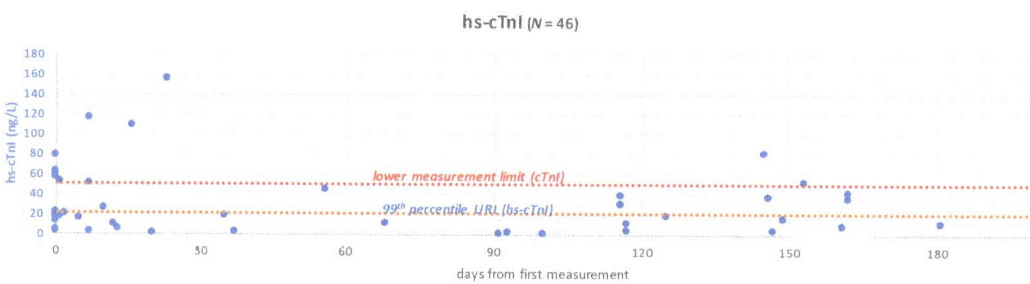

Figure 2. Overall results of hsTnI obtained from 46 children [141].

Finally, the lack of reference values in the pediatric population for all commercially available hs-cTn assays, a gap that we hope will be bridged soon, does not hinder their use for the present application, as chemotherapy-induced cardiac damage should always be monitored following measurement of individual basal values and evaluation of relative variations in the concentration of the biomarker.

5. Conclusions and Future Perspectives

Cardiomyopathy and heart failure are the main causes of death in cancer survivors, especially in children. For this reason, its early detection in cancer survivors is crucial for the prevention of long-term cardiovascular morbidity. Thus, circulating biomarkers are important tools to provide prognostic prediction and to guide cardio-protective therapy during chemotherapy treatment in oncologic patients [142]. Compared to adults, cancer-surviving children are more susceptible to the cardiotoxic effects of anthracycline due to both the life expectancy length and a deficient potential for myocardial growth to compensate for early damage and somatic development. In some survivor ALL doxorubicin-treated children, it has been observed thinner LV walls, increased afterload, and depressed contractility, progressively leading to morbidity or mortality. Early identification of cardiac damage in children after cardiotoxic therapy is crucial to improve clinical practice and benefiting patient care. Finally implementation of preventive measures can limit later myocardial damage. However, so far, no parameters have been identified to predict the possible development of cardiac dysfunction or HF in children.High sensitivity troponin is a very promising tool for early detection of CTRCD, but further prospective studies, particularly in childhood, but also in adulthood are required for its fully entry in clinical practice. Finally, the genetic can explain why some patients develop cardiotoxicity while others with same risk factors do not. This means that, in the future, pharmaco-genetic testing and personalized chemotherapy could be very effective in limiting CTRCD.

Author Contributions: L.M. and M.A. conceived and structured this review paper. M.S., C.M., P.M., P.R. and O.L. wrote the manuscript. All authors have read and agreed to the published version of the manuscript.

Funding: This research received no external funding.

Conflicts of Interest: The authors declare no conflict of interest.

Abbreviations

cTn	cardiac troponin
hs-cTnI or hs-cTnT	high sensitive methods
NGS	next-generation sequencing
HSCT	hematopoietic stem cell transplantation
SMN	secondary malignant neoplasms
CNS	Central Nervous System
CTRCD	Cancer-therapy-related cardiac dysfunction
BNP	brain-type natriuretic peptide
TOP2 (TOP2A and TOP2B)	isoenzymes of topoisomerase II
ROS	reactive oxygen species
LVEF	left ventricular ejection fraction
SNP	single nucleotide polymorphism
ACT	anthracycline-associated cardiotoxicity
CBR3	carbonyl reductase
3′ UTR	3′ Untranslated Region
ABCC1	ATP binding cassette subfamily C member
ALL	Acute Lymphoblastic Leukemia
SULT2B1	sulfotransferase family cytosolic member 2B1
CAT	catalase
GSTP1	glutathione S transferase
GPCR35	G protein-coupled receptor 35
HAS3	Hyaluronan synthase-3
CELF4	Elav-like family member 4
RARG	retinoic acid receptor-γ
hiPSC-CMs	pluripotent stem cell-derived cardiomyocytes
ERK	extracellular regulated kinase
CPNDS	The Canadian Pharmacogenomics Network for Drug Safety
TKIs	Tyrosine kinase inhibitors
CML	chronic myeloid leukemia
GIST	gastrointestinal stromal tumor
ER	endoplasmic reticulum
5-FU	Fluorouracil
RT	radiation therapy
AMI	Acute Myocardial Infarction
CK	creatine kinase
CK-MB	CK isoenzyme MB
NT-proBNP	pro Brain Natriuretic Peptide
ELISA	enzyme linked immunoassay
RIA	radioimmunoassay
C-CB	Cardiac Bio-Markers

NPs	Natriuretic peptides
ANP	atrial natriuretic peptide
B-type	atrial natriuretic peptide or brain
CNP	C-type natriuretic peptide
NPRs	NP receptors
CRP	C-Reactive Protein
AVP	arginine vasopressin
IL-6	Interleukin 6
IL-37	Interleukin 37
Gal-3	Galectin-3
ESC	European Society of Cardiology
ESMO	European Society for Medical Oncology

References

1. Rahal, Z.; Abdulhai, F.; Kadara, H.; Saab, R. Genomics of Adult and Pediatric Solid Tumors. *Am. J. Cancer Res.* **2018**, *8*, 1356–1386. [PubMed]
2. Mardis, E.R. The Impact of Next-Generation Sequencing on Cancer Genomics: From Discovery to Clinic. *Cold Spring Harb. Perspect. Med.* **2019**, *9*, a036269. [CrossRef] [PubMed]
3. Cipri, S.; Abenavoli, L.; Boccuto, L.; Del Baldo, G.; Mastronuzzi, A. How Genetics and Genomics Advances Are Rewriting Pediatric Cancer Research and Clinical Care. *Medicina* **2022**, *58*, 1386. [CrossRef] [PubMed]
4. Saletta, F.; Seng, M.S.; Lau, L.M.S. Advances in Paediatric Cancer Treatment. *Transl. Pediatr.* **2014**, *3*, 156–182. [CrossRef] [PubMed]
5. Choi, D.K.; Helenowski, I.; Hijiya, N. Secondary Malignancies in Pediatric Cancer Survivors: Perspectives and Review of the Literature. *Int. J. Cancer* **2014**, *135*, 1764–1773. [CrossRef] [PubMed]
6. Diagnosis and Management of Cancer Treatment-Related Cardiac Dysfunction and Heart Failure in Children—PMC. Available online: https://www.ncbi.nlm.nih.gov/pmc/articles/PMC9856743/#B5-children-10-00149 (accessed on 29 July 2023).
7. Cheuk, D.K.L.; Sieswerda, E.; van Dalen, E.C.; Postma, A.; Kremer, L.C.M. Medical Interventions for Treating Anthracycline-Induced Symptomatic and Asymptomatic Cardiotoxicity during and after Treatment for Childhood Cancer. *Cochrane Database Syst. Rev.* **2016**, *2016*, CD008011. [CrossRef]
8. Balis, F.M.; Womer, R.B.; Berg, S.; Winick, N.; Adamson, P.C.; Fox, E. Children's Oncology Group Chemotherapy Standardization Task Force Dosing Anticancer Drugs in Infants: Current Approach and Recommendations from the Children's Oncology Group's Chemotherapy Standardization Task Force. *Pediatr. Blood Cancer* **2017**, *64*, e26636. [CrossRef] [PubMed]
9. Armenian, S.H.; Armstrong, G.T.; Aune, G.; Chow, E.J.; Ehrhardt, M.J.; Ky, B.; Moslehi, J.; Mulrooney, D.A.; Nathan, P.C.; Ryan, T.D.; et al. Cardiovascular Disease in Survivors of Childhood Cancer: Insights Into Epidemiology, Pathophysiology, and Prevention. *J. Clin. Oncol.* **2018**, *36*, 2135–2144. [CrossRef]
10. Kang, D.-W.; Wilson, R.L.; Christopher, C.N.; Normann, A.J.; Barnes, O.; Lesansee, J.D.; Choi, G.; Dieli-Conwright, C.M. Exercise Cardio-Oncology: Exercise as a Potential Therapeutic Modality in the Management of Anthracycline-Induced Cardiotoxicity. *Front. Cardiovasc. Med.* **2022**, *8*, 2194. [CrossRef]
11. Lipshultz, S.E.; Adams, M.J.; Colan, S.D.; Constine, L.S.; Herman, E.H.; Hsu, D.T.; Hudson, M.M.; Kremer, L.C.; Landy, D.C.; Miller, T.L.; et al. Long-Term Cardiovascular Toxicity in Children, Adolescents, and Young Adults Who Receive Cancer Therapy: Pathophysiology, Course, Monitoring, Management, Prevention, and Research Directions: A Scientific Statement from the American Heart Association. *Circulation* **2013**, *128*, 1927–1995. [CrossRef]
12. Yester, J.W.; Kühn, B. Mechanisms of Cardiomyocyte Proliferation and Differentiation in Development and Regeneration. *Curr. Cardiol. Rep.* **2017**, *19*, 13. [CrossRef] [PubMed]
13. Di Stefano, V.; Giacca, M.; Capogrossi, M.C.; Crescenzi, M.; Martelli, F. Knockdown of Cyclin-Dependent Kinase Inhibitors Induces Cardiomyocyte Re-Entry in the Cell Cycle. *J. Biol. Chem.* **2011**, *286*, 8644–8654. [CrossRef] [PubMed]
14. Tocchetti, C.G.; Cadeddu, C.; Di Lisi, D.; Femminò, S.; Madonna, R.; Mele, D.; Monte, I.; Novo, G.; Penna, C.; Pepe, A.; et al. From Molecular Mechanisms to Clinical Management of Antineoplastic Drug-Induced Cardiovascular Toxicity: A Translational Overview. *Antioxid. Redox Signal* **2019**, *30*, 2110–2153. [CrossRef] [PubMed]
15. Zhang, S.; Liu, X.; Bawa-Khalfe, T.; Lu, L.-S.; Lyu, Y.L.; Liu, L.F.; Yeh, E.T.H. Identification of the Molecular Basis of Doxorubicin-Induced Cardiotoxicity. *Nat. Med.* **2012**, *18*, 1639–1642. [CrossRef] [PubMed]
16. Maillet, A.; Tan, K.; Chai, X.; Sadananda, S.N.; Mehta, A.; Ooi, J.; Hayden, M.R.; Pouladi, M.A.; Ghosh, S.; Shim, W.; et al. Modeling Doxorubicin-Induced Cardiotoxicity in Human Pluripotent Stem Cell Derived-Cardiomyocytes. *Sci. Rep.* **2016**, *6*, 25333. [CrossRef] [PubMed]
17. Aminkeng, F.; Bhavsar, A.P.; Visscher, H.; Rassekh, S.R.; Li, Y.; Lee, J.W.; Brunham, L.R.; Caron, H.N.; van Dalen, E.C.; Kremer, L.C.; et al. A Coding Variant in RARG Confers Susceptibility to Anthracycline-Induced Cardiotoxicity in Childhood Cancer. *Nat. Genet.* **2015**, *47*, 1079–1084. [CrossRef] [PubMed]
18. Varbiro, G.; Veres, B.; Gallyas, F.; Sumegi, B. Direct Effect of Taxol on Free Radical Formation and Mitochondrial Permeability Transition. *Free Radic. Biol. Med.* **2001**, *31*, 548–558. [CrossRef] [PubMed]

19. Gianni, L.; Zweier, J.L.; Levy, A.; Myers, C.E. Characterization of the Cycle of Iron-Mediated Electron Transfer from Adriamycin to Molecular Oxygen. *J. Biol. Chem.* **1985**, *260*, 6820–6826. [CrossRef]
20. Singal, P.K.; Iliskovic, N.; Li, T.; Kumar, D. Adriamycin Cardiomyopathy: Pathophysiology and Prevention. *FASEB J.* **1997**, *11*, 931–936. [CrossRef]
21. Blanco, J.G.; Sun, C.-L.; Landier, W.; Chen, L.; Esparza-Duran, D.; Leisenring, W.; Mays, A.; Friedman, D.L.; Ginsberg, J.P.; Hudson, M.M.; et al. Anthracycline-Related Cardiomyopathy After Childhood Cancer: Role of Polymorphisms in Carbonyl Reductase Genes—A Report from the Children's Oncology Group. *J. Clin. Oncol.* **2012**, *30*, 1415–1421. [CrossRef]
22. Kim, H.; Kang, H.J.; Park, K.D.; Koh, K.-N.; Im, H.J.; Seo, J.J.; Lee, J.W.; Chung, N.-G.; Cho, B.; Kim, H.K.; et al. Risk Factor Analysis for Secondary Malignancy in Dexrazoxane-Treated Pediatric Cancer Patients. *Cancer Res. Treat.* **2019**, *51*, 357–367. [CrossRef] [PubMed]
23. Eneh, C.; Lekkala, M.R. Dexrazoxane. In *StatPearls*; StatPearls Publishing: Treasure Island, FL, USA, 2023.
24. Langer, S.W. Dexrazoxane for the Treatment of Chemotherapy-Related Side Effects. *Cancer Manag. Res.* **2014**, *6*, 357–363. [CrossRef] [PubMed]
25. Semsei, A.F.; Erdelyi, D.J.; Ungvari, I.; Csagoly, E.; Hegyi, M.Z.; Kiszel, P.S.; Lautner-Csorba, O.; Szabolcs, J.; Masat, P.; Fekete, G.; et al. ABCC1 Polymorphisms in Anthracycline-Induced Cardiotoxicity in Childhood Acute Lymphoblastic Leukaemia. *Cell Biol. Int.* **2012**, *36*, 79–86. [CrossRef] [PubMed]
26. Visscher, H.; Ross, C.J.D.; Rassekh, S.R.; Barhdadi, A.; Dubé, M.-P.; Al-Saloos, H.; Sandor, G.S.; Caron, H.N.; van Dalen, E.C.; Kremer, L.C.; et al. Pharmacogenomic Prediction of Anthracycline-Induced Cardiotoxicity in Children. *J. Clin. Oncol.* **2012**, *30*, 1422–1428. [CrossRef] [PubMed]
27. Visscher, H.; Ross, C.J.D.; Rassekh, S.R.; Sandor, G.S.S.; Caron, H.N.; van Dalen, E.C.; Kremer, L.C.; van der Pal, H.J.; Rogers, P.C.; Rieder, M.J.; et al. Validation of Variants in SLC28A3 and UGT1A6 as Genetic Markers Predictive of Anthracycline-Induced Cardiotoxicity in Children. *Pediatr. Blood Cancer* **2013**, *60*, 1375–1381. [CrossRef] [PubMed]
28. Zhao, Y.; McLaughlin, D.; Robinson, E.; Harvey, A.P.; Hookham, M.B.; Shah, A.M.; McDermott, B.J.; Grieve, D.J. NOX2 NADPH Oxidase Promotes Pathologic Cardiac Remodeling Associated with Doxorubicin Chemotherapy. *Cancer Res.* **2010**, *70*, 9287–9297. [CrossRef] [PubMed]
29. Rajić, V.; Aplenc, R.; Debeljak, M.; Prestor, V.V.; Karas-Kuzelicki, N.; Mlinaric-Rascan, I.; Jazbec, J. Influence of the Polymorphism in Candidate Genes on Late Cardiac Damage in Patients Treated Due to Acute Leukemia in Childhood. *Leuk. Lymphoma* **2009**, *50*, 1693–1698. [CrossRef]
30. Windsor, R.E.; Strauss, S.J.; Kallis, C.; Wood, N.E.; Whelan, J.S. Germline Genetic Polymorphisms May Influence Chemotherapy Response and Disease Outcome in Osteosarcoma: A Pilot Study. *Cancer* **2012**, *118*, 1856–1867. [CrossRef]
31. Min, K.-D.; Asakura, M.; Liao, Y.; Nakamaru, K.; Okazaki, H.; Takahashi, T.; Fujimoto, K.; Ito, S.; Takahashi, A.; Asanuma, H.; et al. Identification of Genes Related to Heart Failure Using Global Gene Expression Profiling of Human Failing Myocardium. *Biochem. Biophys. Res. Commun.* **2010**, *393*, 55–60. [CrossRef]
32. Wang, X.; Liu, W.; Sun, C.-L.; Armenian, S.H.; Hakonarson, H.; Hageman, L.; Ding, Y.; Landier, W.; Blanco, J.G.; Chen, L.; et al. Hyaluronan Synthase 3 Variant and Anthracycline-Related Cardiomyopathy: A Report from the Children's Oncology Group. *J. Clin. Oncol.* **2014**, *32*, 647–653. [CrossRef]
33. Wang, X.; Sun, C.-L.; Quiñones-Lombraña, A.; Singh, P.; Landier, W.; Hageman, L.; Mather, M.; Rotter, J.I.; Taylor, K.D.; Chen, Y.-D.I.; et al. CELF4 Variant and Anthracycline-Related Cardiomyopathy: A Children's Oncology Group Genome-Wide Association Study. *J. Clin. Oncol.* **2016**, *34*, 863–870. [CrossRef] [PubMed]
34. Cooper, T.A.; Ordahl, C.P. A Single Cardiac Troponin T Gene Generates Embryonic and Adult Isoforms via Developmentally Regulated Alternate Splicing. *J. Biol. Chem.* **1985**, *260*, 11140–11148. [CrossRef] [PubMed]
35. Magdy, T.; Jouni, M.; Kuo, H.-H.; Weddle, C.J.; Lyra-Leite, D.; Fonoudi, H.; Romero-Tejeda, M.; Gharib, M.; Javed, H.; Fajardo, G.; et al. Identification of Drug Transporter Genomic Variants and Inhibitors That Protect Against Doxorubicin-Induced Cardiotoxicity. *Circulation* **2022**, *145*, 279–294. [CrossRef] [PubMed]
36. Magdy, T.; Jiang, Z.; Jouni, M.; Fonoudi, H.; Lyra-Leite, D.; Jung, G.; Romero-Tejeda, M.; Kuo, H.-H.; Fetterman, K.A.; Gharib, M.; et al. RARG Variant Predictive of Doxorubicin-Induced Cardiotoxicity Identifies a Cardioprotective Therapy. *Cell Stem Cell* **2021**, *28*, 2076–2089.e7. [CrossRef] [PubMed]
37. Loucks, C.M.; Yan, K.; Tanoshima, R.; Ross, C.J.D.; Rassekh, S.R.; Carleton, B.C. Pharmacogenetic Testing to Guide Therapeutic Decision-Making and Improve Outcomes for Children Undergoing Anthracycline-Based Chemotherapy. *Basic Clin. Pharmacol. Toxicol.* **2022**, *130* (Suppl. S1), 95–99. [CrossRef] [PubMed]
38. Ruiz-Pinto, S.; Pita, G.; Patiño-García, A.; Alonso, J.; Pérez-Martínez, A.; Cartón, A.J.; Gutiérrez-Larraya, F.; Alonso, M.R.; Barnes, D.R.; Dennis, J.; et al. Exome Array Analysis Identifies GPR35 as a Novel Susceptibility Gene for Anthracycline-Induced Cardiotoxicity in Childhood Cancer. *Pharmacogenetics Genom.* **2017**, *27*, 445–453. [CrossRef] [PubMed]
39. Nižnanský, Ľ.; Osinová, D.; Kuruc, R.; Hengerics Szabó, A.; Szórádová, A.; Masár, M.; Nižnanská, Ž. Natural Taxanes: From Plant Composition to Human Pharmacology and Toxicity. *Int. J. Mol. Sci.* **2022**, *23*, 15619. [CrossRef]
40. Gianni, L.; Viganò, L.; Locatelli, A.; Capri, G.; Giani, A.; Tarenzi, E.; Bonadonna, G. Human Pharmacokinetic Characterization and in Vitro Study of the Interaction between Doxorubicin and Paclitaxel in Patients with Breast Cancer. *J. Clin. Oncol.* **1997**, *15*, 1906–1915. [CrossRef]

41. Saad, S.Y.; Najjar, T.A.O.; Alashari, M. Cardiotoxicity of Doxorubicin/Paclitaxel Combination in Rats: Effect of Sequence and Timing of Administration. *J. Biochem. Mol. Toxicol.* **2004**, *18*, 78–86. [CrossRef]
42. Hurwitz, C.A.; Strauss, L.C.; Kepner, J.; Kretschmar, C.; Harris, M.B.; Friedman, H.; Kun, L.; Kadota, R. Paclitaxel for the Treatment of Progressive or Recurrent Childhood Brain Tumors: A Pediatric Oncology Phase II Study. *J. Pediatr. Hematol. Oncol.* **2001**, *23*, 277. [CrossRef]
43. Adinani, H.; Campbell, L.; El-Mallawany, N.K.; Slone, J.; Mehta, P.; Bacha, J. Use of Paclitaxel to Successfully Treat Children, Adolescents, and Young Adults with Kaposi Sarcoma in Southwestern Tanzania. *Children* **2021**, *8*, 275. [CrossRef] [PubMed]
44. Perez-Somarriba, M.; Moreno-Tejero, M.L.; Rozas, M.I.; Pelaez, I.; Madero, L.; Lassaletta, A. Gemcitabine, Paclitaxel, and Oxaliplatin (GEMPOX) in the Treatment of Relapsed/Refractory Intracranial Nongerminomatous Germ Cell Tumors. *Pediatr. Blood Cancer* **2020**, *67*, e28089. [CrossRef] [PubMed]
45. Iwase, K.; Oyama, Y.; Tatsuishi, T.; Yamaguchi, J.; Nishimura, Y.; Kanada, A.; Kobayashi, M.; Maemura, Y.; Ishida, S.; Okano, Y. Cremophor EL Augments the Cytotoxicity of Hydrogen Peroxide in Lymphocytes Dissociated from Rat Thymus Glands. *Toxicol. Lett.* **2004**, *154*, 143–148. [CrossRef] [PubMed]
46. Gutiérrez, M.B.; Miguel, B.S.; Villares, C.; Gallego, J.G.; Tuñón, M.J. Oxidative Stress Induced by Cremophor EL Is Not Accompanied by Changes in NF-kappaB Activation or iNOS Expression. *Toxicology* **2006**, *222*, 125–131. [CrossRef] [PubMed]
47. Rowinsky, E.K.; McGuire, W.P.; Guarnieri, T.; Fisherman, J.S.; Christian, M.C.; Donehower, R.C. Cardiac Disturbances during the Administration of Taxol. *J. Clin. Oncol.* **1991**, *9*, 1704–1712. [CrossRef]
48. Skolnik, J.M.; Adamson, P.C. Tyrosine Kinase Inhibitors in Pediatric Malignancies. *Cancer Investig.* **2007**, *25*, 606–612. [CrossRef] [PubMed]
49. Zhang, X.; Zhu, Y.; Dong, S.; Zhang, A.; Lu, Y.; Li, Y.; Lv, S.; Zhang, J. Role of Oxidative Stress in Cardiotoxicity of Antineoplastic Drugs. *Life Sci.* **2019**, *232*, 116526. [CrossRef] [PubMed]
50. Akam-Venkata, J.; Franco, V.I.; Lipshultz, S.E. Late Cardiotoxicity: Issues for Childhood Cancer Survivors. *Curr. Treat. Options Cardiovasc. Med.* **2016**, *18*, 47. [CrossRef]
51. Iqubal, A.; Iqubal, M.K.; Sharma, S.; Ansari, M.A.; Najmi, A.K.; Ali, S.M.; Ali, J.; Haque, S.E. Molecular Mechanism Involved in Cyclophosphamide-Induced Cardiotoxicity: Old Drug with a New Vision. *Life Sci.* **2019**, *218*, 112–131. [CrossRef]
52. Fabin, N.; Bergami, M.; Cenko, E.; Bugiardini, R.; Manfrini, O. The Role of Vasospasm and Microcirculatory Dysfunction in Fluoropyrimidine-Induced Ischemic Heart Disease. *J. Clin. Med.* **2022**, *11*, 1244. [CrossRef]
53. Bansal, N.; Blanco, J.G.; Sharma, U.; Pokharel, S.; Shisler, S.; Lipshultz, S.E. Cardiovascular Diseases in Survivors of Childhood Cancer. *Cancer Metastasis Rev.* **2020**, *39*, 55–68. [CrossRef] [PubMed]
54. Mitchell, J.D.; Cehic, D.A.; Morgia, M.; Bergom, C.; Toohey, J.; Guerrero, P.A.; Ferencik, M.; Kikuchi, R.; Carver, J.R.; Zaha, V.G.; et al. Cardiovascular Manifestations from Therapeutic Radiation: A Multidisciplinary Expert Consensus Statement from the International Cardio-Oncology Society. *JACC CardioOncol.* **2021**, *3*, 360–380. [CrossRef] [PubMed]
55. Crocco, M.; d'Annunzio, G.; La Valle, A.; Piccolo, G.; Chiarenza, D.S.; Bigatti, C.; Molteni, M.; Milanaccio, C.; Garrè, M.L.; Di Iorgi, N.; et al. Endothelial Dysfunction in Childhood Cancer Survivors: A Narrative Review. *Life* **2021**, *12*, 45. [CrossRef] [PubMed]
56. Ponikowski, P.; Voors, A.A.; Anker, S.D.; Bueno, H.; Cleland, J.G.F.; Coats, A.J.S.; Falk, V.; González-Juanatey, J.R.; Harjola, V.-P.; Jankowska, E.A.; et al. 2016 ESC Guidelines for the Diagnosis and Treatment of Acute and Chronic Heart Failure: The Task Force for the Diagnosis and Treatment of Acute and Chronic Heart Failure of the European Society of Cardiology (ESC)Developed with the Special Contribution of the Heart Failure Association (HFA) of the ESC. *Eur. Heart J.* **2016**, *37*, 2129–2200. [CrossRef] [PubMed]
57. Yancy, C.W.; Jessup, M.; Bozkurt, B.; Butler, J.; Casey, D.E.; Drazner, M.H.; Fonarow, G.C.; Geraci, S.A.; Horwich, T.; Januzzi, J.L.; et al. 2013 ACCF/AHA Guideline for the Management of Heart Failure: A Report of the American College of Cardiology Foundation/American Heart Association Task Force on Practice Guidelines. *Circulation* **2013**, *128*, e240–e327. [CrossRef] [PubMed]
58. Gong, F.F.; Cascino, G.J.; Murtagh, G.; Akhter, N. Circulating Biomarkers for Cardiotoxicity Risk Prediction. *Curr. Treat. Options Oncol.* **2021**, *22*, 46. [CrossRef] [PubMed]
59. Meijers, W.C.; Bayes-Genis, A.; Mebazaa, A.; Bauersachs, J.; Cleland, J.G.F.; Coats, A.J.S.; Januzzi, J.L.; Maisel, A.S.; McDonald, K.; Mueller, T.; et al. Circulating Heart Failure Biomarkers beyond Natriuretic Peptides: Review from the Biomarker Study Group of the Heart Failure Association (HFA), European Society of Cardiology (ESC). *Eur. J. Heart Fail.* **2021**, *23*, 1610–1632. [CrossRef]
60. Karmen, A.; Wróblewski, F.; LaDue, J.S. Transaminase Activity in Human Blood. *J. Clin. Investig.* **1955**, *34*, 126–133. [CrossRef]
61. Laurino, J.P.; Bender, E.W.; Kessimian, N.; Chang, J.; Pelletier, T.; Usategui, M. Comparative Sensitivities and Specificities of the Mass Measurements of CK-MB2, CK-MB, and Myoglobin for Diagnosing Acute Myocardial Infarction. *Clin. Chem.* **1996**, *42*, 1454–1459. [CrossRef]
62. Panteghini, M.; Pagani, F.; Bonetti, G. The Sensitivity of Cardiac Markers: An Evidence-Based Approach. *Clin. Chem. Lab. Med. (CCLM)* **1999**, *37*, 1097–1106. [CrossRef]
63. Garg, P.; Morris, P.; Fazlanie, A.L.; Vijayan, S.; Dancso, B.; Dastidar, A.G.; Plein, S.; Mueller, C.; Haaf, P. Cardiac Biomarkers of Acute Coronary Syndrome: From History to High-Sensitivity Cardiac Troponin. *Intern. Emerg. Med.* **2017**, *12*, 147–155. [CrossRef]
64. Wang, X.-Y.; Zhang, F.; Zhang, C.; Zheng, L.-R.; Yang, J. The Biomarkers for Acute Myocardial Infarction and Heart Failure. *BioMed Res. Int.* **2020**, *2020*, e2018035. [CrossRef] [PubMed]
65. Katrukha, I.A. Human Cardiac Troponin Complex. Structure and Functions. *Biochem. Mosc.* **2013**, *78*, 1447–1465. [CrossRef] [PubMed]

66. Lipshultz, S.E.; Rifai, N.; Sallan, S.E.; Lipsitz, S.R.; Dalton, V.; Sacks, D.B.; Ottlinger, M.E. Predictive Value of Cardiac Troponin T in Pediatric Patients at Risk for Myocardial Injury. *Circulation* **1997**, *96*, 2641–2648. [CrossRef] [PubMed]
67. Kremer, L.C.M.; Bastiaansen, B.A.J.; Offringa, M.; Lam, J.; van Straalen, J.P.; de Winter, R.J.; Voûte, P.A. Troponin T in the First 24 Hours after the Administration of Chemotherapy and the Detection of Myocardial Damage in Children. *Eur. J. Cancer* **2002**, *38*, 686–689. [CrossRef] [PubMed]
68. de Antonio, M.; Lupon, J.; Galan, A.; Vila, J.; Urrutia, A.; Bayes-Genis, A. Combined Use of High-Sensitivity Cardiac Troponin T and N-Terminal pro-B Type Natriuretic Peptide Improves Measurements of Performance over Established Mortality Risk Factors in Chronic Heart Failure. *Am. Heart J.* **2012**, *163*, 821–828. [CrossRef] [PubMed]
69. Cediel, G.; Rueda, F.; García, C.; Oliveras, T.; Labata, C.; Serra, J.; Núñez, J.; Bodí, V.; Ferrer, M.; Lupón, J.; et al. Prognostic Value of New-Generation Troponins in ST-Segment–Elevation Myocardial Infarction in the Modern Era: The RUTI-STEMI Study. *J. Am. Heart Assoc.* **2017**, *6*, e007252. [CrossRef]
70. Lazar, D.R.; Lazar, F.-L.; Homorodean, C.; Cainap, C.; Focsan, M.; Cainap, S.; Olinic, D.M. High-Sensitivity Troponin: A Review on Characteristics, Assessment, and Clinical Implications. *Dis. Markers* **2022**, *2022*, 9713326. [CrossRef]
71. 2023 ESC Guidelines for the Management of Acute Coronary Syndromes | European Heart Journal | Oxford Academic. Available online: https://academic.oup.com/eurheartj/article/44/38/3720/7243210 (accessed on 21 November 2023).
72. Biomarkers Reference Tables. Available online: https://ifcc.org/ifcc-education-division/emd-committees/committee-on-clinical-applications-of-cardiac-bio-markers-c-cb/biomarkers-reference-tables/ (accessed on 21 November 2023).
73. Apple, F.S.; Collinson, P.O. IFCC Task Force on Clinical Applications of Cardiac Biomarkers Analytical Characteristics of High-Sensitivity Cardiac Troponin Assays. *Clin. Chem.* **2012**, *58*, 54–61. [CrossRef]
74. Collinson, P.; Aakre, K.M.; Saenger, A.; Body, R.; Hammarsten, O.; Jaffe, A.S.; Kavsak, P.; Omland, T.; Ordonez-Lianos, J.; Karon, B.; et al. Cardiac Troponin Measurement at the Point of Care: Educational Recommendations on Analytical and Clinical Aspects by the IFCC Committee on Clinical Applications of Cardiac Bio-Markers (IFCC C-CB). *Clin. Chem. Lab. Med. (CCLM)* **2023**, *61*, 989–998. [CrossRef]
75. Alcidi, G.; Goffredo, G.; Correale, M.; Brunetti, N.D.; Iacoviello, M. Brain Natriuretic Peptide Biomarkers in Current Clinical and Therapeutic Scenarios of Heart Failure. *J. Clin. Med.* **2022**, *11*, 3192. [CrossRef] [PubMed]
76. Núñez-Marín, G.; Iraola, D.; Lorenzo, M.; De La Espriella, R.; Villar, S.; Santas, E.; Miñana, G.; Sanchis, J.; Carratalá, A.; Miró, Ò.; et al. An Update on Utilising Brain Natriuretic Peptide for Risk Stratification, Monitoring and Guiding Therapy in Heart Failure. *Expert Rev. Mol. Diagn.* **2023**, *23*, 521–533. [CrossRef] [PubMed]
77. de Lemos, J.A.; Morrow, D.A.; Bentley, J.H.; Omland, T.; Sabatine, M.S.; McCabe, C.H.; Hall, C.; Cannon, C.P.; Braunwald, E. The Prognostic Value of B-Type Natriuretic Peptide in Patients with Acute Coronary Syndromes. *N. Engl. J. Med.* **2001**, *345*, 1014–1021. [CrossRef] [PubMed]
78. McKechnie, D.G.J.; Papacosta, A.O.; Lennon, L.T.; Ramsay, S.E.; Whincup, P.H.; Wannamethee, S.G. Associations between Inflammation, Cardiovascular Biomarkers and Incident Frailty: The British Regional Heart Study. *Age Ageing* **2021**, *50*, 1979–1987. [CrossRef] [PubMed]
79. Reynoso-Villalpando, G.L.; Padilla-Gutiérrez, J.R.; Valdez-Haro, A.; Casillas-Muñoz, F.; Muñoz-Valle, J.F.; Castellanos-Nuñez, E.; Chávez-Herrera, J.C.; Valle, Y. Relationship Between C-Reactive Protein Serum Concentration and the 1846 C>T (Rs1205) Polymorphism in Patients with Acute Coronary Syndrome from Western Mexico. *Genet. Test. Mol. Biomark.* **2017**, *21*, 334–340. [CrossRef] [PubMed]
80. Afzali, D.; Erren, M.; Pavenstädt, H.-J.; Vollert, J.O.; Hertel, S.; Waltenberger, J.; Reinecke, H.; Lebiedz, P. Impact of Copeptin on Diagnosis, Risk Stratification, and Intermediate-Term Prognosis of Acute Coronary Syndromes. *Clin. Res. Cardiol.* **2013**, *102*, 755–763. [CrossRef] [PubMed]
81. Yalta, K.; Yetkin, E.; Yalta, T. Serum Copeptin in Cardiooncology Practice: Review of Pathophysiological and Clinical Implications. *Balk. Med. J.* **2023**, *40*, 82–92. [CrossRef]
82. Folli, C.; Consonni, D.; Spessot, M.; Salvini, L.; Velati, M.; Ranzani, G.; Maiavacca, R.; Monzani, V. Diagnostic Role of Copeptin in Patients Presenting with Chest Pain in the Emergency Room. *Eur. J. Intern. Med.* **2013**, *24*, 189–193. [CrossRef]
83. Jeong, J.H.; Seo, Y.H.; Ahn, J.Y.; Kim, K.H.; Seo, J.Y.; Chun, K.Y.; Lim, Y.S.; Park, P.W. Performance of Copeptin for Early Diagnosis of Acute Myocardial Infarction in an Emergency Department Setting. *Ann. Lab. Med.* **2020**, *40*, 7–14. [CrossRef]
84. Abd El Baky Mahmoud, M.; Shaaban, M.A.A.; Ali Ramzy, A. Clinical Role of Serum Copeptin in Acute Coronary Syndrome. *Egypt. Heart J.* **2018**, *70*, 155–159. [CrossRef]
85. Nickel, C.H.; Bingisser, R.; Morgenthaler, N.G. The Role of Copeptin as a Diagnostic and Prognostic Biomarker for Risk Stratification in the Emergency Department. *BMC Med.* **2012**, *10*, 7. [CrossRef] [PubMed]
86. Kamińska, J.; Koper, O.M.; Siedlecka-Czykier, E.; Matowicka-Karna, J.; Bychowski, J.; Kemona, H. The Utility of Inflammation and Platelet Biomarkers in Patients with Acute Coronary Syndromes. *Saudi J. Biol. Sci.* **2018**, *25*, 1263–1271. [CrossRef] [PubMed]
87. Liebetrau, C.; Hoffmann, J.; Dörr, O.; Gaede, L.; Blumenstein, J.; Biermann, H.; Pyttel, L.; Thiele, P.; Troidl, C.; Berkowitsch, A.; et al. Release Kinetics of Inflammatory Biomarkers in a Clinical Model of Acute Myocardial Infarction. *Circ. Res.* **2015**, *116*, 867–875. [CrossRef] [PubMed]

88. Held, C.; White, H.D.; Stewart, R.A.H.; Budaj, A.; Cannon, C.P.; Hochman, J.S.; Koenig, W.; Siegbahn, A.; Steg, P.G.; Soffer, J.; et al. Inflammatory Biomarkers Interleukin-6 and C-Reactive Protein and Outcomes in Stable Coronary Heart Disease: Experiences from the STABILITY (Stabilization of Atherosclerotic Plaque by Initiation of Darapladib Therapy) Trial. *J. Am. Heart Assoc.* **2017**, *6*, e005077. [CrossRef] [PubMed]
89. Fanola, C.L.; Morrow, D.A.; Cannon, C.P.; Jarolim, P.; Lukas, M.A.; Bode, C.; Hochman, J.S.; Goodrich, E.L.; Braunwald, E.; O'Donoghue, M.L. Interleukin-6 and the Risk of Adverse Outcomes in Patients After an Acute Coronary Syndrome: Observations from the SOLID-TIMI 52 (Stabilization of Plaque Using Darapladib—Thrombolysis in Myocardial Infarction 52) Trial. *J. Am. Heart Assoc.* **2017**, *6*, e005637. [CrossRef] [PubMed]
90. Nold, M.F.; Nold-Petry, C.A.; Zepp, J.A.; Palmer, B.E.; Bufler, P.; Dinarello, C.A. IL-37 Is a Fundamental Inhibitor of Innate Immunity. *Nat. Immunol.* **2010**, *11*, 1014–1022. [CrossRef] [PubMed]
91. Boraschi, D.; Lucchesi, D.; Hainzl, S.; Leitner, M.; Maier, E.; Mangelberger, D.; Oostingh, G.J.; Pfaller, T.; Pixner, C.; Posselt, G.; et al. IL-37: A New Anti-Inflammatory Cytokine of the IL-1 Family. *Eur. Cytokine Netw.* **2011**, *22*, 127–147. [CrossRef]
92. Ye, Z.; Wang, C.; Tang, J.; Zhou, Y.; Bai, L.; Liu, Y.; Kijlstra, A.; Yang, P. Decreased Interleukin-37 Expression in Vogt-Koyanagi-Harada Disease and Upregulation Following Immunosuppressive Treatment. *J. Interferon Cytokine Res.* **2015**, *35*, 265–272. [CrossRef]
93. Chai, M.; Ji, Q.; Zhang, H.; Zhou, Y.; Yang, Q.; Zhou, Y.; Guo, G.; Liu, W.; Han, W.; Yang, L.; et al. The Protective Effect of Interleukin-37 on Vascular Calcification and Atherosclerosis in Apolipoprotein E-Deficient Mice with Diabetes. *J. Interferon Cytokine Res.* **2015**, *35*, 530–539. [CrossRef]
94. Liu, H.; Zheng, R.; Wang, P.; Yang, H.; He, X.; Ji, Q.; Bai, W.; Chen, H.; Chen, J.; Peng, W.; et al. IL-37 Confers Protection against Mycobacterial Infection Involving Suppressing Inflammation and Modulating T Cell Activation. *PLoS ONE* **2017**, *12*, e0169922. [CrossRef]
95. Yang, T.; Fang, F.; Chen, Y.; Ma, J.; Xiao, Z.; Zou, S.; Zheng, N.; Yan, D.; Liao, S.; Chen, S.; et al. Elevated Plasma Interleukin-37 Playing an Important Role in Acute Coronary Syndrome through Suppression of ROCK Activation. *Oncotarget* **2017**, *8*, 9686–9695. [CrossRef] [PubMed]
96. Xiao, H.; Wang, X.; Li, S.; Liu, Y.; Cui, Y.; Deng, X. Advances in Biomarkers for Detecting Early Cancer Treatment-Related Cardiac Dysfunction. *Front. Cardiovasc. Med.* **2021**, *8*, 753313. [CrossRef] [PubMed]
97. French, B.; Wang, L.; Ky, B.; Brandimarto, J.; Basuray, A.; Fang, J.C.; Sweitzer, N.K.; Cappola, T.P. Prognostic Value of Galectin-3 for Adverse Outcomes in Chronic Heart Failure. *J. Card. Fail.* **2016**, *22*, 256–262. [CrossRef] [PubMed]
98. Zivlas, C.; Triposkiadis, F.; Psarras, S.; Giamouzis, G.; Skoularigis, I.; Chryssanthopoulos, S.; Kapelouzou, A.; Ramcharitar, S.; Barnes, E.; Papasteriadis, E.; et al. Cystatin C and Galectin-3 as Therapeutic Targets in Heart Failure. *Ther. Adv. Cardiovasc. Dis.* **2018**, *12*, 233–235. [CrossRef] [PubMed]
99. D'Alessandra, Y.; Devanna, P.; Limana, F.; Straino, S.; Di Carlo, A.; Brambilla, P.G.; Rubino, M.; Carena, M.C.; Spazzafumo, L.; De Simone, M.; et al. Circulating microRNAs Are New and Sensitive Biomarkers of Myocardial Infarction. *Eur. Heart J.* **2010**, *31*, 2765–2773. [CrossRef] [PubMed]
100. Vausort, M.; Wagner, D.R.; Devaux, Y. Long Noncoding RNAs in Patients with Acute Myocardial Infarction. *Circ. Res.* **2014**, *115*, 668–677. [CrossRef] [PubMed]
101. Devaux, Y. Transcriptome of Blood Cells as a Reservoir of Cardiovascular Biomarkers. *Biochim. Et Biophys. Acta (BBA)—Mol. Cell Res.* **2017**, *1864*, 209–216. [CrossRef]
102. Ikeda, S.; Pu, W.T. Expression and Function of microRNAs in Heart Disease. *Curr. Drug Targets* **2010**, *11*, 913–925. [CrossRef]
103. Li, M.; Duan, L.; Li, Y.; Liu, B. Long Noncoding RNA/Circular Noncoding RNA-miRNA-mRNA Axes in Cardiovascular Diseases. *Life Sci.* **2019**, *233*, 116440. [CrossRef]
104. Li Santi, A.; Gorrasi, A.; Alfieri, M.; Montuori, N.; Ragno, P. A Novel Oncogenic Role for Urokinase Receptor in Leukemia Cells: Molecular Sponge for Oncosuppressor microRNAs. *Oncotarget* **2018**, *9*, 27823–27834. [CrossRef]
105. Alfieri, M.; Meo, L.; Ragno, P. Posttranscriptional Regulation of the Plasminogen Activation System by Non-Coding RNA in Cancer. *Int. J. Mol. Sci.* **2023**, *24*, 962. [CrossRef]
106. Adachi, T.; Nakanishi, M.; Otsuka, Y.; Nishimura, K.; Hirokawa, G.; Goto, Y.; Nonogi, H.; Iwai, N. Plasma MicroRNA 499 as a Biomarker of Acute Myocardial Infarction. *Clin. Chem.* **2010**, *56*, 1183–1185. [CrossRef] [PubMed]
107. Kuwabara, Y.; Ono, K.; Horie, T.; Nishi, H.; Nagao, K.; Kinoshita, M.; Watanabe, S.; Baba, O.; Kojima, Y.; Shizuta, S.; et al. Increased MicroRNA-1 and MicroRNA-133a Levels in Serum of Patients with Cardiovascular Disease Indicate Myocardial Damage. *Circ. Cardiovasc. Genet.* **2011**, *4*, 446–454. [CrossRef] [PubMed]
108. Li, M.; Wang, L.-F.; Yang, X.-C.; Xu, L.; Li, W.-M.; Xia, K.; Zhang, D.-P.; Wu, R.-N.; Gan, T. Circulating Long Noncoding RNA LIPCAR Acts as a Novel Biomarker in Patients with ST-Segment Elevation Myocardial Infarction. *Med. Sci. Monit.* **2018**, *24*, 5064–5070. [CrossRef] [PubMed]
109. Kumarswamy, R.; Bauters, C.; Volkmann, I.; Maury, F.; Fetisch, J.; Holzmann, A.; Lemesle, G.; de Groote, P.; Pinet, F.; Thum, T. Circulating Long Noncoding RNA, LIPCAR, Predicts Survival in Patients with Heart Failure. *Circ. Res.* **2014**, *114*, 1569–1575. [CrossRef]
110. Gao, L.; Liu, Y.; Guo, S.; Yao, R.; Wu, L.; Xiao, L.; Wang, Z.; Liu, Y.; Zhang, Y. Circulating Long Noncoding RNA HOTAIR Is an Essential Mediator of Acute Myocardial Infarction. *Cell. Physiol. Biochem.* **2017**, *44*, 1497–1508. [CrossRef] [PubMed]

111. Zamorano, J.L.; Lancellotti, P.; Rodriguez Munoz, D.; Aboyans, V.; Asteggiano, R.; Galderisi, M.; Habib, G.; Lenihan, D.J.; Lip, G.Y.H.; Lyon, A.R.; et al. 2016 ESC Position Paper on Cancer Treatments and Cardiovascular Toxicity Developed under the Auspices of the ESC Committee for Practice Guidelines: The Task Force for Cancer Treatments and Cardiovascular Toxicity of the European Society of Cardiology (ESC). *Eur. Heart J.* **2016**, *37*, 2768–2801. [CrossRef] [PubMed]
112. Curigliano, G.; Lenihan, D.; Fradley, M.; Ganatra, S.; Barac, A.; Blaes, A.; Herrmann, J.; Porter, C.; Lyon, A.R.; Lancellotti, P.; et al. Management of Cardiac Disease in Cancer Patients throughout Oncological Treatment: ESMO Consensus Recommendations. *Ann. Oncol.* **2020**, *31*, 171–190. [CrossRef]
113. Leong, D.P.; Lenihan, D.J. Clinical Practice Guidelines in Cardio-Oncology. *Heart Fail. Clin.* **2022**, *18*, 489–501. [CrossRef]
114. Katsurada, K.; Ichida, M.; Sakuragi, M.; Takehara, M.; Hozumi, Y.; Kario, K. High-Sensitivity Troponin T as a Marker to Predict Cardiotoxicity in Breast Cancer Patients with Adjuvant Trastuzumab Therapy. *Springerplus* **2014**, *3*, 620. [CrossRef]
115. Cheung, Y.; Li, V.W.; Lai, C.T.; Shin, V.Y.; Keung, W.; Cheuk, D.K.; Kwong, A.; Li, R.A.; Chan, G.C. Circulating High-Sensitivity Troponin T and microRNAs as Markers of Myocardial Damage during Childhood Leukaemia Treatment. *Pediatr. Res.* **2021**, *89*, 1245–1252. [CrossRef] [PubMed]
116. Díaz-Antón, B.; Madurga, R.; Zorita, B.; Wasniewski, S.; Moreno-Arciniegas, A.; López-Melgar, B.; Ramírez Merino, N.; Martín-Asenjo, R.; Barrio, P.; Amado Escañuela, M.G.; et al. Early Detection of Anthracycline- and Trastuzumab-induced Cardiotoxicity: Value and Optimal Timing of Serum Biomarkers and Echocardiographic Parameters. *ESC Heart Fail.* **2022**, *9*, 1127–1137. [CrossRef] [PubMed]
117. Prayogo, A.A.; Suryantoro, S.D.; Savitri, M.; Hendrata, W.M.; Wijaya, A.Y.; Pikir, B.S. High Sensitivity Troponin T as Complementary Modality for Determining Doxorubicin Regimen Cardiotoxicity in Non-Hodgkin Lymphoma Patients. *Adv. Pharm. Bull.* **2022**, *12*, 163–168. [CrossRef] [PubMed]
118. Bisoc, A.; Ciurescu, D.; Rădoi, M.; Tântu, M.M.; Rogozea, L.; Sweidan, A.J.; Bota, D.A. Elevations in High-Sensitive Cardiac Troponin T and N-Terminal Prohormone Brain Natriuretic Peptide Levels in the Serum Can Predict the Development of Anthracycline-Induced Cardiomyopathy. *Am. J. Ther.* **2020**, *27*, e142–e150. [CrossRef] [PubMed]
119. Finke, D.; Romann, S.W.; Heckmann, M.B.; Hund, H.; Bougatf, N.; Kantharajah, A.; Katus, H.A.; Müller, O.J.; Frey, N.; Giannitsis, E.; et al. High-Sensitivity Cardiac Troponin T Determines All-Cause Mortality in Cancer Patients: A Single-Centre Cohort Study. *ESC Heart Fail.* **2021**, *8*, 3709–3719. [CrossRef] [PubMed]
120. Petricciuolo, S.; Delle Donne, M.G.; Aimo, A.; Chella, A.; De Caterina, R. Pre-Treatment High-Sensitivity Troponin T for the Short-Term Prediction of Cardiac Outcomes in Patients on Immune Checkpoint Inhibitors. *Eur. J. Clin. Investig.* **2021**, *51*, e13400. [CrossRef] [PubMed]
121. Demissei, B.G.; Hubbard, R.A.; Zhang, L.; Smith, A.M.; Sheline, K.; McDonald, C.; Narayan, V.; Domchek, S.M.; DeMichele, A.; Shah, P.; et al. Changes in Cardiovascular Biomarkers with Breast Cancer Therapy and Associations with Cardiac Dysfunction. *J. Am. Heart Assoc.* **2020**, *9*, e014708. [CrossRef] [PubMed]
122. Clerico, A.; Zaninotto, M.; Passino, C.; Padoan, A.; Migliardi, M.; Plebani, M. Chapter Six—High-Sensitivity Methods for Cardiac Troponins: The Mission Is Not over Yet. In *Advances in Clinical Chemistry*; Makowski, G.S., Ed.; Elsevier: Amsterdam, The Netherlands, 2021; Volume 103, pp. 215–252.
123. Caselli, C.; Cangemi, G.; Masotti, S.; Ragusa, R.; Gennai, I.; Del Ry, S.; Prontera, C.; Clerico, A. Plasma Cardiac Troponin I Concentrations in Healthy Neonates, Children and Adolescents Measured with a High Sensitive Immunoassay Method: High Sensitive Troponin I in Pediatric Age. *Clin. Chim. Acta* **2016**, *458*, 68–71. [CrossRef]
124. Bohn, M.K.; Higgins, V.; Kavsak, P.; Hoffman, B.; Adeli, K. High-Sensitivity Generation 5 Cardiac Troponin T Sex- and Age-Specific 99th Percentiles in the CALIPER Cohort of Healthy Children and Adolescents. *Clin. Chem.* **2019**, *65*, 589–591. [CrossRef]
125. Jehlicka, P.; Rajdl, D.; Sladkova, E.; Sykorova, A.; Sykora, J. Dynamic Changes of High-Sensitivity Troponin T Concentration During Infancy: Clinical Implications. *Physiol. Res.* **2021**, *70*, 27–32. [CrossRef]
126. Lam, L.; Ha, L.; Heron, C.; Chiu, W.; Kyle, C. Identification of Macrotroponin T: Findings from a Case Report and Non-Reproducible Troponin T Results. *Clin. Chem. Lab. Med.* **2021**, *59*, 1972–1980. [CrossRef] [PubMed]
127. Mondal, T.; Ryan, P.M.; Gupta, K.; Radovanovic, G.; Pugh, E.; Chan, A.K.C.; Hill, S. Cord-Blood High-Sensitivity Troponin-I Reference Interval and Association with Early Neonatal Outcomes. *Am. J. Perinatol.* **2022**, *29*, 1548–1554. [CrossRef] [PubMed]
128. Soldin, S.J.; Murthy, J.N.; Agarwalla, P.K.; Ojeifo, O.; Chea, J. Pediatric Reference Ranges for Creatine Kinase, CKMB, Troponin I, Iron, and Cortisol. *Clin. Biochem.* **1999**, *32*, 77–80. [CrossRef] [PubMed]
129. Engin, Y.; Ustün, Y.; Kurtay, G. Cardiac Troponin I Levels in Umbilical Cord Blood. *Int. J. Gynaecol. Obs.* **2002**, *77*, 239–241. [CrossRef] [PubMed]
130. Trevisanuto, D.; Pitton, M.; Altinier, S.; Zaninotto, M.; Plebani, M.; Zanardo, V. Cardiac Troponin I, Cardiac Troponin T and Creatine Kinase MB Concentrations in Umbilical Cord Blood of Healthy Term Neonates. *Acta Paediatr.* **2003**, *92*, 1463–1467. [CrossRef] [PubMed]
131. Nie, J.; George, K.P.; Tong, T.K.; Gaze, D.; Tian, Y.; Lin, H.; Shi, Q. The Influence of a Half-Marathon Race upon Cardiac Troponin T Release in Adolescent Runners. *Curr. Med. Chem.* **2011**, *18*, 3452–3456. [CrossRef] [PubMed]
132. Nie, J.; George, K.P.; Tong, T.K.; Tian, Y.; Shi, Q. Effect of Repeated Endurance Runs on Cardiac Biomarkers and Function in Adolescents. *Med. Sci. Sports Exerc.* **2011**, *43*, 2081–2088. [CrossRef]
133. Peretti, A.; Mauri, L.; Masarin, A.; Annoni, G.; Corato, A.; Maloberti, A.; Giannattasio, C.; Vignati, G. Cardiac Biomarkers Release in Preadolescent Athletes After an High Intensity Exercise. *High. Blood Press. Cardiovasc. Prev.* **2018**, *25*, 89–96. [CrossRef]

134. Pompa, A.G.; Arora, G.; Harris, T.H. Effect of Treadmill Exercise Stress Testing on Troponin Levels in Children and Adolescents. *Cardiol. Young* **2023**, *33*, 380–382. [CrossRef]
135. Cirer-Sastre, R.; Legaz-Arrese, A.; Corbi, F.; López-Laval, I.; Puente-Lanzarote, J.; Hernández-González, V.; Reverter-Masià, J. Effect of Training Load on Post-Exercise Cardiac Troponin T Elevations in Young Soccer Players. *Int. J. Environ. Res. Public. Health* **2019**, *16*, 4853. [CrossRef]
136. Cirer-Sastre, R.; Legaz-Arrese, A.; Corbi, F.; López-Laval, I.; George, K.; Reverter-Masia, J. Influence of Maturational Status in the Exercise-Induced Release of Cardiac Troponin T in Healthy Young Swimmers. *J. Sci. Med. Sport.* **2021**, *24*, 116–121. [CrossRef] [PubMed]
137. McEvoy, J.W.; Wang, D.; Brady, T.; Tang, O.; Ndumele, C.E.; Coresh, J.; Christenson, R.H.; Selvin, E. Myocardial Injury Thresholds for 4 High-Sensitivity Troponin Assays in a Population-Based Sample of US Children and Adolescents. *Circulation* **2023**, *148*, 7–16. [CrossRef] [PubMed]
138. Patel, T.; Kelleman, M.; West, Z.; Peter, A.; Dove, M.; Butto, A.; Oster, M.E. Comparison of Multisystem Inflammatory Syndrome in Children-Related Myocarditis, Classic Viral Myocarditis, and COVID-19 Vaccine-Related Myocarditis in Children. *J. Am. Heart Assoc.* **2022**, *11*, e024393. [CrossRef] [PubMed]
139. Dionne, A.; Kheir, J.N.; Sleeper, L.A.; Esch, J.J.; Breitbart, R.E. Value of Troponin Testing for Detection of Heart Disease in Previously Healthy Children. *J. Am. Heart Assoc.* **2020**, *9*, e012897. [CrossRef] [PubMed]
140. Belhadjer, Z.; Méot, M.; Bajolle, F.; Khraiche, D.; Legendre, A.; Abakka, S.; Auriau, J.; Grimaud, M.; Oualha, M.; Beghetti, M.; et al. Acute Heart Failure in Multisystem Inflammatory Syndrome in Children in the Context of Global SARS-CoV-2 Pandemic. *Circulation* **2020**, *142*, 429–436. [CrossRef]
141. Alfieri, M.; Munno, C.; Savarese, M.; Pollice, A.; Antignani, A.; Leone, O. Upgrading to a High-Sensitivity Troponin Bedside Assay to Monitor Chemotherapy-Induced Cardiotoxicity in 15 Paediatric Patients. *Ligand Assay* **2022**, *27*, 233.
142. Lv, X.; Pan, C.; Guo, H.; Chang, J.; Gao, X.; Wu, X.; Zhi, X.; Ren, C.; Chen, Q.; Jiang, H.; et al. Early Diagnostic Value of High-Sensitivity Cardiac Troponin T for Cancer Treatment-Related Cardiac Dysfunction: A Meta-Analysis. *ESC Heart Fail.* **2023**, *10*, 2170–2182. [CrossRef]

pharmaceutics

MDPI

Review

Off-Label Prescribing in Pediatric Population—Literature Review for 2012–2022

Valentina Petkova [1,*], Dilyana Georgieva [2], Milen Dimitrov [2] and Irina Nikolova [3]

[1] Department of Social Pharmacy, Faculty of Pharmacy, Medical University of Sofia, 1000 Sofia, Bulgaria
[2] Department of Pharmaceutical Technology, Faculty of Pharmacy, Medical University of Sofia, 1000 Sofia, Bulgaria; dgeorgieva@pharmfac.mu-sofia.bg (D.G.); mdimitrov@pharmfac.mu-sofia.bg (M.D.)
[3] Department of Pharmacology, Pharmacotherapy and Toxicology, Faculty of Pharmacy, Medical University of Sofia, 1000 Sofia, Bulgaria; inikolova@pharmfac.mu-sofia.bg
* Correspondence: vpetkova@pharmfac.mu-sofia.bg

Abstract: Off-label prescribing is widespread among pediatricians, and it is unlikely that this trend will soon be bound by a uniform legal framework. This is necessitated by the fact that there are four variables: the patient's health condition, the physician's experience and knowledge, the legislative measures (laws, directives, guidelines, and recommendations), and finally, the pharmaceutical industry. There is considerable concern worldwide about the use of off-label medicines in children. We may call it an enormous global problem that is much talked about and written about; however, we should not forget that the goal around which everyone should unite is the patient's life. For healthcare providers, the most important thing will always be the health and preservation of the patient's life, particularly when it comes to children with life-threatening conditions in neonatal and pediatric intensive care units (NICU and PICU). The study aimed to examine the prevalence of off-label drug use in pediatrics. Literature research was conducted, and we included studies from 2012 to 2022 that evaluated off-label drug prevalence in various pediatric patient populations.

Keywords: off-label use; children; neonates; pediatrics; safety; prescription; legislation

1. Introduction

Off-label use is very common and generally legal unless it violates ethical guidelines or safety regulations. Often the reason is to respond to patients' medical needs or enable access to innovative medicines, especially when there is no alternative option [1,2]. Compared to the drugs that are authorized for adults, those licensed for pediatric use are comparatively a much smaller fraction. In addition, off-label use of medicines is in general not supported by the same level of evidence as medicines licensed for adults [3]. This may result in increased uncertainty on efficacy as well as the risk for adverse drug reactions (ADRs).

Once a medicinal product is licensed, it is the prescribers who assess the benefit–risk ratio and decide whether that medicinal product should be prescribed. All prescriptions that do not comply with the licensed Summary of Product Characteristics (SmPC), whether indication, age, dose or dosage regime, route of administration, mode of use, etc., fall under 'off-label use' [4]. The SmPC is a legal document, approved by national regulatory agencies, EMA, FDA, TGA, etc., as part of the marketing authorization of each medicine. However, for better or worse, 'off-label' is a real fact, a working phenomenon, despite not completely legitimate, that slowly paved its way into therapeutic regimens, and we already accepted it as a regular practice [5,6].

Medicines regulation controls how medicinal products are marketed, not how they are prescribed [4]. Regulatory approval is a costly and time-consuming process. It is obvious that not every drug will be tested for every eventual indication in its entirety. Thus, the regulation of therapeutic freedom adopts "an anything not explicitly prohibited is permitted" approach and assumes that medicines can be used in ways not specified in the label as long as they are prescribed by a competent professional based on scientific knowledge [4,7]. Healthcare providers are not required to limit prescriptions or recommendations to the indications approved by their country's drug regulatory body. Despite the risk, healthcare professionals often prescribe various medications that do not contain regulatory labels for use in pediatrics. The standard of care for many conditions involves off-label uses. When this process is unavoidable, it should always be guided by a rigorous benefit/risk assessment since healthcare professionals are solely responsible for off-label use [8]. In other words, properly understanding why off-label use is common and "usually appropriate, rather than rare and usually inappropriate", requires understanding [9].

The reason that many medications in children are administered in an off-label manner, is: (1) there are not enough legalized medicines for the pediatric population, and (2) there are not enough pharmaceutical dosage forms suitable for use in children [10]. The existence of many legal restrictions on the conduct of clinical trials in children further leads to a lag in the regulation of medicines for pediatric use, and hence the development of pediatric dosage forms suitable for both parenteral and oral use [11,12].

The current review aims to evaluate the worldwide prevalence frequency of off-label prescriptions in children in the last decade (2012–2022) and to identify the key determinants for the future aspects of enhancing the proper treatment of the pediatric population. The legislative attempts and their role are briefly explored. The current review article identifies and summarizes the existing issues for off-label treatment in the pediatric population and the recent achievements in this area.

2. The Need for Pediatric Drugs

2.1. Features of the Children

Childhood is characterized by periods of rapid growth, maturation, and development. It is widely acknowledged that children constitute a diverse and heterogeneous population, encompassing preterm neonates to post-pubertal adolescents, and are not simply miniature versions of adults [13]. The characteristics of children, in terms of physiology and development, differ from those of adults, and these also differ in the age range from newborn to adolescence [14,15]. The pharmacokinetics (PKs) and pharmacodynamics (PDs) of drugs may be altered by age and development and can be significantly affected by different factors to an extent that is not well studied to date [16,17]. In addition, the age groups of children themselves differ from each other [18].

In neonates, it is particularly difficult to detect small but significant effects as outcome measures are more difficult to assess [15]. Developmental stages can also alter the action and response to a drug. This is true for the desired action and ADRs [19]. Unfortunately, history taught us that different drug effects seen in children can be toxic, as seen with chloramphenicol, valproate, and tetracycline, or enhanced, as seen with some treatments for leukemia [20]. In addition, the natural course of disease in children may differ from that seen in adults, and they may suffer from diseases not common in adults [21]. Understanding the differences in physiology at different stages of development assists with designing drug formulations and dose regimens [22]. Age-related periods in a child's development are defined as neonate/newborn (ages 0–29 days); infant (>28 days–12 months); toddler (>12–23 months); preschool child (2–5 years); school-aged child (6–11 years); and adolescent/teen (12–18 years).

2.2. Drug Formulations for Children

The development of age-appropriate dosage forms and strengths is a major challenge for the pharmaceutical industry [23]. Our knowledge of child-appropriate formulations has many gaps, and the industry faces many challenges in the process of creating appropriate formulations for all age groups [24,25]. The availability of suitable dosage forms is also limited even when the drug is approved for use by children. The complexity comes from the fact that accurate dosing is needed for different age groups [26]. It is unlikely that a single formulation will be appropriate across the pediatric population, necessitating multiple product variants [27]. Pediatric dosage forms must also be adapted to the chemical–pharmaceutical properties of the active substance and excipients, taste masking, the quantity taken, acceptability, and convenience to the patient as well as to caregivers [28]. The excipients used in pediatric formulations need to be appropriate for the age group [29,30] to avoid the consequences of excipient toxicity [31]. All these factors further complicate the manufacturing process.

The oral route of administration remains the most preferred due to its convenience and stability [32]. Recent advances in pharmaceutical technology led to the development of various types of tablets, such as melts [33], chewable and orodispersible tablets, oral lyophilizates and oral films, powders, granules [34], and pellets or sprinkles for reconstitution; however, generally, liquid products are preferred, especially in children under 6 years old [35]. The major barrier in the development of oral liquid formulations is the taste-masking of drugs, a hurdle that can be very costly and may not be totally achievable [36].

Drug acceptability is of great importance for receiving adequate therapy [37]. Pediatric formulations must be appropriate for the child to ensure compliance with the medication [28]. Different pharmaceutical forms may differ in their pharmacokinetic profile, highlighting the risks associated with the use of drugs that are not intended for use in children or were manipulated. The manipulation or extemporaneous preparation of medicines by pharmacists has its risks due to the lack of sufficient data on the quality of the final product [38,39]. Frequently, additional adjustments to medications are made by parents and caregivers to enhance adherence, especially in the pediatric demographic, where 19% of administered medications undergo manipulation [40,41].

Due to the diverse factors that influence the development of pediatric dosage forms, not forgetting the high manufacturing cost, it is lagging in pace compared to the development of adult dosage forms [42].

2.3. Dosing in Children

Drug dosage determination is challenging in children since traditional pharmacokinetic studies are difficult to conduct and are subject to a greater number of ethical considerations [22]. Modifications related to typical growth and development necessitate the use of evidence-based approaches to determine safe and efficient medication doses for children at various developmental stages. Additionally, it is crucial to design suitable delivery systems for these medications. Due to the lack of sufficient studies related to PKs in children, it is still a common practice to calculate pediatric doses from data obtained from the adult population [27]. However, dosage adjustments are often more complex than simply reducing the dose set for adults based on the child's age or weight [43].

The US Food and Drug Administration (FDA) and the European Medicines Agency (EMA) emphasized the absence of pediatric clinical trials and dosing details as critical clinical gaps. There is now a demand for increased pediatric data in the assessment of new drugs [44]. Recently, Shaniv et al. [45] identified eight different neonatal formularies worldwide (Europe, the USA, Australia-New Zealand, Middle East), and six of them were compared. Each formulary varies in style and monograph template, drug information, dosing information, and update routine. Healthcare professionals may retrieve required drug dose details; however, institutions usually give access to only one formulary (if any), thus limiting the amount of essential information. For example, Suwa et al. [46] compared 72 products with pediatric indications in the USA and found that only 83% (60/72) and 43% (32/72) of the products had pediatric indications in the UK and Japan, respectively.

Most pediatric drug dosing is usually based on weight (mg/kg) or body surface area (BSA; mg/cm^2) [47]. Utilizing total body weight (TBW) is a widespread and suitable method for calculating drug doses in children. Nevertheless, it is important to note that pediatric drug dosages cannot be directly standardized from an adult dose based solely on TBW (i.e., 60 kg adult is not equal to 60 kg child) when pediatric dosing data are unavailable [48]. Additionally of note is a very pressing issue in the last 15–20 years about drug dosing in obese children [49]. In obese children, dosing based on body weight and

BSA might result in doses exceeding the maximum recommended for adults. To address this, alternative weight measures, such as ideal body weight (IBW) and adjusted body weight (ABW), were devised to better accommodate these variations. This is because the volume of distribution (Vd) and clearance (Cl) are mostly affected by physiological changes (body mass, extracellular water, tissue perfusion, and proportions of lean and fat tissue) that occur during childhood development [50,51]. Generally, hydrophilic active substances should be dosed on IBW, partly lipophilic on ABW, and lipophilic on TBW [52]. Collectively, the physiological and pharmacokinetic changes in children with obesity may require adjustments to the loading and maintenance dose, dose interval, and time to reach a steady state in certain medications—a severely hampered process when it comes to off-label use [53].

2.4. Conducting Clinical Research with Children

Well-designed controlled clinical trials provide reliable evidence of treatment efficacy through rigorously controlled testing of human interventions. Conducting pediatric trials is challenging due to the heterogeneity of the population and specific ethical issues [54,55]. Ethical concerns about the inclusion of children in clinical trials are disproportionately high, resulting in strict laws and ethical guidelines [56,57]. The safeguarding of children traces back to the Nüremberg code, which permits clinical investigations only in individuals capable of giving informed consent [58], followed by the "Belmont Report" [59], ICH Guideline For GCP [60] and ICH Topic E11 [61], Directive 2001/20/EC, Ref. [62], and others. In the USA, the National Institute of Health (NIH) considers, under a legal framework, the inclusion of children in clinical trials unless there are "scientific or ethical reasons to exclude them". Furthermore, in 1998, the FDA approved a requirement that new drugs intended for use in children entering the market must undergo prior evaluation on "clinical tests in the pediatric population to determine their security, effectiveness and correct dose" [63,64].

In Canada, the revised version of the Tri-Council Policy Statement: Ethical Conduct for Research Involving Humans—TCPS 2 (2022) stipulates that the inclusion of pediatric patients in clinical trials is permissible only when the study's objectives cannot be achieved through alternative means, informed consent is secured from parents or legal representatives, and the research poses no more than minimal risk to the children [65]. Moreover, numerous countries formulated ethical guidelines and regulatory frameworks for conducting clinical research involving children [1].

The number of clinical trials conducted in children is relatively small worldwide [66]. There exist neither mandatory requirements nor enough financial drivers for the development of pediatric medicines. The high development costs and low expected returns of new medicines for children do not usually attract the pharmaceutical industry to invest in this area. Globally, the population of children aged 0 to 14 is declining. For 2022, they comprise 25%, in comparison to 30% and 35% in 2000 and 1980, respectively. In 2022, in the EU, children under 14 years only account for 15% of the total population [67].

A high level of evidence is a prerequisite that seriously limits available drug treatment for children, as the underlying evidence is low across ages and drug classes. In a recent analysis by van der Zanden [68], findings revealed that only 14% of all off-label records (n = 2718) were substantiated by high-quality evidence, with 4% stemming from meta-analyses or systematic reviews and 10% from high-quality randomized controlled trials (RCTs). Furthermore, ethical, harmful, and consent concerns often pose challenges in obtaining institutional review board approval for clinical trials involving children [69]. Some researchers advocate for concurrently conducting phase I/II clinical trials for both adults and children, emphasizing the importance of interim reports from adult trials to inform and enhance clinical studies involving children [70–73]. This approach aims to minimize the time required to gather valuable and valid data on pediatric treatment while safeguarding children from exposure to ineffective and harmful treatments [74]. Consequently, the scientific community bears the responsibility of encouraging clinical trials in children to uncover novel and effective treatments. Viewing pediatric clinical research from a broader perspective, it underscores both the right of children to access efficient, evidence-based treatments and the obligation of health authorities and regulatory agencies to provide high-quality, evidence-based medical care.

3. Legislative and Ethical Measures for Off-Label Restriction

Over the past two decades, changes in drug regulation generated by the FDA and EMA resulted in substantial changes in how new drugs with potential use in children are studied and labeled [75,76]. To achieve child's health protection and to ensure that medications are used ethically, in 2007, the European Union (EU) issued legislation for the development and authorization of pediatric drugs [77,78]. In addition, pharmaceutical companies are required to submit a pediatric investigation plan (PIP) to the EMA's Pediatric Committee (PDCO) for every new medicine unless an exemption (waiver) is granted [79]. Ten years after Pediatric Regulation came into force, a total of 273 new medicines and 43 additional pharmaceutical forms appropriate for use in children were authorized in the EU [80].

Several governmental regulations were established to address off-label use in children. For example, the Pediatric Research Equity Act (PREA) of 2003 mandates pharmaceutical companies to investigate the impacts of new drugs on children when these drugs have the potential for pediatric prescriptions [81]. Studies conducted under PREA are obligatory, while those under the Best Pharmaceuticals for Children Act (BPCA) are voluntary. BPCA incentivizes pharmaceutical companies with an additional six months of patent exclusivity for drugs already on the market if they conduct clinical trials involving children [82]. These regulations not only underscore the importance of obtaining pediatric safety, efficacy, and dosing information but also contribute to the transparency of the drug approval process.

In the United States, once a drug receives approval for a specific purpose, physicians have the liberty to prescribe it for any other purpose they deem safe and effective in their professional judgment, irrespective of official FDA-approved indications [4]. The FDA lacks legal authority to regulate medical practice, allowing physicians to prescribe drugs off-label. Contrary to common belief, the use of drugs off-label is legal in the USA and many other countries. In 2014, the American Academy of Pediatrics issued a statement addressing the off-label use of pharmaceuticals in children [83]. The statement advises pediatricians that "Off-label use is neither incorrect nor investigational if based on sound scientific evidence, expert medical judgment, or published literature". Moreover, the statement advocates for increased support and incentives for clinical testing of drugs in children and the publication of all results, regardless of positive outcomes [83]. Therefore, for doctors to be able to treat their patients safely and avoid experimental treatments, their choices should be based on scientific evidence [84]. This leads to the conclusion that for such evidence to be available, doctors and manufacturers should be incentivized to collect and publish data on off-label use. This would contribute to driving the off-label use process.

In the United Kingdom, physicians are permitted to prescribe medications off-label. In line with guidance from the General Medical Council, the physician must ensure there is ample evidence or experience supporting the medicine's safety and efficacy. Off-label prescribing may be deemed necessary when no appropriately licensed medicine is accessible to address the patient's requirements or when the prescription is part of approved research [85].

In China, a guideline was introduced in 2022 with the aim of aiding the management of pediatricians, pharmacists, medical managers, policymakers, and primary care physicians in handling the off-label use of drugs in pediatric cases. Additionally, the guideline offers recommendations for shaping future healthcare policies [86].

An important ethical issue in this context is determining the responsible party for informing parents or caregivers when a child is prescribed an off-label drug. Occasionally, physicians do not provide this information, while on the other hand, the pharmacist is obligated to give it [87]. Hence, two possibilities follow: (1) the parents are stressed and refuse to give their child a drug with no established efficacy and safety and (2) the parents return to the doctor in search of another alternative drug [88]. In our view, to avoid complications, it is a physician's obligation (evidenced by giving informed consent), later confirmed by the pharmacist.

4. Methods

4.1. Search Strategy for the Prevalence of Off-Label Use

A literature search for the prevalence of off-label drug use was conducted in PubMed, Scopus, ScienceDirect, and Web of Science. Medical subject headings and free text searches were identical in all databases ("off-label use", "prevalence", "pediatric", "children", "neonates", and/or "study"). Identified article titles and abstracts were reviewed, and articles were included if evaluating off-label drug uses, with a clear description of the health care setting and studied population. The duplicates were removed from the identified papers with the help of Zotero software (v6.0.26), and the rest were browsed for relevance. The search strategy, flow diagram, and retrieved articles are presented in Figure 1.

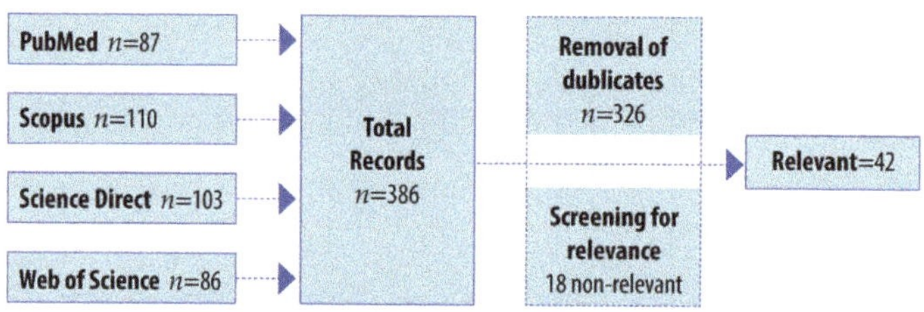

Figure 1. Flow diagram of the search strategy.

Only full-text research articles published in English, between January 2012 and December 2022, and reporting on the prevalence of off-label prescribing in children were included in this review. All papers considered relevant and meeting the selected criteria (n = 42) were original articles discussing the off-label treatment in the pediatric population.

4.2. Inclusion and Exclusion Criteria

Reference lists were searched to identify any relevant articles. Therapeutic and clinical guidelines, conference proceedings, book chapters, therapeutic strategies, and updates, as well as all systematic or other reviews, were excluded.

Two review authors independently conducted the quality assessment of the eligible studies. Owing to disparities in study design, children's age, study duration, and outcome measures, statistical pooling of data was not performed. Instead, a thematic analysis of the included studies was undertaken, involving a meticulous examination and reexamination to identify emerging themes and groupings of similar themes from the articles.

Data extracted included: the country where the study was performed, a clear description of the health care setting, the studied population, the number of patients included in the study, the duration of the study, the number of prescriptions, and off-label drug prescriptions as a percent. The included articles were divided into three age groups: from 0 to 18 years old; from 0 to 15 years old; and neonates. Further, the articles were browsed for the most often off-label prescribed drug groups.

5. Results

5.1. Overall Prevalence of Off-Label Drug Prescribing in Pediatrics

We reviewed published literature from 2012 to 2022 to provide an up-to-date summary of the extent of off-label use in pediatric patients. The proportion of off-label prescriptions in our survey ranged from 3.3% (non-clinical settings; Italy) [89] to 94% (for NICU patients; Ireland) [90]. Comparing our review with some previously published literature, Moulis et al. [91] and Gore et al. [92] reported 7.0–78.7% and 36.3–97.0%, respectively. Magalhães et al. [93] retrieved 34 studies in which off-label prescriptions ranged from

12.2% to 70.6%. Balan et al. [94] reported a more extensive range of off-label prescriptions (i.e., 1.2–99.7%). Experience in several countries showed that despite it being almost impossible to estimate real-world data, especially in outpatients [95], many published retrospective and prospective trials studies estimate a high proportion of off-label pediatric prescribing [6]. As might reasonably be expected, patients treated out-of-hospital are less likely to be prescribed off-label medications [89,96–98]. In a hospital setting, the disease and patient's condition are of primary importance. Oshikoya et al. [99] reported a low rate of off-label prescriptions in the chronic treatment of epilepsy, asthma, and sickle cell anemia, while in the most vulnerable group of NICU patients, the percentage skyrocketed to 94% [90]. Comparative data on the extent of off-label prescribing in children 0 to 18 years in different countries and regions, published in medical literature from 2012 to 2022, are summarized in Table 1.

Table 1. Data on off-label prescribing in children 0 to 18 years by countries.

Country	% Off-Label Prescriptions (Total Prescriptions)	Type of Study (Number of Patients and Age)	Studied Period
Italy [89]	3.3% (4,027,119)	Retrospective (n = 1,708,755 non-clinical setting; 0–18 years)	12 months (January–December 2011)
Finland [100]	71% (1054)	Retrospective (n = 123; inpatients; 0–18 years)	0.5 months (April–May 2011)
Norway [101]	44% (930)	Prospective cross-sectional (n = 400 inpatients; 0–17 years)	6 months (September–October 2013 and (September–December 2014)
Sweden [102]	41% (11 294)	Prospective (n = 2947 inpatients; 0–18 years)	4 days (2 days in May and 2 days in October 2008)
Portugal [96]	28.1% (724)	Retrospective descriptive (n = 700 outpatient; 0–18 years)	12 months (January–October 2010)
Croatia [103]	19.7% (1643)	Prospective (n = 531 inpatients; 0–18 years)	12 months (May 2010–April 2011)
Slovakia [104]	15.7% (267)	Prospective (n = 68 inpatients; 2–18 years)	1 month (February–March 2011)
USA [105]	36% (1090)	Retrospective cohort (n = 82 inpatients; 0–18 years)	3 months (June 2008–August 2008)
Canada [106]	38.2% (2145)	Retrospective cross-sectional (n = 308 inpatients; 0–18 years)	A day (5 March 2014)
Australia [107]	25.7% (2654)	Retrospective (n = 699 ED *, in- and outpatients; 0–18 years)	24 months (January–December 2008)
Australia [108]	30.5% (6786)	Retrospective observational (n = 3343 ED patients; 0–17 years)	12 months (July 2011–June 2012)
Australia [109]	53.9% (1160)	Retrospective cross-sectional study (n = 190 inpatients; 0–18 years)	1 month (June 2013)
Malaysia [110]	34.1% (1295)	Prospective (n = 194 inpatients; 28 days–18 years)	3 months (April–June 2012)
Indonesia [111]	71.5% (1961)	Retrospective cross-sectional (n = 200 inpatients; 1 month–18 years)	3 months (August–October 2014)
Malaysia [112]	35.6% (508)	Prospective (n = 220 outpatients; 1 month–17 years)	6 months (July 2011–December 2011)
Nigeria [99]	7.7% (1746)	Retrospective descriptive (n = 477 inpatients; 0–16 years)	12 months (January–October 2015)

* ED = emergency department.

In the group of studies involving children up to 15 years of age (Table 2), the differences in age and dose are the main reasons for off-label use. It is noteworthy that many drugs were in off-label use for many years [113]. The most often prescribed drugs, as off-label use, are from groups of drugs for the treatment of the respiratory system, anti infectives, nervous system, and alimentary system. Different studies give varying reasons for off-label use, such as dosage/frequency [114,115], age [116], and formulation [117]. All the reported ranges are considerably wide. The prevalence rate of off-label medicine use in Germany, especially for children aged 3 to 6 years, is 48.7% [95]. In 1998, Conroy [118] performed a prospective study of off-label use in five European countries (United Kingdom, Sweden, Germany, Italy, and the Netherlands) and found that off-label prescriptions were 39%. Schaffer, Ref. [119] reported only 12.2% of prescriptions, based on age, to be off-label in Australia.

Table 2. Data on off-label prescribing in children 0 to ≤15 years by countries.

Country	% Off-Label Prescriptions (Total Prescriptions)	Type of Study (Number of Patients and Age)	Studied Period
Czech Republic [97]	9.02% (8559)	Prospective observational (n = 4282 outpatients; 0–15 years)	6 months (January–June 2012)
Slovakia [104]	21% (206)	Prospective (n = 49 inpatients; 0–6 years)	1 month (February–March 2011)
USA [120]	57% (240)	Prospective observational (n = 40 inpatients; 3 weeks–15 years)	4.5 months (November 2011–April 2012)
Brazil [121]	31.7% (731)	Retrospective cross-sectional (n = 705 outpatients; 0–12 years)	5 months (August–December 2012
Brazil [122]	39% (342)	Prospective cross-sectional (n = 342 inpatients; 0–14 years)	3 months (November 2007–January 2008)
Brazil [123]	77.8% (1158)	Prospective (n = 320 inpatients; 2–14 years)	6 months (September 2012–February 2013
Brazil [117]	45% (1328)	Prospective observational (n = 157 inpatients; 1 month–12 years)	A week period Phase 1 (August 2014) Phase 2 (January 2015)
Australia [114]	31.8% (887)	Retrospective (n = 300 inpatients; 0–12 years) Group 1—150 consecutive patients Group 2—150 consecutive patients	2 months Group 1 (1 July 2009–5 August 2009). Group 2 (1 January 2010–22 February 2010)
India [113]	41.25% (1789)	Prospective observational (n = 482 PICU patients; 1 month–12 years)	12 months (April 2012–March 2013)
India [98]	10.1% (405)	Prospective cross-sectional (n = 170 outpatients; 15 days–12 years)	2 months (July 2012–August 2012)
Indonesia [116]	18.6% (4936)	Retrospective population-based (n = 4936 outpatients; 0–5 years)	12 months (January–December 2012)
Pakistan [124]	48.6% (3168)	Prospective, observational (n = 895 inpatients; 1 month–15 years)	12 months (March 2014–February 2015)
Malta [115]	51.7% (209)	Prospective (n = 209 outpatients; 0–14 years)	A month period Phase 1 (September 2006) Phase 2 (January 2007)

5.2. Prevalence of Off-Label Drug Prescribing in Neonates

Generally, neonates receive more prescriptions (mean = 5–7) per patient [117,125,126]. For instance, Langerová et al. [97] reported the lowest rate of off-label use (9.019%; n = 4282 patients) in children 0 to 15 years; however, the data on neonates are 40.9%, just as the other reports for this age group (Table 3).

Table 3. Data on off-label prescribing in neonates by countries.

Country	% Off-Label Prescriptions (Total Prescriptions)	Type of Study (Number of Patients and Age)	Studied Period
Spain [127]	22.5% (564)	A Prospective, observational study (*n* = 84 NICU * patients)	6 months (April–September 2018)
Slovakia [128]	43% (962)	Prospective cross-sectional (*n* = 202 NICU patients)	6 months (April–September 2012)
Portugal [129]	52.7% (1011)	Retrospective cross-sectional study (*n* = 218 NICU patients)	6 months (January–June 2013)
France [130]	59.5% (8891)	Prospective, observational (*n* = 910 NICU patients)	12 months (January–December 2012)
Italy [131]	59% (720)	Prospective (*n* = 220 NICU patients)	1-day survey (May–July 2014)
Ireland [90]	94% (900)	Prospective (*n* = 110 NICU patients)	2 months (February–March 2012)
Brazil [132]	27.7% (318)	Observational cohort study (*n* = 61 NICU patients)	1.5 months (July–August 2011)
Brazil [133]	49.3% (3935)	Prospective cohort study (*n* = 220 NICU patients)	12 months (August 2015–July 2016)
Brazil [134]	79.0% (16,143)	A nonconcurrent, hospital-based cohort study (*n* = 592 NICU preterm patients)	24 months (January 2016–December 2017)
India [135]	50% (568)	Prospective (*n* = 156 NICU patients)	3 months (June–August 2009)
India [136]	12.3% (2642)	Prospective descriptive (*n* = 460 NICU patients)	9 months (July 2014–March 2015)
Pakistan [137]	52.14% (3448)	Prospective, observational (*n* = 1300 inpatients)	12 months (May 2014–April 2015)
Israel [138]	64.8% (1064)	Prospective (*n* = 134 NICU patients)	2 months (December 2015–January 2016)

* NICU = neonatal intensive care unit.

Gore et al. [92], Cuzzolin and Agostino [131], Gonçalves and Heineck [121], and Aamir et al. [137] also reported a higher percentage of off-label prescriptions in pediatric intensive care units (PICU), pediatric medical and surgical wards, and neonatal intensive care units (NICU). In the study of Gore et al. [92], the number of patients studied ranged from 34 in NICU to 355,409 hospitalized children. Gonçalves and Heineck [121] found that 95.5% of newborns were prescribed at least 1 off-label drug, and the studied newborns were admitted to the NICU of a university hospital in Brazil. The condition's severity and the need for intensive care in the NICU may explain the considerable number of prescriptions per patient [121,134]. Lindell-Osuagwu et al. [139] reported that in Finland, the proportion of off-label prescriptions increased from 50% in the 2001 [139] to 71% in 2011 [100]. In Mumbai, India, Chauthankar et al. [136] reported that 38% of neonates received at least one off-label drug, and overall off-label use was 12.3%. Similarly, in Brazil, Carvalho et al. [132] reported 27.7%, while Vieira et al. [134] reported 79% of off-label use. The great difference is not due to the year the study was performed, but rather to the definition of off-label, gestational age, inclusion and exclusion criteria, severity of medical condition, and variety of drugs used. This indicates that both the low and the high percentages may be accepted as valid. In contrast, a study performed in Norway [101] reported no difference between neonates (42%) and total off-label prescriptions (44%; 0–17 years).

An aspect in which we found notable differences between studies is the reason why the drug was used in off-label conditions. Such differences may be due to the definition of off-label use and varying reasons for off-label use (Table 4).

Table 4. Most common reasons for off-label use in the NICU.

Reason for Off-Label Determination	Prevalence of the Reason (%)	Reference
Dosage	25.7–40–52–61.29	[129,136–138]
Indication	13.68–36	[137,138]
Frequency	32	[138]
Age	10.79–15–44.8	[130,137,138]
Route of administration	14	[138]
Combined (more than one reason)	0.11–8.12–15	[136–138]
Contraindication	13.8	[128]

5.3. *Prevalence of Off-Label Drug Prescribing by Drug Groups*

Prevalence of off-label prescribing also varies widely with the class of drugs: off-label use was highest among anti-infectives [99,106,108,111,114,116,122,126,128–130,134–136,138], CNS drug group [99,102,106,108,109,111,114,122,126,133–136], respiratory [104,107,108,111, 112,115,121,122,133], alimentary tract medicines [103,104,106–108,111,122,126,128,134], and cardiovascular medications [107,113,119,126,133,134]. This order was also observed in other studies [89,91,96,140–142], while the lowest off-label use was noted in antidiabetic drugs [143].

Four of the studies reported the dose, age, and indication as major contributors to off-label prescribing [99,106,111,112]. It is not possible to isolate individual, most commonly prescribed off-label medications, as studies vary widely from one another. Most recently, Oishi et al. [144] reported a surprisingly high (18.8%) level of off-label prescriptions of asthma inhalers in pediatric patients aged 0–14 years in Japan. Despite the fact that Carnovale et al. [89] reported that 12.8% of off-label prescriptions are contraindicated drugs, any of the above-mentioned drug classes have well-established use in protocols, clinical trials, and meta-analyses, but were not investigated in controlled clinical trials that meet regulatory agency's criteria [132].

Different studies give varying reasons for off-label use, such as dosage/frequency [114,115], age [116], and formulation [117]. Likewise, in some studies [106,108], the existence of published scientific evidence was analyzed as well. Smeets et al. [145] described that only 14% of all off-label records (n = 2718) were supported by high-quality evidence based on randomized clinical trials. This indicates that data should be presented by age-related periods in a child's development, from neonates to adolescents, rather than overall, as well as those inpatients, ED patients, and outpatients must be considered separately. The benefit of these reviews is that it can be noted that most off-label prescriptions were prescribed in neonates/infants, and especially in emergency settings [146], which is most likely due to the extreme vulnerability of this group of patients and the lack of clinical studies, including pharmacokinetic studies. These findings are supported by an EU report [79] and corroborated by systematic reviews by Balan et al. [147] and Allen et al. [6]. By providing fresh insights into the practice of off-label drug prescribing, these findings aim to contribute to the generation of novel and more effective knowledge, addressing the demand for high-quality drugs that are both safe and efficacious in the pediatric population.

In NICU, the most often off-label prescribed drug groups were anti-infectives (such as amikacin, gentamicin, vancomycin, meropenem, cefepime, and cefazoline), followed by drugs acting on the nervous system, the respiratory system, gastrointestinal system, and cardiovascular agents in [128–136,138].

A comparison between included studies, regarding the most commonly off-label prescribed active principles and the reason for it, was not performed in our study, due to the sheer variety of drugs used and polypharmacy, especially where NICU or PICU are concerned, different study periods, and the broad definition of off-label use, i.e., anything beyond the official approved SmPC (mode of use, age group, indication, dose and dosage regime, route of administration, contraindications, and precautions/warnings). The main variations in the studies are due to: (1) the broad definition of off-label use, which includes all the information in the SmPC, such as dose and dose regimen, including lower or higher dose, patient age and weight, route of administration, indications, and precautions and contraindications [104,111,148]; (2) the drug information included in the SmPC of the specific product or other products with the same active ingredient, as well as the use of databases and formularies (national and international) when looking for product information; (3) the patient's condition (acute or chronic), as well as the duration of the disease; (4) the physician's experience and the availability of national therapeutic recommendations for the disease; (5) the season in which the study was conducted; and (6) inpatient or ambulatory treatment. All these factors are equal in severity.

6. Discussion

In a recent collaborative position statement, the European Academy of Pediatrics and the European Society for Developmental Perinatal and Pediatric Pharmacology recommend considering off-label prescribing for children as rational and clinically appropriate, provided that the benefits outweigh the risks [149,150]. However, there is a lack of specific guidance on how to evaluate the benefits and risks of off-label use. The application of the Grading of Recommendations Assessment, Development, and Evaluation (GRADE) methodology [151], commonly used in evidence-based medicine for assessing the benefits and risks of an intervention, has limitations in this context. Crucial areas that are not adequately addressed include appropriate dose selection, evaluation of the availability of suitable drug formulations, and considerations of safety [152,153]. Special emphasis on dose selection is crucial, as detailed in Section 2, considering that age-specific alterations in pharmacokinetics (PKs) and pharmacodynamics (PDs) could significantly influence the required dose to achieve the target exposure [50,154]. In addressing the inherent challenges of off-label prescribing in children, a practical framework named Benefit and Risk Assessment for Off-label Use (BRAvO) was introduced in 2021 for healthcare professionals and guideline working groups. This framework provides guidance on whether and how to conduct a benefit–risk analysis for off-label pediatric prescribing, encompassing dose selection to ultimately enhance both drug efficacy and safety [150]. The conclusions regarding the balance and acceptance of benefits and risks are, therefore, subject to the judgment of healthcare professionals. While a standardized scoring system could objectify the assessment outcome, it may also compromise ease of use. The framework, by ensuring a structured and documented approach, promotes transparency and verifiability in the decision-making process. Additionally, it is crucial to recognize that a benefit–risk assessment is an ongoing and dynamic process. As new insights surface, the equilibrium between benefits and risks may undergo significant shifts, potentially leading to different conclusions [150]. Moreover, drug information is continually evolving with the emergence of new formulations as technology advances. This dynamic nature means that studies published at different times might have varying definitions of off-label prescription, even for the same drug.

Over the past two decades, there were significant advances in policy and legislation that support the development of medicines used from neonates to adolescents [155–157]. Since the introduction of the US and European legislation, we witnessed the most substantial advances in pediatric drug development, resulting in the incorporation of pediatric use labeling information in almost 700 product labels [158,159]. The Pediatric Regulation was enacted in the European Union (EU) on 26 January 2007, with the primary goal of enhancing the health of children in Europe by simplifying the development and accessibility of medicines for individuals aged 0 to 17 years. In October 2017, the European Commission released a comprehensive ten-year report on the implementation of the Pediatric Regulation [160]. The report indicates a notable increase in the availability of medicines for children across various therapeutic areas over the past decade, particularly in rheumatology and infectious diseases. However, it also highlights limited progress in conditions exclusively affecting children or those exhibiting biological distinctions between adults and children, especially in the case of rare diseases. Subsequently, the European Commission, along with the European Medicines Agency (EMA) and its Pediatric Committee (PDCO), devised an action plan to enhance the implementation of the Regulation [161].

The longstanding use of off-label medications in children is a common global phenomenon and remains a concern, persisting despite heightened awareness and enacted legislation. It is noteworthy that many drugs were in off-label use for many years [113]. A typical example is paracetamol, which is often mentioned as off-label use [96,102,109,111, 118,122,124,127,129,132,136,137], despite it being on the market for nearly 70 years. The lack of pediatric information or if it is insufficient or unclear in the SmPCs emerges as one of the main factors for classifying a drug as off-label in many cases. Our literature review demonstrates that off-label use of medications in pediatric patients is a common practice accounting for inpatients and outpatients. We evaluated the problems and achievements in the off-label treatment of children. A wide range of results were detected between studies. The number of products identified varies greatly between the studies, depending on the country, the studied period (from one day [106] to two years [134]), and the number and kind of units included. Such difference may be due to the inequalities in drug therapies dependent on geographic areas and updates in SmPC. This may lead to some of the off-label uses being considered as such, because despite the experience with a drug, it is introduced in the clinical guidelines but not in the drug's SmPC. Hence, off-label use could be associated with increased safety concerns, and under or overdosing due to insufficient or unclear information for use in children [92,162,163]. Despite various international regulatory initiatives and achievements over the past 20 years, many challenges remain in the development and evaluation of the safety and efficacy of pediatric medicines [164]. The review showed the complexity of the matter. More age-specific research is needed to provide adequate drug safety and efficacy for children. Until more data are provided, clinical decision-making should be guided by the best available scientific evidence and closely monitored while authorities, academics, and manufacturers collaborate to foster trials and authorize adequate drugs for this population. Therefore, we agree with Yamashiro et al. [165], van der Zanden et al., [150], and Kaguelidou et al. [164] that the most important thing is the compliance with the off-label prescription algorithm and the creation of a professional network of off-label prescriptions and their implications so that healthcare providers have a foundation to stand on when deciding whether to prescribe an off-label drug or not.

The problem of pediatric clinical trials existed for many years. Although there were great achievements in the last two decades, clinical trials in children will always lag behind those in adults because of the enormous diversity and specificity of this category of patients [164]. Off-label use in pediatrics is ubiquitous and primarily based on physicians' experience, collaboration, knowledge, and existing published scientific literature.

The key determinants and interactions between the patient's state of health, the doctor's knowledge and experience, legislative measures, and the influence of the pharmaceutical industry on the prescription of off-label drugs in pediatrics are, first of all, the different age groups in children, characterized by their anatomical, morphological, and the psychological condition, that makes the creation of medicines for children a great challenge for the industry. Secondly, it is evidence-based medicine, which allows the medical practitioners, based on their experience, to prescribe a drug that is not intended, but which they are afraid to promote because of the risk of a possible error. The next determinant is the various legislative measures and initiatives around the world that seek to facilitate children's access to medicines, but which are not uniform, which in turn leads to confusion in an industry characterized by globalization rather than segmentation, and this versatility leads to choosing the easiest step—avoiding development of medicines for children. Conversely, variations in regulatory criteria among national agencies can contribute to the prevalence of off-label prescriptions. Overly stringent criteria may result in reduced access to medications [166]. Given the prevalence of off-label drug use, the cooperation of health and regulatory authorities on one hand, and the pharmaceutical industry on the other side, is integral to instituting individual measures to provide safe and comprehensive pharmacotherapy for pediatric patients. Enforcement of legislation in the drug development process, along with subsequent pharmacovigilance, has the potential to enhance the quality of information and increase accountability within the pharmaceutical industry. This, in turn, could aid and streamline drug research in children [92]. Where it is common and evidence-based, the marketing authorization holder and the relevant regulatory authorities should have a shared responsibility to take appropriate measures to address legal uncertainties and safety concerns, including updating the SmPC. Health authorities and health insurance should support and thus reimburse therapeutic practices that are evidence-based or recommended by a respected and responsible professional body, regardless of labeling status. Legislation should be enacted to effectively encourage research into off-label medicines and facilitate the registration of off-label uses with a favorable balance between benefits and harms [149].

To summarize, the evidence, as shown in our study, is that different countries have different extents of off-label prescriptions (from 3.3% for non-clinical settings to 94% for NICU patients). A major problem arises that depending on the clinical setting and the region, different drugs may be prioritized for various periods, which is especially certain for antibiotics. The lack of pediatric information or if it is insufficient or unclear in the SmPC emerges as one of the main factors for classifying a drug as off-label in many of the cases. We posit that the considerable variability in the observed ranges stems from significant heterogeneity among the studies under review, likely attributed to differences in methodology and the diverse patient populations studied (ranging from general ward to ICU patients). The varying perspectives among prescribers, influenced by their experience and the availability of drugs in their local contexts, could also contribute to this heterogeneity. Notably, ICU patients, being generally more unwell, may receive a higher volume of prescriptions compared to patients in general wards. Additionally, hospitalized patients present a spectrum of diagnoses, leading to diverse drug prescriptions with variations in frequencies, formulations, dosages, and routes of administration. Because significantly more off-label medicines are prescribed at NICU and PICU, it is of paramount importance to provide the best possible information to prescribers on the appropriate use of medicines for children, especially concerning age and dose.

7. Conclusions

7.1. Achievements

In conclusion, though much progress in pediatric drug development was made over the past several years, further efforts are necessary to improve the availability of pediatric medications. Unless there is an increase in the availability of sufficient pediatric clinical trials and licensed drugs, the practice of off-label drug prescriptions should not be discouraged, but rather encouraged in a systematic manner. Our review offers recommendations for expanding scientific knowledge and understanding of the off-label use. The results are not directly comparable but provide valuable information on the issue. To allow results comparability, the need to unify the presentation of clinical studies on the prevalence of off-label use in pediatrics is highlighted. Equally, prescribers should (1) refer to authorized drug databases/formularies or drug information in the Summary of Product Characteristics (SmPC) before prescribing; (2) contemplate prescribing an off-label drug only when essential, following discussions with the patients' parents or caregivers regarding associated risks and benefits; (3) inform the parents or caregivers and sign a consent form; and (4) closely monitor the patient, taking necessary steps to address adverse reactions following an off-label drug prescription, and ensure proper documentation while submitting the report to the country's drug authority. In our opinion, off-label use should be accepted as an already established practice, but on the assumption that it is based on evidence-based medicine, especially when it comes to old medicines that are of particular importance for young patients.

7.2. Limitations

Our study had several limitations. We do not distinguish between in- and outpatients, age groups, and active principles used because of the vast divergencies (study design methodologies, terms of participants, and different study periods) between reviewed studies. We do not comment on the most often used medicines as well as the consequences of off-label prescriptions, as the present paper is a narrative review of the literature on the prevalence of off-label drug use in children for the period of 2012 to 2022.

Author Contributions: Conceptualization, V.P. methodology, I.N. and M.D. investigation, V.P., M.D., I.N. and D.G. writing—original draft preparation, M.D.; writing—review and editing, M.D. and D.G. visualization, V.P. and M.D. supervision, V.P. project administration. All authors have read and agreed to the published version of the manuscript.

Funding: The authors would like to acknowledge the financial support by the European Union-NextGenerationEU, through the National Recovery and Resilience Plan of the Republic of Bulgaria, project › BG-RRP-2.004-0004-C01.

Institutional Review Board Statement: Not applicable.

Informed Consent Statement: Not applicable.

Data Availability Statement: Not applicable.

Conflicts of Interest: The authors declare no conflict of interest.

References

1. Rusz, C.-M.; Ősz, B.-E.; Jîtcă, G.; Miklos, A.; Bătrînu, M.-G.; Imre, S. Off-Label Medication: From a Simple Concept to Complex Practical Aspects. *Int. J. Environ. Res. Public Health* **2021**, *18*, 10447. [CrossRef]
2. Wu, H.; Wu, G. Strategy to address innovative off-label medication use in China: Grading management. *Eur. J. Clin. Pharmacol.* **2014**, *70*, 1271–1273. [CrossRef]
3. Kaley, V.R.; Aregullin, E.O.; Samuel, B.P.; Vettukattil, J.J. Trends in the off-label use of β-blockers in pediatric patients. *Pediatr. Int.* **2019**, *61*, 1071–1080. [CrossRef]
4. Aronson, J.K.; Ferner, R.E. Unlicensed and off-label uses of medicines: Definitions and clarification of terminology. *Br. J. Clin. Pharmacol.* **2017**, *83*, 2615–2625. [CrossRef]
5. Oni, L.; Hawcutt, D.; Turner, M.; Beresford, M.; McWilliam, S.; Barton, C.; Park, B.; Murray, P.; Wilm, B.; Copple, I.; et al. Optimising the use of medicines to reduce acute kidney injury in children and babies. *Pharmacol. Ther.* **2017**, *174*, 55–62. [CrossRef]
6. Allen, H.C.; Garbe, M.C.; Lees, J.; Aziz, N.; Chaaban, H.; Miller, J.L.; Johnson, P.; DeLeon, S. Off-Label Medication use in Children, More Common than We Think: A Systematic Review of the Literature. *J. Okla. State Med. Assoc.* **2018**, *111*, 776–783.
7. Zhang, L.L.; Li, Y.P.; Linan, Z.; Iang, Y.; Hu, D.; Liu, Y.; Lv, J. Evidence-based evaluation on off-label drug use policies in 15 countries. Chin. *J. Evid.-Based Med.* **2012**, *12*, 426–435.
8. Nardini, C. The ethics of clinical trials. *Ecancermedicalscience* **2014**, *8*, 387. [CrossRef]
9. Seale, J.P. Off-label prescribing. *Med. J. Aust.* **2014**, *200*, 65. [CrossRef]
10. Khan, D.; Kirby, D.; Bryson, S.; Shah, M.; Mohammed, A.R. Paediatric specific dosage forms: Patient and formulation considerations. *Int. J. Pharm.* **2022**, *616*, 121501. [CrossRef]
11. Lenk, C. Off-label drug use in paediatrics: A world-wide problem. *Curr. Drug Targets* **2012**, *13*, 878–884. [CrossRef]
12. McCune, S.; Portman, R.J. Accelerating Pediatric Drug Development: A 2022 Special Issue of Therapeutic Innovation & Regulatory Science. *Ther. Innov. Regul. Sci.* **2022**, *56*, 869–872. [CrossRef]
13. Klassen, T.P.; Hartling, L.; Craig, J.C.; Offringa, M. Children Are Not Just Small Adults: The Urgent Need for High-Quality Trial Evidence in Children. *PLOS Med.* **2008**, *5*, e172. [CrossRef]
14. Martinez-Castaldi, C.; Silverstein, M.; Bauchner, H. Child Versus Adult Research: The Gap in High-Quality Study Design. *Pediatrics* **2008**, *122*, 52–57. [CrossRef]
15. Allegaert, K.; Anker, J.v.D. Neonates are not just little children and need more finesse in dosing of antibiotics. *Acta Clin. Belg.* **2019**, *74*, 157–163. [CrossRef]
16. Batchelor, H.K.; Marriott, J.F. Paediatric pharmacokinetics: Key considerations. *Br. J. Clin. Pharmacol.* **2015**, *79*, 395–404. [CrossRef]
17. Ku, L.C.; Smith, P.B. Dosing in neonates: Special considerations in physiology and trial design. *Pediatr. Res.* **2015**, *77*, 2–9. [CrossRef]
18. Mulugeta, Y.; Barrett, J.S.; Nelson, R.; Eshete, A.T.; Mushtaq, A.; Yao, L.; Glasgow, N.; Mulberg, A.E.; Gonzalez, D.; Green, D.; et al. Exposure Matching for Extrapolation of Efficacy in Pediatric Drug Development. *J. Clin. Pharmacol.* **2016**, *56*, 1326–1334. [CrossRef]

19. Jimenez, R.; Smith, A.; Carleton, B. New Ways of Detecting ADRs in Neonates and Children. *Curr. Pharm. Des.* **2015**, *21*, 5643–5649. [CrossRef]
20. Stephenson, T. How children's responses to drugs differ from adults. *Br. J. Clin. Pharmacol.* **2005**, *59*, 670–673. [CrossRef]
21. Raymond, A.S.; Brasseur, D. Development of medicines for children in Europe: Ethical implications. *Paediatr. Respir. Rev.* **2005**, *6*, 45–51. [CrossRef]
22. O'Hara, K. Paediatric pharmacokinetics and drug doses. *Aust. Prescr.* **2016**, *39*, 208–210. [CrossRef]
23. Milne, C.-P.; Bruss, J.B. The economics of pediatric formulation development for off-patent drugs. *Clin. Ther.* **2008**, *30*, 2133–2145. [CrossRef]
24. Ogbonna, J.D.N.; Cunha, E.; Attama, A.A.; Ofokansi, K.C.; Ferreira, H.; Pinto, S.; Gomes, J.; Marx, M.G.; Peres, A.M.; Lobo, J.M.S.; et al. Overcoming Challenges in Pediatric Formulation with a Patient-Centric Design Approach: A Proof-of-Concept Study on the Design of an Oral Solution of a Bitter Drug. *Pharmaceuticals* **2022**, *15*, 1331. [CrossRef]
25. Nunn, T.; Williams, J. Formulation of medicines for children. *Br. J. Clin. Pharmacol.* **2005**, *59*, 674–676. [CrossRef]
26. Duncan, J.C.; Bracken, L.E.; Nunn, A.J.; Peak, M.; Turner, M.A. Development and evaluation of an assessment of the age-appropriateness/inappropriateness of formulations used in children. *Int. J. Clin. Pharm.* **2022**, *44*, 1394–1405. [CrossRef]
27. Batchelor, H.K.; Marriott, J.F. Formulations for children: Problems and solutions. *Br. J. Clin. Pharmacol.* **2015**, *79*, 405–418. [CrossRef]
28. Ranmal, S.R.; Cram, A.; Tuleu, C. Age-appropriate and acceptable paediatric dosage forms: Insights into end-user perceptions, preferences and practices from the Children's Acceptability of Oral Formulations (CALF) Study. *Int. J. Pharm.* **2016**, *514*, 296–307. [CrossRef]
29. Souza, A.; Santos, D.; Fonseca, S.; Medeiros, M.; Batista, L.; Turner, M.; Coelho, H. Toxic excipients in medications for neonates in Brazil. *Eur. J. Pediatr.* **2014**, *173*, 935–945. [CrossRef]
30. Fabiano, V.; Mameli, C.; Zuccotti, G.V. Paediatric pharmacology: Remember the excipients. *Pharmacol. Res.* **2011**, *63*, 362–365. [CrossRef]
31. Saito, J.; Agrawal, A.; Patravale, V.; Pandya, A.; Orubu, S.; Zhao, M.; Andrews, G.P.; Petit-Turcotte, C.; Landry, H.; Croker, A.; et al. The Current States, Challenges, Ongoing Efforts, and Future Perspectives of Pharmaceutical Excipients in Pediatric Patients in Each Country and Region. *Children* **2022**, *9*, 453. [CrossRef]
32. Alessandrini, E.; Brako, F.; Scarpa, M.; Lupo, M.; Bonifazi, D.; Pignataro, V.; Cavallo, M.; Cullufe, O.; Enache, C.; Nafria, B.; et al. Children's Preferences for Oral Dosage Forms and Their Involvement in Formulation Research via EPTRI (European Paediatric Translational Research Infrastructure). *Pharmaceutics* **2021**, *13*, 730. [CrossRef]
33. Li, J.; Li, C.; Zhang, H.; Gao, X.; Wang, T.; Wang, Z.; Zheng, A. Preparation of Azithromycin Amorphous Solid Dispersion by Hot-Melt Extrusion: An Advantageous Technology with Taste Masking and Solubilization Effects. *Polymers* **2022**, *14*, 495. [CrossRef]
34. Huynh, D.T.M.; Hai, H.T.; Hau, N.M.; Lan, H.K.; Vinh, T.P.; De Tran, V.; Pham, D.T. Preparations and characterizations of effervescent granules containing azithromycin solid dispersion for children and elder: Solubility enhancement, taste-masking, and digestive acidic protection. *Heliyon* **2023**, *9*, e16592. [CrossRef]
35. Cornilă, A.; Iurian, S.; Tomuță, I.; Porfire, A. Orally Dispersible Dosage Forms for Paediatric Use: Current Knowledge and Development of Nanostructure-Based Formulations. *Pharmaceutics* **2022**, *14*, 1621. [CrossRef]
36. Van Riet-Nales, D.A.; Kozarewicz, P.; Aylward, B.; de Vries, R.; Egberts, T.C.G.; Rademaker, C.M.A.; Schobben, A.F.A.M. Paediatric Drug Development and Formulation Design—A European Perspective. *AAPS Pharmscitech.* **2017**, *18*, 241–249. [CrossRef]
37. Baguley, D.; Lim, E.; Bevan, A.; Pallet, A.; Faust, S.N. Prescribing for children—Taste and palatability affect adherence to antibiotics: A review. *Arch. Dis. Child.* **2012**, *97*, 293–297. [CrossRef]
38. Yuliani, S.H.; Putri, D.C.A.; Virginia, D.M.; Gani, M.R.; Riswanto, F.D.O. Prevalence, Risk, and Challenges of Extemporaneous Preparation for Pediatric Patients in Developing Nations: A Review. *Pharmaceutics* **2023**, *15*, 840. [CrossRef]
39. MacArthur, R.B.; Ashworth, L.D.; Zhan, K.; Parrish, R.H., 2nd. How Compounding Pharmacies Fill Critical Gaps in Pediatric Drug Development Processes: Suggested Regulatory Changes to Meet Future Challenges. *Children* **2022**, *9*, 1885. [CrossRef]
40. Mennella, J.A.; Spector, A.C.; Reed, D.R.; Coldwell, S.E. The bad taste of medicines: Overview of basic research on bitter taste. *Clin. Ther.* **2013**, *35*, 1225–1246. [CrossRef]
41. Smith, L.; Leggett, C.; Borg, C. Administration of medicines to children: A practical guide. *Aust. Prescr.* **2022**, *45*, 188–192. [CrossRef]
42. Vieira, I.; Sousa, J.J.; Vitorino, C. Paediatric Medicines—Regulatory Drivers, Restraints, Opportunities and Challenges. *J. Pharm. Sci.* **2021**, *110*, 1545–1556. [CrossRef]
43. Kearns, G.L.; Abdel-Rahman, S.M.; Alander, S.W.; Blowey, D.L.; Leeder, J.S.; Kauffman, R.E. Developmental Pharmacology—Drug Disposition, Action, and Therapy in Infants and Children. *N. Engl. J. Med.* **2003**, *349*, 1157–1167. [CrossRef]
44. Rahimzadeh, V.; Wolfert, S.; Buenger, V.; Campbell, C.; French, R.; Ludwinski, D.; Weinstein, A.; Barrett, C. A systematic literature review to identify ethical, legal, and social responsibilities of nonprofit organizations when funding clinical trials in pediatric cancer. *Pediatr. Blood Cancer* **2022**, *69*, e29854. [CrossRef]
45. Shaniv, D.; Bolisetty, S.; Young, T.E.; Mangum, B.; Ainsworth, S.; Elbers, L.; Schultz, P.; Cucchi, M.; de Wildt, S.N.; van der Zanden, T.M.; et al. Neonatal Drug Formularies—A Global Scope. *Children* **2023**, *10*, 848. [CrossRef]

46. Suwa, M.; Miyake, S.; Urushihara, H. Comparison of Regulations and Status of Promoting Drug Development and Authorization of Pediatric Indications among Japan, the United States and the United Kingdom. *Rinsho yakuri/Jpn. J. Clin. Pharmacol. Ther.* **2022**, *53*, 225–234. [CrossRef]
47. Le, J.; Bradley, J.S. Optimizing Antibiotic Drug Therapy in Pediatrics: Current State and Future Needs. *J. Clin. Pharmacol.* **2018**, *58* (Suppl. 10), S108–S122. [CrossRef]
48. Mahmood, I. A comparison of different methods for the first-in-pediatric dose selection. *J. Clin. Translat. Res.* **2022**, *8*, 369–381.
49. Gaeta, F.; Conti, V.; Pepe, A.; Vajro, P.; Filippelli, A.; Mandato, C. Drug dosing in children with obesity: A narrative updated review. *Ital. J. Pediatr.* **2022**, *48*, 168. [CrossRef]
50. van den Anker, J.; Reed, M.D.; Allegaert, K.; Kearns, G.L. Developmental Changes in Pharmacokinetics and Pharmacodynamics. *J. Clin. Pharmacol.* **2018**, *58* (Suppl. 10), S10–S25. [CrossRef]
51. Anderson, B.J.; Holford, N.H.G. Understanding dosing: Children are small adults, neonates are immature children. *Arch. Dis. Child.* **2013**, *98*, 737–744. [CrossRef]
52. Roy, H.; Bertoldi, C.; Farrell, C.; Rousseau, E. Prescribing drugs to overweight and obese children: Balancing efficacy and safety. *Paediatr. Child Health* **2021**, *26*, e236–e239. [CrossRef]
53. Kendrick, J.G.; Carr, R.R.; Ensom, M.H. Pediatric Obesity: Pharmacokinetics and Implications for Drug Dosing. *Clin. Ther.* **2015**, *37*, 1897–1923. [CrossRef]
54. Joseph, P.D.; Craig, J.C.; Caldwell, P.H. Clinical trials in children. *Br. J. Clin. Pharmacol.* **2015**, *79*, 357–369. [CrossRef]
55. Pawar, G.; Wu, F.; Zhao, L.; Fang, L.; Burckart, G.J.; Feng, K.; Mousa, Y.M.; Naumann, F.; Batchelor, H.K. Development of a Pediatric Relative Bioavailability/Bioequivalence Database and Identification of Putative Risk Factors Associated with Evaluation of Pediatric Oral Products. *AAPS J.* **2021**, *23*, 57. [CrossRef]
56. Matsui, K.; Ibuki, T.; Tashiro, S.; Nakamura, H.; Study Group on Regulatory Science for Early Clinical Application of Pediatric Pharmaceuticals. Principles of ethical consideration required for clinical research involving children. *Pediatr. Int.* **2021**, *63*, 248–259. [CrossRef]
57. Krishna, S.; Fuloria, M. Ethical Considerations in Neonatal Research. *NeoReviews* **2022**, *23*, e151–e158. [CrossRef]
58. Declaration of Helsinki. Ethical Principles for Medical Research Involving Human Subjects. Available online: https://www.wma.net/policies-post/wma-declaration-of-helsinki-ethical-principles-for-medical-research-involving-human-subjects (accessed on 30 July 2023).
59. The Belmont Report: Ethical Principles and Guidelines for the Protection of Human Subject of Research. Available online: https://www.hhs.gov/ohrp/sites/default/files/the-belmont-report-508c_FINAL.pdf (accessed on 24 August 2023).
60. Guideline for Good Clinical Practice E6(R2). Available online: https://www.ema.europa.eu/en/documents/scientific-guideline/ich-guideline-good-clinical-practice-e6r2-step-5_en.pdf (accessed on 25 August 2023).
61. ICH Topic E11. Clinical Investigation of Medicinal Products in the Paediatric Population. CPMP/ICH/2711/99. Available online: https://www.ema.europa.eu/en/documents/scientific-guideline/e-11-clinical-investigation-medicinal-products-paediatric-population-step-5_en.pdf (accessed on 5 August 2023).
62. Directive 2001/20/EC of the European Parliament and the Council on the Approximation of the Laws, Regulations and Administrative Provisions of the Member States Relating to Implementation of Good Clinical Practice-GCP-In the Conduct of Clinical Trials on Medicinal Products for Human Use. Available online: https://health.ec.europa.eu/system/files/2016-11/dir_2001_20_en_0.pdf (accessed on 12 August 2023).
63. Code for Federal Regulations (CFR), Title 45, Part 46, Subpart D. Additional Protections for Children Involved as Subjects in Research. Available online: https://www.ecfr.gov/current/title-45/subtitle-A/subchapter-A/part-46/subpart-D (accessed on 15 August 2023).
64. NHI Policy and Guidelines on the Inclusion of Children as Participants in Research Involving Human Subjects. March 1998. Available online: https://grants.nih.gov/grants/guide/notice-files/not98-024.html (accessed on 15 August 2023).
65. Tri-Council Policy Statement: Ethical Conduct for Research Involving Humans—TCPS 2. 2022. Available online: https://ethics.gc.ca/eng/documents/tcps2-2022-en.pdf (accessed on 21 August 2023).
66. Thompson, G.; Barker, C.I.; Folgori, L.; Bielicki, J.A.; Bradley, J.S.; Lutsar, I.; Sharland, M. Global shortage of neonatal and paediatric antibiotic trials: Rapid review. *BMJ Open* **2017**, *7*, e016293. [CrossRef]
67. The World Bank. Population Ages 0–14 (% of Total Population). Available online: https://data.worldbank.org/indicator/SP.POP.0014.TO.ZS (accessed on 25 August 2023).
68. van der Zanden, T.M.; Smeets, N.J.; de Hoop-Sommen, M.; Schwerzel, M.F.; Huang, H.J.; Barten, L.J.; van der Heijden, J.E.; Freriksen, J.J.; Horstink, A.A.; Holsappel, I.H.; et al. Off-Label, but on-Evidence? A Review of the Level of Evidence for Pediatric Pharmacotherapy. *Clin. Pharmacol. Ther.* **2022**, *112*, 1243–1253. [CrossRef]
69. Fung, A.; Yue, X.; Wigle, P.R.; Guo, J.J. Off-label medication use in rare pediatric diseases in the United States. *Intractable Rare Dis. Res.* **2021**, *10*, 238–245. [CrossRef]
70. Lagler, F.B.; Hirschfeld, S.; Kindblom, J.M. Challenges in clinical trials for children and young people. *Arch. Dis. Child.* **2021**, *106*, 321–325. [CrossRef]
71. Tsukamoto, K.; Carroll, K.A.; Onishi, T.; Matsumaru, N.; Brasseur, D.; Nakamura, H. Improvement of Pediatric Drug Development: Regulatory and Practical Frameworks. *Clin. Ther.* **2016**, *38*, 574–581. [CrossRef]

72. Song, L.; Jia, Y.; Ran, S.; Li, B.; Xu, J.; Huo, B.; Yin, N.; Ai, M.; Liu, Y. Current situation of pediatric clinical trials in China: Focus on trials for drug marketing application and administrative approval. *BMC Pediatr.* **2022**, *22*, 144. [CrossRef]
73. Siapkara, A.; Fracasso, C.; Egger, G.F.; Rizzari, C.; Trasorras, C.S.; Athanasiou, D.; Turner, M.A.; Working Group Membership. Recommendations by the European Network of Paediatric Research at the European Medicines Agency (Enpr-EMA) Working Group on preparedness of clinical trials about paediatric medicines process. *Arch. Dis. Child.* **2021**, *106*, 1149–1154. [CrossRef]
74. Subramanian, D.; Cruz, C.V.; Garcia-Bournissen, F. Systematic Review of Early Phase Pediatric Clinical Pharmacology Trials. *J. Pediatr. Pharmacol. Ther.* **2022**, *27*, 609–617. [CrossRef]
75. Moore-Hepburn, C.; Rieder, M. Paediatric pharmacotherapy and drug regulation: Moving past the therapeutic orphan. *Br. J. Clin. Pharmacol.* **2022**, *88*, 4250–4257. [CrossRef]
76. Guidi, B.; Parziale, A.; Nocco, L.; Maiese, A.; La Russa, R.; Di Paolo, M.; Turillazzi, E. Regulating pediatric off-label uses of medicines in the EU and USA: Challenges and potential solutions: Comparative regulation framework of off label prescriptions in pediatrics: A review. *Int. J. Clin. Pharm.* **2021**, *44*, 264–269. [CrossRef]
77. Carvalho, M.L. Challenges on off label medicine use. *Rev. Paul. Pediatr.* **2016**, *34*, 1–2. [CrossRef]
78. Regulation (EC) No. 1901/2006 of the European Parliament and of the Council of 12 December 2006 on Medicinal Products for Paediatric Use. Available online: https://eur-lex.europa.eu/legal-content/EN/TXT/PDF/?uri=CELEX:32006R1901 (accessed on 15 August 2023).
79. European Commission, Directorate-General for Health and Food Safety; Marjolein, W.; Hoebert, J.; Vertvloet, M.; Puigmarti, C.M.; Damen, N.; Marchange, S.; Langedijk, J.; Lisman, J.; van Dijk, L. Study on Off-Label Use of Medicinal Products in the European Union. 2019. Available online: https://data.europa.eu/doi/10.2875/464022 (accessed on 27 August 2023).
80. Tomasi, P.A.; Egger, G.F.; Pallidis, C.; Saint-Raymond, A. Enabling Development of Paediatric Medicines in Europe: 10 Years of the EU Paediatric Regulation. *Pediatr. Drugs* **2017**, *19*, 505–513. [CrossRef]
81. Pediatric Research Equity Act of 2003. Public Law, 108–155, 2003. Available online: https://www.govinfo.gov/content/pkg/PLAW-108publ155/pdf/PLAW-108publ155.pdf (accessed on 12 August 2023).
82. Best Pharmaceuticals for Children Act. Public Law, 107–109, 2002. Available online: https://www.congress.gov/107/plaws/publ109/PLAW-107publ109.pdf (accessed on 25 August 2023).
83. Neville, K.A.; Frattarelli, D.A.; Galinkin, J.L.; Green, T.P.; Johnson, T.D.; Paul, I.M.; Anker, J.N.V.D.; American Academy of Pediatrics Committee on Drugs. Off-Label Use of Drugs in Children. *Pediatrics* **2014**, *133*, 563–567. [CrossRef]
84. de Wildt, S.N.; Foeldvari, I.; Siapkara, A.; Lepola, P.; Kriström, B.; Ruggieri, L.; Eichler, I.; Egger, G.F. Off-label is not always off-evidence: Authorising paediatric indications for old medicines. *Lancet Child Adolesc. Health* **2023**, *7*, 371–372. [CrossRef]
85. General Medical Council. Good Practice in Prescribing and Managing Medicines and Devices. General Medical Council (5 April 2021). 2021. Available online: https://www.gmc-uk.org/-/media/documents/prescribing-guidance-updated-english-20210405_pdf-85260533.pdf (accessed on 28 August 2023).
86. Meng, M.; Zhou, Q.; Lei, W.; Tian, M.; Wang, P.; Liu, Y.; Sun, Y.; Chen, Y.; Li, Q. Recommendations on Off-Label Drug Use in Pediatric Guidelines. *Front. Pharmacol.* **2022**, *13*, 892574. [CrossRef]
87. Balan, S.; Hassali, M.A.; Mak, V.S.L. Awareness, knowledge and views of off-label prescribing in children: A systematic review. *Br. J. Clin. Pharmacol.* **2015**, *80*, 1269–1280. [CrossRef]
88. Tsujii, N.; Saito, T.; Izumoto, Y.; Usami, M.; Okada, T.; Negoro, H.; Iida, J. Experiences with Patient Refusal of Off-Label Prescribing of Psychotropic Medications to Children and Adolescents in Japan. *J. Child Adolesc. Psychopharmacol.* **2016**, *26*, 642–645. [CrossRef]
89. Carnovale, C.; Conti, V.; Perrone, V.; Antoniazzi, S.; Pozzi, M.; Merlino, L.; Venegoni, M.; Clementi, E.; Radice, S. Paediatric drug use with focus on off-label prescriptions in Lombardy and implications for therapeutic approaches. *Eur. J. Pediatr.* **2013**, *172*, 1679–1685. [CrossRef]
90. Kieran, E.A.; O'Callaghan, N.; O'Donnell, C. Unlicensed and off-label drug use in an Irish neonatal intensive care unit: A prospective cohort study. *Acta Paediatr.* **2014**, *103*, e139–e142. [CrossRef]
91. Moulis, F.; Durrieu, G.; Lapeyre-Mestre, M. Off-label and unlicensed drug use in children population. *Therapies* **2018**, *73*, 135–149. [CrossRef]
92. Gore, R.; Chugh, P.K.; Tripathi, C.D.; Lhamo, Y.; Gautam, S. Pediatric Off-Label and Unlicensed Drug Use and Its Implications. *Curr. Clin. Pharmacol.* **2017**, *12*, 18–25. [CrossRef]
93. Magalhães, J.; Rodrigues, A.T.; Roque, F.; Figueiras, A.; Falcão, A.; Herdeiro, M.T. Use of off-label and unlicenced drugs in hospitalised paediatric patients: A systematic review. *Eur. J. Clin. Pharmacol.* **2015**, *71*, 1–13. [CrossRef]
94. Balan, S.; Hassali, M.; Mak, V. Non-regulatory related factors leading to off-label prescribing in children: A concept map. *Res. Soc. Adm. Pharm.* **2017**, *13*, 1219–1221. [CrossRef]
95. Knopf, H.; Wolf, I.-K.; Sarganas, G.; Zhuang, W.; Rascher, W.; Neubert, A. Off-label medicine use in children and adolescents: Results of a population-based study in Germany. *BMC Public Health* **2013**, *13*, 631. [CrossRef]
96. Ribeiro, M.; Jorge, A.; Macedo, A.F. Off-label drug prescribing in a Portuguese Paediatric Emergency Unit. *Int. J. Clin. Pharm.* **2012**, *35*, 30–36. [CrossRef]
97. Langerová, P.; Vrtal, J.; Urbánek, K. Incidence of unlicensed and off-label prescription in children. *Ital. J. Pediatr.* **2014**, *40*, 12. [CrossRef]
98. Bhadiyadara, S.N.; Rana, D.A.; Malhotra, S.D.; Patel, V.J. Off-label and Unlicensed Drug Use in Paediatric Outpatient Department—A Prospective Study at a Tertiary Care Teaching Hospital. *J. Young Pharm.* **2015**, *7*, 164. [CrossRef]

99. Oshikoya, K.A.; Oreagba, I.A.; Godman, B.; Fadare, J.; Orubu, S.; Massele, A.; Senbanjo, I.O. Off-label prescribing for children with chronic diseases in Nigeria; findings and implications. *Expert Opin. Drug Saf.* **2017**, *16*, 981–988. [CrossRef]
100. Lindell-Osuagwu, L.; Hakkarainen, M.; Sepponen, K.; Vainio, K.; Naaranlahti, T.; Kokki, H. Prescribing for off-label use and unauthorized medicines in three paediatric wards in Finland, the status before and after the European Union Paediatric Regulation. *J. Clin. Pharm. Ther.* **2014**, *39*, 144–153. [CrossRef]
101. Teigen, A.; Wang, S.; Truong, B.T.; Bjerknes, K. Off-label and unlicensed medicines to hospitalised children in Norway. *J. Pharm. Pharmacol.* **2017**, *69*, 432–438. [CrossRef]
102. Kimland, E.; Nydert, P.; Odlind, V.; Böttiger, Y.; Lindemalm, S. Paediatric drug use with focus on *off-label* prescriptions at Swedish hospitals—A nationwide study. *Acta Paediatr.* **2012**, *101*, 772–778. [CrossRef]
103. Palčevski, G.; Skočibušić, N.; Vlahović-Palčevski, V. Unlicensed and off-label drug use in hospitalized children in Croatia: A cross-sectional survey. *Eur. J. Clin. Pharmacol.* **2012**, *68*, 1073–1077. [CrossRef]
104. Slažneva, J.; Kovács, L.; Kuželová, M. Off-label drug use among hospitalized children: Identifying extent and nature. *Eur. Pharm. J.* **2012**, *59*, 48–54. [CrossRef]
105. Maltz, L.A.; Klugman, D.; Spaeder, M.C.; Wessel, D.L. Off-Label Drug Use in a Single-Center Pediatric Cardiac Intensive Care Unit. *World J. Pediatr. Congenit. Heart Surg.* **2013**, *4*, 262–266. [CrossRef]
106. Corny, J.; Bailey, B.; Lebel, D.; Bussières, J.-F. Unlicensed and off-label drug use in paediatrics in a mother-child tertiary care hospital. *Paediatr. Child Health* **2016**, *21*, 83–87. [CrossRef]
107. Czarniak, P.; Bint, L.; Favié, L.; Parsons, R.; Hughes, J.; Sunderland, B. Clinical Setting Influences Off-Label and Unlicensed Prescribing in a Paediatric Teaching Hospital. *PLoS ONE* **2015**, *10*, e0120630. [CrossRef]
108. Taylor, D.M.; Joffe, P.; Taylor, S.E.; Jones, A.; Cheek, J.A.; Craig, S.S.; Graudins, A.; Dhir, R.; Krieser, D.; Babl, F.E. Off-label and unlicenced medicine administration to paediatric emergency department patients. *Emerg. Med. Australas.* **2015**, *27*, 440–446. [CrossRef]
109. Landwehr, C.; Richardson, J.; Bint, L.; Parsons, R.; Sunderland, B.; Czarniak, P. Cross-sectional survey of off-label and unlicensed prescribing for inpatients at a paediatric teaching hospital in Western Australia. *PLoS ONE* **2019**, *14*, e0210237. [CrossRef]
110. Lee, J.L.; Redzuan, A.M.; Shah, N.M. Unlicensed and off-label use of medicines in children admitted to the intensive care units of a hospital in Malaysia. *Int. J. Clin. Pharm.* **2013**, *35*, 1025–1029. [CrossRef]
111. Tukayo, B.L.A.; Sunderland, B.; Parsons, R.; Czarniak, P. High prevalence of off-label and unlicensed paediatric prescribing in a hospital in Indonesia during the period Aug.—Oct. 2014. *PLoS ONE* **2020**, *15*, e0227687. [CrossRef]
112. Mohamad, N.F.; Ali, A.M.; Shah, N.M. Respiratory drugs prescribed off-label among children in the outpatient clinics of a hospital in Malaysia. *Int. J. Clin. Pharm.* **2014**, *37*, 127–132. [CrossRef]
113. Jobanputra, N.; Save, S.U.; Bavdekar, S.B. Off-label and unlicensed drug use in children admitted to Pediatric Intensive Care Units (PICU). *Int. J. Risk Saf. Med.* **2015**, *27*, 113–121. [CrossRef]
114. Ballard, C.D.; Peterson, G.M.; Thompson, A.J.; Beggs, S.A. Off-label use of medicines in paediatric inpatients at an Australian teaching hospital. *J. Paediatr. Child Health* **2013**, *49*, 38–42. [CrossRef]
115. Ellul, I.C.; Grech, V. Off-label and unlicensed paediatric prescribing in a community setting: A prospective longitudinal cohort study in Malta. *Paediatr. Int. Child Health* **2014**, *34*, 12–18. [CrossRef]
116. Abdulah, R.; Khairinisa, M.A.; Pratiwi, A.A.; Barliana, M.I.; Pradipta, I.S.; Halimah, E.; Diantini, A.; Lestari, K. Off-label paediatric drug use in an Indonesian community setting. *J. Clin. Pharm. Ther.* **2015**, *40*, 409–412. [CrossRef]
117. Dornelles, A.D.; Calegari, L.H.; de Souza, L.; Ebone, P.; Tonelli, T.S.; Carvalho, C.G. The Unlicensed and Off-label Prescription of Medications in General Paediatric Ward: An Observational Study. *Curr. Pediatr. Rev.* **2019**, *15*, 62–66. [CrossRef]
118. Conroy, S.; Choonara, I.; Impicciatore, P.; Mohn, A.; Arnell, H.; Rane, A.; Knoeppel, C.; Seyberth, H.; Pandolfini, C.; Raffaelli, M.P.; et al. Survey of unlicensed and off label drug use in paediatric wards in European countries. European Network for Drug Investigation in Children. *BMJ* **2000**, *320*, 79–82. [CrossRef]
119. Schaffer, A.L.; Bruno, C.; Buckley, N.A.; Cairns, R.; Litchfield, M.; Paget, S.; Zoega, H.; Nassar, N.; Pearson, S. Prescribed medicine use and extent of off-label use according to age in a nationwide sample of Australian children. *Paediatr. Périnat. Epidemiol.* **2022**, *36*, 726–737. [CrossRef]
120. Luedtke, K.E.; Buck, M.L. Evaluation of Off-label Prescribing at a Children's Rehabilitation Center. *J. Pediatr. Pharmacol. Ther.* **2014**, *19*, 296–301. [CrossRef]
121. Gonçalves, M.G.; Heineck, I. Frequency of prescriptions of off-label drugs and drugs not approved for pediatric use in primary health care in a southern municipality of Brazil. *Rev. Paul Pediatr.* **2016**, *34*, 11–17. [CrossRef]
122. Dos Santos, L.; Heineck, I. Drug utilization study in pediatric prescriptions of a university hospital in southern brazil: Off-label, unlicensed and high-alert medications. *Farm. Hosp.* **2012**, *36*, 180–186. [CrossRef]
123. Pereira Gomes, V.; Melo da Silva, K.; Oliveira Chagas, S.; dos Santos Magalhães, I.R. Off-label and unlicensed utilization of drugs in a Brazilian pediatric hospital. *Farm. Hosp.* **2015**, *39*, 176–180. [CrossRef]
124. Aamir, M.; Khan, J.A.; Shakeel, F.; Asim, S.M. Unlicensed and off-label use of drugs in pediatric surgical units at tertiary care hospitals of Pakistan. *Int. J. Clin. Pharm.* **2017**, *39*, 860–866. [CrossRef]
125. Saito, J.; Nadatani, N.; Setoguchi, M.; Nakao, M.; Kimura, H.; Sameshima, M.; Kobayashi, K.; Matsumoto, H.; Yoshikawa, N.; Yokoyama, T.; et al. Potentially harmful excipients in neonatal medications: A multicenter nationwide observational study in Japan. *J. Pharm. Health Care Sci.* **2021**, *7*, 23. [CrossRef]

126. Flint, R.B.; van Beek, F.; Andriessen, P.; Zimmermann, L.J.; Liem, K.D.; Reiss, I.K.; de Groot, R.; Tibboel, D.; Burger, D.M.; Simons, S.H.; et al. Large differences in neonatal drug use between NICUs are common practice: Time for consensus? *Br. J. Clin. Pharmacol.* **2018**, *84*, 1313–1323. [CrossRef]
127. Alonso, A.S.; Avila-Alvarez, A.; Eiriz, M.C.; Roca, C.M.; Gómez, P.Y.; López, A.C.; Trisac, J.L.F.; Díaz, S.P. Use of off-label drugs in neonatal intensive care. *Anal. Pediatr.* **2019**, *91*, 237–243. [CrossRef]
128. Schweigertova, J.; Durisova, A.; Dolnikova, D.; Ondriasova, E.; Balazova, M.; Slezakova, V.; Kuzelova, M. Off-label and unlicensed use of medicinal products in the neonatal setting in the Slovak Republic. *Pediatr. Int.* **2016**, *58*, 126–131. [CrossRef]
129. Silva, J.; Flor-De-Lima, F.; Soares, H.; Guimarães, H. Off-Label and Unlicensed Drug Use in Neonatology: Reality in a Portuguese University Hospital. *Acta Med. Portug.* **2015**, *28*, 297–306. [CrossRef]
130. Riou, S.; Plaisant, F.; Boulch, D.M.; Kassai, B.; Claris, O.; Nguyen, K.-A. Unlicensed and off-label drug use: A prospective study in French NICU. *Acta Paediatr.* **2015**, *104*, e228–e231. [CrossRef]
131. Cuzzolin, L.; Agostino, R. Off-label and unlicensed drug treatments in Neonatal Intensive Care Units: An Italian multicentre study. *Eur. J. Clin. Pharmacol.* **2016**, *72*, 117–123. [CrossRef]
132. Carvalho, C.G.; Ribeiro, M.R.; Bonilha, M.M.; Fernandes, M., Jr.; Procianoy, R.S.; Silveira, R.C. Use of off-label and unlicensed drugs in the neonatal intensive care unit and its association with severity scores. *J. Pediatr.* **2012**, *88*, 465–470. [CrossRef]
133. Costa, H.T.M.d.L.; Costa, T.X.; Martins, R.R.; Oliveira, A.G. Use of off-label and unlicensed medicines in neonatal intensive care. *PLoS ONE* **2018**, *13*, e0204427. [CrossRef]
134. Vieira, V.C.; Costa, R.S.; Lima, R.C.G.; Queiroz, D.B.; de Medeiros, D.S. Prescription of off-label and unlicensed drugs for preterm infants in a neonatal intensive care unit. *Rev. Brasil. Ter. Intens.* **2021**, *33*, 266–275. [CrossRef]
135. Jain, S.; Saini, S.S.; Chawla, D.; Kumar, P.; Dhir, S. Off-label use of drugs in neonatal intensive care units. *Indian Pediatr.* **2014**, *51*, 644–646. [CrossRef]
136. Chauthankar, S.A.; Marathe, P.A.; Potey, A.V.; Nanavati, R.N. Drug utilization in neonatal intensive care unit of a tertiary-care hospital in Mumbai, India. *Indian Pediatr.* **2017**, *54*, 931–934. [CrossRef]
137. Aamir, M.; Khan, J.A.; Shakeel, F.; Shareef, R.; Shah, N. Drug utilization in neonatal setting of Pakistan: Focus on unlicensed and off label drug prescribing. *BMC Pediatr.* **2018**, *18*, 242. [CrossRef]
138. Nir-Neuman, H.; Abu-Kishk, I.; Toledano, M.; Heyman, E.; Ziv-Baran, T.; Berkovitch, M. Unlicensed and Off-Label Medication Use in Pediatric and Neonatal Intensive Care Units: No Change Over a Decade. *Adv. Ther.* **2018**, *35*, 1122–1132. [CrossRef]
139. Lindell-Osuagwu, L.; Korhonen, M.J.; Saano, S.; Helin-Tanninen, M.; Naaranlahti, T.; Kokki, H. Off-label and unlicensed drug prescribing in three paediatric wards in Finland and review of the international literature. *J. Clin. Pharm. Ther.* **2009**, *34*, 277–287. [CrossRef]
140. Belayneh, A.; Abatneh, E.; Abebe, D.; Getachew, M.; Kebede, B.; Dessie, B. Off-label medication use in pediatrics and associated factors at public hospitals in east Gojjam zone, Ethiopia. *SAGE Open Med.* **2022**, *10*, 20503121221096534. [CrossRef]
141. Czaja, A.S.; Reiter, P.D.; Schultz, M.L.; Valuck, R.J. Patterns of Off-Label Prescribing in the Pediatric Intensive Care Unit and Prioritizing Future Research. *J. Pediatr. Pharmacol. Ther.* **2015**, *20*, 186–196. [CrossRef]
142. Blanco-Reina, E.; Medina-Claros, A.; Vega-Jiménez, M.; Ocaña-Riola, R.; Márquez-Romero, E.; Ruiz-Extremera, Á. Drug utilization pattern in children and off-label use of medicines in a pediatric intensive care unit. *Med. Intensiv.* **2015**, *40*, 1–8. [CrossRef]
143. Arocas Casañ, V.; Cabezuelo Escribano, B.; Garrido-Corro, B.; De la Cruz Murie, P.; Blázquez Álvarez, M.J.; De la Rubia Nieto, M.A. Off-label and unlicensed drug use in a Spanish Neonatal Intensive Care Unit. *Farm. Hosp.* **2017**, *41*, 371–381. [CrossRef]
144. Oishi, K.; Inage, E.; Kojima, M.; Yamada, H.; Tanaka, Y.; Yoneyama, T.; Yamazaki, S.; Honjo, A.; Baba, Y.; Kudo, T.; et al. Evidence of off-label inhalation therapy on pediatric asthma practice in Japan. *Pediatr. Int.* **2023**, *65*, e15595. [CrossRef]
145. Smeets, N.J.L.; Raaijmakers, L.P.M.; van der Zanden, T.M.; Male, C.; de Wildt, S.N. Guiding future paediatric drug studies based on existing pharmacokinetic and efficacy data: Cardiovascular drugs as a proof of concept. *Br. J. Clin. Pharmacol.* **2023**, *89*, 2888–2901. [CrossRef]
146. Zodidi, M. Off Label and Unlicensed Drug Use in Neonatal Wards (Excluding Neonatal ICU) at Tygerberg Children's Hospital (TBH). Master's Thesis, (MMed)-Stellenbosch University, Stellenbosch, South Africa, December 2019. Available online: http://hdl.handle.net/10019.1/106987 (accessed on 20 August 2023).
147. Balan, S.; Hassali, M.A.A.; Mak, V.S.L. Two decades of off-label prescribing in children: A literature review. *World J. Pediatr.* **2018**, *14*, 528–540. [CrossRef]
148. Le Jeunne, C.; Billon, N.; Dandon, A.; Berdaï, D.; Adgibi, Y.; Bergmann, J.-F.; Bordet, R.; Carpentier, A.; Cohn, E.; Courcier, S.; et al. Off-label Prescriptions: How to Identify Them, Frame Them, Announce Them and Monitor Them in Practice? *Therapies* **2013**, *68*, 233–239. [CrossRef]
149. Schrier, L.; Hadjipanayis, A.; Stiris, T.; Ross-Russell, R.I.; Valiulis, A.; Turner, M.A.; Zhao, W.; De Cock, P.; De Wildt, S.N.; Allegaert, K.; et al. Off-label use of medicines in neonates, infants, children, and adolescents: A joint policy statement by the European Academy of Paediatrics and the European society for Developmental Perinatal and Pediatric Pharmacology. *Eur. J. Pediatr.* **2020**, *179*, 839–847. [CrossRef]
150. van der Zanden, T.M.; Mooij, M.G.; Vet, N.J.; Neubert, A.; Rascher, W.; Lagler, F.B.; Male, C.; Grytli, H.; Halvorsen, T.; de Hoog, M.; et al. Benefit-Risk Assessment of Off-Label Drug Use in Children: The Bravo Framework. *Clin. Pharmacol. Ther.* **2021**, *110*, 952–965. [CrossRef]

151. Guyatt, G.H.; Oxman, A.D.; Vist, G.E.; Kunz, R.; Falck-Ytter, Y.; Alonso-Coello, P.; Schünemann, H.J.; GRADE Working Group. GRADE: An emerging consensus on rating quality of evidence and strength of recommendations. *BMJ* **2008**, *336*, 924–926. [CrossRef]
152. Kalra, A.; Goindi, S. Issues Impacting Therapeutic Outcomes in Pediatric Patients: An Overview. *Curr. Pediatr. Rev.* **2014**, *10*, 184–193. [CrossRef]
153. Ivanovska, V.; Rademaker, C.M.; van Dijk, L.; Mantel-Teeuwisse, A.K. Pediatric Drug Formulations: A Review of Challenges and Progress. *Pediatrics* **2014**, *134*, 361–372. [CrossRef]
154. Richey, R.H.; Hughes, C.; Craig, J.V.; Shah, U.U.; Ford, J.L.; Barker, C.E.; Peak, M.; Nunn, A.J.; Turner, M.A. A systematic review of the use of dosage form manipulation to obtain required doses to inform use of manipulation in paediatric practice. *Int. J. Pharm.* **2017**, *518*, 155–166. [CrossRef]
155. Greenberg, R.G.; McCune, S.; Attar, S.; Hovinga, C.; Stewart, B.; Lacaze-Masmonteil, T. Pediatric Clinical Research Networks: Role in Accelerating Development of Therapeutics in Children. *Ther. Innov. Regul. Sci.* **2022**, *56*, 934–947. [CrossRef]
156. Green, D.J.; Zineh, I.; Burckart, G.J. Pediatric Drug Development: Outlook for Science-Based Innovation. *Clin. Pharmacol. Ther.* **2018**, *103*, 376–378. [CrossRef]
157. Samuels, S.; Park, K.; Bhatt-Mehta, V.; Sun, H.; Mulugeta, Y.; Yao, L.; Green, D.J.; Burckart, G.J. Pediatric Efficacy Extrapolation in Drug Development Submitted to the US Food and Drug Administration 2015–2020. *J. Clin. Pharmacol.* **2023**, *63*, 307–313. [CrossRef]
158. Dunn, A.; Jung, D.; Bollinger, L.L.; Krams, M.; Smith, B.P.; Gobburu, J.V.S. Accelerating the Availability of Medications to Pediatric Patients by Optimizing the Use of Extrapolation of Efficacy. *Ther. Innov. Regul. Sci.* **2022**, *56*, 873–882. [CrossRef]
159. Ward, R.M.; Benjamin, D.K.; Davis, J.M.; Gorman, R.L.; Kauffman, R.; Kearns, G.L.; Murphy, M.D.; Sherwin, C.M. The Need for Pediatric Drug Development. *J. Pediatr.* **2018**, *192*, 13–21. [CrossRef]
160. State of Paediatric Medicines in the EU. Available online: https://health.ec.europa.eu/system/files/2017-11/2017_childrensmedicines_report_en_0.pdf (accessed on 28 August 2023).
161. Boosting the Development of Medicines for Children. Closing Report of the European Medicines Agency and European Commission (DG Health and Food Safety) Action Plan on Paediatrics. EMA/635567/2022. Available online: https://www.ema.europa.eu/en/documents/report/boosting-development-medicines-children-closing-report-european-medicines-agency-european-commission_en.pdf (accessed on 26 August 2023).
162. Bellis, J.R.; Kirkham, J.J.; Nunn, A.J.; Pirmohamed, M. Adverse drug reactions and off-label and unlicensed medicines in children: A prospective cohort study of unplanned admissions to a paediatric hospital. *Br. J. Clin. Pharmacol.* **2014**, *77*, 545–553. [CrossRef]
163. Saiyed, M.M.; Lalwani, T.; Rana, D. Is off-label use a risk factor for adverse drug reactions in pediatric patients? A prospective study in an Indian tertiary care hospital. *Int. J. Risk Saf. Med.* **2015**, *27*, 45–53. [CrossRef]
164. Kaguelidou, F.; Ouèdraogo, M.; Treluyer, J.-M.; Le Jeunne, C.; Annereau, M.; Blanc, P.; Bureau, S.; Ducassou, S.; Fiquet, B.; Flamein, F.; et al. Paediatric drug development and evaluation: Existing challenges and recommendations. *Therapie* **2023**, *78*, 105–114. [CrossRef]
165. Yamashiro, Y.; Martin, J.; Gazarian, M.; Kling, S.; Nakamura, H.; Matsui, A.; Cucchiara, S.; Aloi, M.; Wynn, E.L.; Mulberg, A.E. Drug Development: The use of unlicensed/off-label medicines in pediatrics. *J. Pediatr. Gastroenterol. Nutr.* **2012**, *55*, 506–510. [CrossRef]
166. Costa, H.T.M.L.; Florencio, A.P.; Bezerra, P.K.D.V.; Cavalcanti, J.E.C.; Costa, T.X.; Fernandes, F.E.M.; Martins, R.R. Comparative assessment of off-label and unlicensed drug prescription in neonatal intensive care: FDA versus Brazilian guidelines. *An. Pediatr.* **2021**, *94*, 153–160. [CrossRef]

pharmaceutics

MDPI

Review

Expanding the Availability of Onasemnogene Abeparvovec to Older Patients: The Evolving Treatment Landscape for Spinal Muscular Atrophy

Charlotte A. René [1,2,3] and Robin J. Parks [1,2,3,4,*]

1 Regenerative Medicine Program, Ottawa Hospital Research Institute, Ottawa, ON K1H 8L6, Canada; chrene@ohri.ca
2 Department of Biochemistry, Microbiology, and Immunology, University of Ottawa, Ottawa, ON K1H 8M5, Canada
3 Centre for Neuromuscular Disease, University of Ottawa, Ottawa, ON K1H 8M5, Canada
4 Department of Medicine, The Ottawa Hospital, Ottawa, ON K1H 8L6, Canada
* Correspondence: rparks@ohri.ca

Abstract: Spinal muscular atrophy (SMA) is a devastating neuromuscular disorder caused by mutations in the survival of motor neuron 1 (*SMN1*) gene, which leads to a reduced level in the SMN protein within cells. Patients with SMA suffer from a loss of alpha motor neurons in the spinal cord leading to skeletal muscle atrophy in addition to deficits in other tissues and organs. Patients with severe forms of the disease require ventilator assistance and typically succumb to the disease due to respiratory failure. Onasemnogene abeparvovec is an adeno-associated virus (AAV)-based gene therapeutic that has been approved for infants and young children with SMA, and it is delivered through intravenous administration using a dose based on the weight of the patient. While excellent outcomes have been observed in treated patients, the greater viral dose necessary to treat older children and adults raises legitimate safety concerns. Recently, onasemnogene abeparvovec use was investigated in older children through a fixed dose and intrathecal administration, a route that provides a more direct delivery to affected cells in the spinal cord and central nervous system. The promising results observed in the STRONG trial may support approval of onasemnogene abeparvovec for a greater proportion of patients with SMA.

Keywords: gene therapy; onasemnogene abeparvovec; neuromuscular disease; motor neuron disease; spinal muscular atrophy

1. Introduction

Spinal muscular atrophy (SMA) is a genetic neuromuscular disorder that was initially described at the end of the nineteenth century by Werdnig [1] and by Hoffmann [2]. SMA is characterized by a degeneration of the alpha motor neurons of the spinal cord, which leads to atrophy of skeletal muscle, although primary defects also occur in many other tissues and organs [3–5]. SMA is caused by the homozygous mutation or deletion of the survival of motor neuron 1 (*SMN1*) gene [6], resulting in inadequate levels of survival of motor neuron (SMN) protein within cells [7]. Humans have a paralogous gene, termed *SMN2*, that contains a key C-to-T base transition relative to *SMN1* that induces a skipping of exon 7 in the majority of the messenger RNA (mRNA) transcripts that are derived from this gene, leading to the production of only ~10% full-length SMN protein [8,9]. *SMN2* is variably amplified in humans, and more copies of the gene result in the production of a greater amount of the full-length SMN protein within cells [10]. Thus, more copies of *SMN2* commonly leads to less severe disease for a patient with SMA [11].

Fortunately, several treatments have been approved for this devastating disorder, including nusinersen and risdiplam, both of which promote the inclusion of exon 7 in the

SMN2-derived mRNA, and thus a greater production of the full-length SMN protein [12–14]. Arguably, the most promising therapy, onasemnogene abeparvovec, an adeno-associated virus (AAV)-based vector that encodes the *SMN1* gene, has only been approved for use in infants and young children [15–18]. Onasemnogene abeparvovec is currently administered intravenously (IV) using a dose based on patient weight, and it is presently unavailable to older children with SMA due to safety concerns related to high absolute doses of vector [15–19]. However, a recent trial has explored the use of administering fixed-dose onasemnogene abeparvovec in children who are up to 5 years of age through intrathecal (IT) administration [20]—a more direct route through which to deliver the therapy to the cells of the spinal cord and central nervous system (CNS). In this review, we will provide background and context for this recent trial.

2. Onasemnogene Abeparvovec

Onasemnogene abeparvovec, marketed as Zolgensma, is a self-complementary AAV serotype 9 (scAAV9) vector that encodes a functional copy of *SMN1* that is under the control of a hybrid cytomegalovirus (CMV) enhancer-chicken beta-actin promoter (CBA) [21]. The safety and efficacy of onasemnogene abeparvovec has been explored in several clinical trials, as detailed in Table 1.

Table 1. Onasemnogene abeparvovec clinical trials.

Clinical Trial	Patient Age	*SMN2* Copy #	*n*	Administration Method	Dose	Status *
START Phase 1 NCT02122952	<8 months	2	15	Intravenous	Low: 6.7×10^{13} vg/kg High: 1.1×10^{14} vg/kg	Completed
STR1VE-US Phase 3 NCT03306277	<6 months	1 or 2	22	Intravenous	1.1×10^{14} vg/kg	Completed
STR1VE-EU Phase 3 NCT03461289	<6 months	1 or 2	33	Intravenous	1.1×10^{14} vg/kg	Completed
SPR1NT Phase 3 NCT03505099	<6 weeks	1, 2, or 3	30	Intravenous	1.1×10^{14} vg/kg	Completed
STRONG Phase 1 NCT03381729	6–60 months	3	32	Intrathecal	Low: 6.0×10^{13} vg Medium: 1.2×10^{14} vg High: 2.4×10^{14} vg	Terminated
SMART Phase 3b NCT04851873	<17 years	N/A	24	Intravenous	N/A (likely 1.1×10^{14} vg/kg)	Active
STEER Phase 3 NCT05089656	≥2–<18 years	N/A	125 (estimated)	Intrathecal	1.2×10^{14} vg	Recruiting

* as of June 2023.

Initially, the safety and efficacy of a single IV infusion of onasemnogene abeparvovec was examined in the phase 1 START trial (NCT02122952), which involved symptomatic infants <8 months of age with SMA type 1 and who possessed two copies of *SMN2*. A total of 15 infants received either a low (6.7×10^{13} viral genomes (vg)/kg; $n = 3$) or a high (1.1×10^{14} vg/kg; $n = 12$) dose of IV onasemnogene abeparvovec. All 15 infants were alive without the need for mechanical ventilation at 20 months of age, a dramatic improvement from the 8% survival rate observed in the historical control cohort. Among 11/12 children in the high-dose cohort, an increase in survival was accompanied by improvements in the Children's Hospital of Philadelphia Infant Test of Neuromuscular Disorders (CHOP-INTEND) scores compared to their baseline. A total of 13 patients from the START trial were enrolled in a long-term follow-up (LTFU) study (NCT03421977) in which all 10 children from the high-dose group were alive without the need for permanent ventilation and maintained previously achieved motor milestones for up to 7.5 years post-treatment, demonstrating the longevity of onasemnogene abeparvovec [22,23]. Without treatment, children with SMA type 1 with two copies of *SMN2* rarely survive past the age of two, typically succumbing to respiratory failure [24,25].

The follow-up phase 3 trials, STR1VE-US (NCT03306277) and STR1VE-EU (NCT03461289), treated children < 6 months of age with SMA type I and up to two copies of *SMN2* with the high dose used in the START trial [21,26,27]. Both of these trials demonstrated that over 90% of infants survived free of the need for permanent ventilation at 14 months compared to 26% in the natural history cohort; furthermore, approximately half achieved independent sitting at 18 months, a milestone that was not achieved in the natural history cohort. Both STR1VE trials showed a very good benefit–risk profile for the IV administration of onasemnogene abeparvovec in symptomatic infants with SMA that were younger than 6 months, thus supporting the case for the drug's approval [15]. This favourable benefit–risk profile was also demonstrated in the SPR1NT trial (NCT03505099), which treated pre-symptomatic infants less than 6 weeks of age with 2 ($n = 14$) or 3 ($n = 15$) copies of *SMN2* [28,29]. The START, STR1VE, and SPR1NT trials examined the safety of onasemnogene abeparvovec in both symptomatic and pre-symptomatic infants with SMA; however, all the infants who participated in these studies weighed < 8.5 kg. The Global Managed Access Program (GMAP) launched by Novartis in January 2020 provided treatment to all patients with SMA under the age of 24 months and weighing $\leq$ 21 kg [30]. As of 2022, 5 out of 102 children who were treated through this program were $\geq$13.5 kg, the heaviest of which was 17 kg (this patient received a dose of 1.87×10^{15} total vg). The GMAP data showed that the safety findings of patients that were $\geq$8.5 kg at the time of infusion were consistent with the previous data of patients who were <8.5 kg.

As of January 2023, IV onasemnogene abeparvovec was approved in 45 countries [31], although the maximum patient age and/or weight varies between countries. In the United States and Japan, the first countries to approve onasemnogene abeparvovec, the drug is approved for use in children with SMA up to two years old, regardless of weight [15,16]. In Canada and Europe, onasemnogene abeparvovec is used for the treatment of pediatric patients with 5q SMA that have bi-allelic mutations in the *SMN1* gene, and who are either clinically diagnosed as SMA type 1, or possess three or fewer copies of the *SMN2* gene [17,18,32]. This regulatory approval includes dosing guidance for babies and young children up to 21 kg. Based on natural history studies, the majority of untreated children 5 years old or younger with SMA type 1 or type 2 would likely be $\leq$21 kg, and this could include children as old as 8 years of age [33].

To further explore the efficacy and safety of IV onasemnogene abeparvovec in heavier children, the SMART phase 3b trial (NCT04851873) is investigating the use of IV onasemnogene abeparvovec in children with SMA who were <18 years of age and who weighed $\geq$ 8.5 kg to $\leq$21 kg. Although recruitment criteria for this trial permit participants to be up to 17 years of age, it is unlikely that participants over 8 years of age would meet the weight requirement of $\leq$21 kg at the time of infusion [33].

Following the success of the STR1VE and SPR1NT trials, there was an obvious desire to examine the efficacy of onasemnogene abeparvovec in an older patient population. However, there are inherent challenges in treating older, and thus larger, patients with SMA. To date, the therapeutic dose has been calculated based on weight at 1.1×10^{14} vg/kg. Larger patients would require larger absolute doses of vector. A very high dose of vector is required because IV administration is a relatively inefficient method through which to deliver vector to the CNS—only a small portion of the vector actually transits through the blood–brain barrier (BBB) and transduces the target tissues located within the CNS [34,35]. The majority of the IV-administered vector actually accumulates in the liver and peripheral tissues [36]. No gene therapy vector is completely "safe"; thus, administering a greater quantity of vector raises legitimate safety concerns. Use of AAV, such as onasemnogene abeparvovec, can cause serious adverse events, including acute liver failure in large animal models [34] and in human trials [19], as well as thrombotic microangiopathy (TMA) in human trials [37]—the risk of which increases as more viral genomes are administered. Indeed, trends toward greater elevations in liver transaminases have been reported amongst heavier children who were administered onasemnogene abeparvovec [38,39]; however, this was not the case in all studies [30]. Tragically, two children have died of acute liver failure within 5 to 6 weeks following IV administration of onasemnogene abeparvovec [40,41]. Novartis released a statement following the patient fatalities, highlighting that acute liver failure is a known side effect of onasemnogene abeparvovec; however, the benefit-risk profile is still favourable [41]. Similarly, four children in a clinical trial for the genetic neuromuscular disorder X-linked myotubular myopathy (XLMTM) died following the IV administration of AAV8-MTM1, three of which received a dose of 3.5×10^{14} vg/kg and were confirmed to have died from complications of liver failure [42–45]. AAV may not have been the sole cause of liver failure in these children; it is possible that the administration of the vector could have exacerbated pre-existing liver dysfunction, as intrahepatic cholestasis has been found to be a clinically significant feature of XLMTM [46]. Finally, although the majority of delivered AAV genomes remain episomal, AAV can insert in the cell's genome, which has been associated with hepatocellular carcinoma in humans [47] and mice [48–50] (although not in all studies [51–54]). In short, although AAV-mediated gene therapy can be very effective, it does not come without risk. For SMA, an alternative approach to achieve efficient delivery to the CNS using less vector is greatly desired.

3. Intrathecal Administration of Onasemnogene Abeparvovec

To circumvent the need for the extremely high numbers of vg required for IV treatment in older, and thus larger, patients, IT administration of onasemnogene abeparvovec has been explored with the aim of providing a more efficient transduction of the CNS. In mice and nonhuman primates, IT administration of scAAV9-SMN results in widespread transgene expression throughout the spinal cord, and this is achieved using 10-fold less vector compared to IV administration [55].

Initiated in 2017, the phase 1 STRONG trial (NCT03381729) evaluated a single IT fixed-dose administration of onasemnogene abeparvovec in non-ambulatory children with SMA type 2 and who were 6 to <60-months of age with three copies of *SMN2*. Unlike the previous trials that investigated onasemnogene abeparvovec, there was no weight limit in the eligibility criteria for the STRONG trial. This phase I dose escalation study used doses ranging from 6.0×10^{13} to 2.4×10^{14} total vg, which is significantly less than the highest dose administered to patients in the IV phase 1 START trial (which administered 1.69×10^{15} total vg to the largest patient [21]). Unfortunately, a partial clinical hold was placed on the STRONG trial by the FDA in October 2019, citing concern due to dorsal root ganglia (DRG) mononuclear cell inflammation observed in animals treated with IT onasemnogene abeparvovec [56,57]. Following further long-term preclinical safety studies, the partial clinical hold was lifted in August of 2021 [58].

Recently, results of the completed STRONG trial were published [20]. 32 children were divided into two groups based on age at dosing: younger (6 to <24 months) and older (24 to <60 months). Patients in the younger children grouping were enrolled into one of three fixed-dose cohorts: low- (6.0×10^{13} total vg, $n = 3$), medium- (1.2×10^{14} total vg, $n = 13$), and high-dose (2.4×10^{14} total vg, $n = 4$). The older group all received the medium dose (1.2×10^{14} total vg, $n = 12$). Amongst the younger patients, 1/3 (33.3%) in the low-dose cohort and 1/13 (7.7%) in the medium-dose cohort (or 12.5% (2/16 treated patients) when combining the two dosing groups) achieved independent standing. Based on natural history studies, 13.7% would have been predicted to achieve this milestone. Again, amongst the younger children cohort, two children that received the low dose gained a total of four motor Bayley-III milestones (crawls, $n = 2$; pulls to stand, $n = 1$;

and stands alone, $n = 1$), while six children in the medium-dose cohort gained a total of 15 motor milestones (rolls, $n = 4$; crawls, $n = 2$; pulls to a stand $n = 2$; stands with assistance, $n = 3$; stands alone, $n = 1$; walks with assistance $n = 2$; and walks alone, $n = 1$). Three children in the high-dose cohort achieved 3 motor milestones (rolls, $n = 1$; pulls to a stand, $n = 1$; and stands with assistance $n = 1$). Older children who received the medium dose (1.2×10^{14} total vg, $n = 12$) showed a mean change of 6.0 points in their Hammersmith Functional Motor Scale Expanded (HFMSE) scores at month 12 when compared to baseline, which was significantly different from the natural history cohort, who only saw a 0.5-point change. Furthermore, 11/12 (91.7%) of treated children achieved a clinically meaningful ($\geq$3-point) increase in their HFMSE score compared to their initial score at baseline visit, which is far greater than the 13.3% who achieved a similar improvement in the natural history cohort. Three children in this group achieved a total of four Bayley-III motor milestones (rolling, $n = 1$; standing with assistance, $n = 2$; and walking with assistance, $n = 1$). No deaths were reported in this study. Several adverse events of special interest (AESI) were reported, including nine hepatotoxicity events in seven children (21.9%), including one patient in the medium-dose cohort who experienced elevated alanine aminotransferase (ALT) and aspartate aminotransferase (AST)—which was deemed a treatment-related serious adverse event. There were also five thrombocytopenia events observed in five children (15.6%, one of which was deemed probably treatment related), twelve cardiac events in nine children (28.1%, including one instance each of sinus tachycardia and increased creatinine phosphokinase-MB, which were deemed to possibly be treatment related), and one instance of hepatomegaly (deemed probably treatment related). Overall, the investigators concluded that IT onasemnogene abeparvovec is safe and well-tolerated, and the therapy showed efficacy in children aged 2 to 5 years. Unfortunately, the primary efficacy endpoint of independent standing for $\geq$3 s in children aged 6 to 24 months was not met during the post-dose observation period of this study.

Patients enrolled in the STRONG trial could participate in LT-002 (NCT04042025), a voluntary phase 4, 15-year follow-up safety and efficacy study, which also enrolled patients from the STR1VE and SPR1NT studies. Novartis provided an update on LT-002 at the 2023 Muscular Dystrophy Association Clinical and Scientific Conference. All children who participated in the STRONG trial had maintained or achieved new developmental gains at a mean follow-up length of 3.6 years [23]. In addition, 5/16 (31.3%) had achieved a new motor milestone; 6 of 12 (50%) had a $\geq$3-point increase in HFMSE score; and 3 of 12 (25%) had a >10-point increase [59]. However, interpretation of the data is somewhat complicated by the fact that some of the patients also received add-on therapy (nusinersen or risdiplam) [23,59]. Of the 18 patients from the STRONG trial who were enrolled in LT-002, 50% were also receiving add-on therapy [59]. This is far greater than the 24.6% of patients who received add-on therapy following treatment with IV onasemnogene abeparvovec in the STR1VE or SPRINT trials. It is unclear why a larger proportion of patients that received the IT treatment also sought add-on therapy compared to the IV-treated group. Perhaps the systemic distribution of onasemnogene abeparvovec to all tissues of the body during IV treatment provides a better outcome than delivering vector only to the CNS. While combining therapies may be in the best interest of the patient, it does complicate interpretation of the data from the clinical trial as any improvement in motor function may be attributed to more than just onasemnogene abeparvovec. As more data become available, it will be interesting to see if there is a correlation between dose, age, and performance in tests of motor function among those who received add-on therapy compared to onasemnogene abeparvovec alone.

As the medium-dose of IT onasemnogene abeparvovec was well-tolerated and demonstrated efficacy, it was selected for use in the ongoing phase 3 STEER trial (NCT05089656), which is exploring the use of IT fixed-dose onasemnogene abeparvovec in patients aged $\geq$2 to <18 years old. Unlike the SMART trial—in which patients were only eligible if they were $\leq$21 kg in weight at the time of infusion—all treated patients in the STEER trial will be administered 1.2×10^{14} total vg, regardless of weight. Exploring the efficacy of onasemnogene abeparvovec in the oldest population to date through an IT administration of a fixed dose has the potential to satisfy the unmet need for gene therapy for children and adolescent patients with SMA.

Although IT onasemnogene abeparvovec may be a promising therapeutic option for the treatment of SMA in older children, it is important to note that the most dramatic improvement with IV onasemnogene abeparvovec were observed in pre-symptomatic infants treated at less than 6 weeks of age [28,29]. In the SPR1NT trial, infants with three copies of *SMN2* all achieved independent sitting, and most achieved independent walking, within the normal development window, which is typically not seen in patients with SMA [29]. Amongst infants with two copies of *SMN2*, most sat independently for ≥30 s within the normal development window, and all achieved this milestone by 18 months, while none in the natural history cohort achieved this milestone [28]. In the STRONG trial, children in the younger group gained more Bayley-III motor milestones than those in the older group [20]. Treatment is likely most effective when supplied before the irreversible loss of motor neurons has occurred. These data emphasize the urgent need for universal newborn screening to identify at-risk children as early as possible in order to initiate treatment early. Fortunately, newborn screening has been adopted in many countries around the world [60]. The early treatment of individuals at high risk of developing SMA, prior to symptom onset, results in improved outcomes and greater functional independence, leading to improved quality of life.

4. Onasemnogene Abeparvovec versus Nusinersen or Risdiplam

The results of the STRONG trial should be compared to similar trials involving nusinersen, marketed as Spinraza, which is currently available for the treatment of SMA in patients of all ages. Nusinersen is an antisense oligonucleotide (ASO) delivered IT that modulates the splicing of *SMN2* pre-mRNA to promote the inclusion of exon 7, thereby increasing the production of the full-length SMN protein [13,61,62]. As opposed to onasemnogene abeparvovec, which is delivered with a one-time infusion, nusinersen is administered IT through a series of four loading doses over the course of the first two months, followed by maintenance doses every four months [15,63]. All patients receive the same dose (12 mg of the ASO in a 5 mL volume), regardless of age, size, or severity of disease. The CHERISH trial (NCT02292537) used nusinersen to treat 84 children with SMA between 2 and 12 years of age and who had between two and four copies of *SMN2*, with 42 children in a sham control group [64]. At 15 months, 57% of children in the treated group had achieved a change in their HFMSE score of ≥3 points compared to 27% in the sham control group [64]. This is far less than the 91.7% of children who were 2 to 5 years of age and were treated with the medium dose of onasemnogene abeparvovec in the STRONG trial, and who achieved the same increase in HMFSE score at month 12 [20]. Overall, the mean increases in HMFSE scores were not as pronounced in the CHERISH trial at 15 months than in the STRONG trial at 12 months [20,64]. Nevertheless, the CHERISH trial concluded that significant improvement in motor function was observed in children with later-onset SMA compared to the sham control group [64]. Complications associated with lumbar puncture were significantly higher in the treated group than in the control group (15% versus 3%, respectively), and these included back pain, headache, and vomiting. Pyrexia and epistaxis were also ≥5 percentage points higher in the treated group relative to the control group (pyrexia: 43% versus 36%; epistaxis: 7% versus 0%, respectively). This study reported no elevations in ALT or AST as adverse events, unlike in some patients who were treated with onasemnogene abeparvovec [19,20,64].

The use of ASOs such as nusinersen comes with some associated risks, such as renal toxicity, thrombocytopenia, and coagulation abnormalities [63]. Recently, delivery of ASOs into the cerebrospinal fluid (CSF) have been linked to neurotoxicity in mice, which is caused by changes in the intercellular levels of calcium [65]. In several studies in mice, ASO delivery to the CNS has led to behavioural abnormalities, such as decreased desire to explore the cage, reduced responsiveness to stimulation, unusual postures, disrupted breathing patterns, and reduced consciousness [65–68]. However, this phenomenon has not been reported in any human patients to date.

Importantly, up to 50% of patients in some clinical trials have failed to respond to nusinersen for unknown reasons [64]. Regardless of these drawbacks, nusinersen is considered to be reasonably safe, reasonably effective, and is approved for a wider age group than onasemnogene abeparvovec. Indeed, treatment with nusinersen has demonstrated a stabilization of disease progression and even clinically meaningful improvements in the motor function in some adult patients with SMA [69,70].

Risdiplam, marketed as Evrysdi, is a small molecule splicing modifier approved to treat patients with SMA of all ages [71,72]. It also acts on *SMN2* by stabilizing the *SMN2* transcript and promoting the inclusion of exon 7 to increase the cellular levels of full-length SMN protein [14]. The drug is taken once daily in an oral solution and is dosed based on patient age and weight at 0.15 mg–0.25 mg/kg up to 20 kg, and 5 mg is the maximum recommended dose for all patients above 20 kg [73]. In clinical trials, the use of risdiplam improved HMFSE scores, although to a lesser degree than that observed for nusinersen and IT onasemnogene abeparvovec [20,64,74,75]. Patients between 2 to 11 years of age only achieved a mean 1.7-point increase in HMFSE score at month 24 following treatment with risdiplam [74]. Unlike nusinersen, which is designed to interact with only *SMN2* pre-mRNA, risdiplam does not necessarily target only *SMN2*. Indeed, in animal models risdiplam has been associated with alternative splicing of the off-target genes *FOXM1* and *MADD*, which are associated with the cell cycle and apoptosis, respectively [14]. Whether the off-target splicing of *FOXM1*, *MADD*, or other genes has long-term, adverse consequences in treated patients has yet to be determined. The degree of off-target splicing (if any) in patients has not yet been reported [74,75]. The easy administration of risdiplam makes the drug attractive to patients with SMA; however, the clinical benefits do not appear to be as pronounced as onasemnogene abeparvovec or nusinersen.

5. Conclusions

For children with SMA between the ages of 2 and 5, the results of the STRONG trial propose treatment with IT onasemnogene abeparvovec as a therapeutic option as it has a favourable benefit-risk profile. Although there have been some adverse events associated with onasemnogene abeparvovec, this treatment appears more effective than nusinersen in older children with SMA (91.7% versus 57% of children attaining a $\geq$3-point increase in HFMSE score for IT onasemnogene abeparvovec versus nusinersen, respectively) [20,64]. A $\geq$3-point change in HFMSE score is considered a clinically meaningful change involving two or three skills [76,77]. Attaining these skills may translate into significant improvements in the quality of life for children with SMA. For example, an improvement in the HFMSE test item "one hand to head in sitting task" may mean that a patient could assist in their feeding or do so independently. IV onasemnogene abeparvovec has been proven to be effective for at least 7 years [22,23]; thus, it is possible the older children who were IT-treated may also maintain achieved motor milestones for many years after treatment. All of the approved treatments for SMA are exceedingly expensive, but a single dose of onasemnogene abeparvovec is reported to be more cost effective than the chronic dosing of nusinersen [78], and thus may ultimately save health care costs.

Some patients with SMA who previously were treated with onasemnogene abeparvovec have started an additional add-on therapy (nusinersen or risdiplam) [23,59]. In fact, there are dedicated clinical trials exploring the safety and efficacy of treatment with either nusinersen (NCT04488133) or risdiplam (NCT05861986) following treatment with onasemnogene abeparvovec. In most cases, add-on therapy is initiated due to a perceived or real plateauing of motor function improvement following the initial onasemnogene abeparvovec treatment [79–81]. Results from combinatorial therapies have previously been reported, but these are typically of small sample size or have relatively short follow-up duration [79–81]. Onasemnogene abeparvovec, nusinersen, and risdiplam all aim to increase SMN protein concentration, but they use different mechanisms of action to do so [12–18]. Although the use of multiple drugs will obviously increase the already high cost of treatment, a combinatorial approach to treatment may provide an improved outcome compared to monotherapy for some patients with SMA.

In recent years, the prognosis for SMA has been transformed by the availability of life-changing therapeutics. Most notably, the availability of a gene therapy drug restoring a functional copy of *SMN1* through a single intravenous infusion has allowed infants to not only achieve previously unattainable motor milestones, but to also live far beyond the average lifespan of untreated infants. Now, efforts are focusing on expanding the availability of this transformative drug to other age groups. The results of the STRONG clinical trial investigatingIT administration of onasemnogene abeparvovec in older children provides optimism for the field, and positive outcomes from the STEER trial may support broadening the availability of onasemnogene abeparvovec for patients up to the age of 18. Clinically meaningful improvements in motor function from this and other therapies will hopefully improve the quality of life for a wider group of patients with SMA.

Author Contributions: Conceptualization, C.A.R. and R.J.P.; literature search, C.A.R.; resources, R.J.P.; writing—original draft, C.A.R.; writing—review and editing, C.A.R. and R.J.P.; supervision, R.J.P.; funding acquisition, C.A.R. and R.J.P.; project administration, R.J.P. All authors have read and agreed to the published version of the manuscript.

Funding: Research in the Parks lab was supported by grants to R.J.P. from the Canadian Institutes of Health Research (FRN-142316, PJT-178120, FRN-175428, PJT-186267), the Natural Sciences and Engineering Research Council (RGPIN-2019-04786), and Cure SMA/Cure SMA Canada. C.A.R. was supported by a Queen Elizabeth II Graduate Scholarship in Science and Technology from the Ontario Provincial Government (Canada).

Institutional Review Board Statement: Not applicable.

Informed Consent Statement: Not applicable.

Data Availability Statement: Not applicable.

Conflicts of Interest: The authors declare no conflict of interest.

References

1. Werdnig, G. Zwei frühinfantile hereditäre Fälle von progressiver Muskelatrophie unter dem Bilde der Dystrophie, aber anf neurotischer Grundlage. *Arch. Psychiatr. Nervenkrankh.* **1891**, *22*, 437–480. [CrossRef]
2. Hoffmann, J. Ueber chronische spinale Muskelatrophie im Kindesalter, auf familiärer Basis. *Dtsch. Z. Nervenheilkd.* **1893**, *3*, 427–470. [CrossRef]
3. Yeo, C.J.J.; Darras, B.T. Overturning the Paradigm of Spinal Muscular Atrophy as Just a Motor Neuron Disease. *Pediatr. Neurol.* **2020**, *109*, 12–19. [CrossRef]
4. Deguise, M.O.; Baranello, G.; Mastella, C.; Beauvais, A.; Michaud, J.; Leone, A.; De Amicis, R.; Battezzati, A.; Dunham, C.; Selby, K.; et al. Abnormal fatty acid metabolism is a core component of spinal muscular atrophy. *Ann. Clin. Transl. Neurol.* **2019**, *6*, 1519–1532. [CrossRef] [PubMed]
5. Nery, F.C.; Siranosian, J.J.; Rosales, I.; Deguise, M.O.; Sharma, A.; Muhtaseb, A.W.; Nwe, P.; Johnstone, A.J.; Zhang, R.; Fatouraei, M.; et al. Impaired kidney structure and function in spinal muscular atrophy. *Neurol. Genet.* **2019**, *5*, e353. [CrossRef] [PubMed]
6. Lefebvre, S.; Bürglen, L.; Reboullet, S.; Clermont, O.; Burlet, P.; Viollet, L.; Benichou, B.; Cruaud, C.; Millasseau, P.; Zeviani, M. Identification and characterization of a spinal muscular atrophy-determining gene. *Cell* **1995**, *80*, 155–165. [CrossRef]
7. Lefebvre, S.; Burlet, P.; Liu, Q.; Bertrandy, S.; Clermont, O.; Munnich, A.; Dreyfuss, G.; Melki, J. Correlation between severity and SMN protein level in spinal muscular atrophy. *Nat. Genet.* **1997**, *16*, 265–269. [CrossRef]
8. Lorson, C.L.; Hahnen, E.; Androphy, E.J.; Wirth, B. A single nucleotide in the SMN gene regulates splicing and is responsible for spinal muscular atrophy. *Proc. Natl. Acad. Sci. USA* **1999**, *96*, 6307–6311. [CrossRef]
9. Monani, U.R.; Lorson, C.L.; Parsons, D.W.; Prior, T.W.; Androphy, E.J.; Burghes, A.H.; McPherson, J.D. A single nucleotide difference that alters splicing patterns distinguishes the SMA gene SMN1 from the copy gene SMN2. *Hum. Mol. Genet.* **1999**, *8*, 1177–1183. [CrossRef]
10. Wadman, R.I.; Jansen, M.D.; Stam, M.; Wijngaarde, C.A.; Curial, C.A.D.; Medic, J.; Sodaar, P.; Schouten, J.; Vijzelaar, R.; Lemmink, H.H.; et al. Intragenic and structural variation in the SMN locus and clinical variability in spinal muscular atrophy. *Brain Commun.* **2020**, *2*, fcaa075. [CrossRef]

11. Feldkötter, M.; Schwarzer, V.; Wirth, R.; Wienker, T.F.; Wirth, B. Quantitative analyses of SMN1 and SMN2 based on real-time lightCycler PCR: Fast and highly reliable carrier testing and prediction of severity of spinal muscular atrophy. *Am. J. Hum. Genet.* **2002**, *70*, 358–368. [CrossRef] [PubMed]
12. Singh, R.N.; Singh, N.N. Mechanism of Splicing Regulation of Spinal Muscular Atrophy Genes. *Adv. Neurobiol.* **2018**, *20*, 31–61. [CrossRef] [PubMed]
13. Chiriboga, C.A.; Swoboda, K.J.; Darras, B.T.; Iannaccone, S.T.; Montes, J.; De Vivo, D.C.; Norris, D.A.; Bennett, C.F.; Bishop, K.M. Results from a phase 1 study of nusinersen (ISIS-SMN(Rx)) in children with spinal muscular atrophy. *Neurology* **2016**, *86*, 890–897. [CrossRef] [PubMed]
14. Ratni, H.; Ebeling, M.; Baird, J.; Bendels, S.; Bylund, J.; Chen, K.S.; Denk, N.; Feng, Z.; Green, L.; Guerard, M.; et al. Discovery of Risdiplam, a Selective Survival of Motor Neuron-2 (SMN2) Gene Splicing Modifier for the Treatment of Spinal Muscular Atrophy (SMA). *J. Med. Chem.* **2018**, *61*, 6501–6517. [CrossRef]
15. AveXis. AveXis Receives FDA Approval for Zolgensma®, the First and Only Gene Therapy for Pediatric Patients with Spinal Muscular Atrophy (SMA). 2019. Available online: https://www.novartis.com/news/media-releases/avexis-receives-fda-approval-zolgensma-first-and-only-gene-therapy-pediatric-patients-spinal-muscular-atrophy-sma (accessed on 11 October 2022).
16. Novartis. Novartis Receives Approval from Japanese Ministry of Health, Labour and Welfare for Zolgensma®the Only Gene Therapy for Patients with Spinal Muscular Atrophy (SMA). 2020. Available online: https://www.novartis.com/news/media-releases/novartis-receives-approval-from-japanese-ministry-health-labour-and-welfare-zolgensma-only-gene-therapy-patients-spinal-muscular-atrophy-sma#:~:text=(%E2%80%9CNovartis%20Pharma%E2%80%9D)%20today,are%20pre%2Dsymptomatic%20at%20diagnosis (accessed on 18 April 2023).
17. Health-Canada. Summary Basis of Decision—Zolgensma—Health Canada. 2021. Available online: https://hpr-rps.hres.ca/reg-content/summary-basis-decision-detailTwo.php?linkID=SBD00521#AClinBasisTitle (accessed on 18 April 2023).
18. European-Medicines-Agency. New Gene Therapy to Treat Spinal Muscular Atrophy. 2020. Available online: https://www.ema.europa.eu/en/news/new-gene-therapy-treat-spinal-muscular-atrophy-corrected (accessed on 14 June 2023).
19. Chand, D.; Mohr, F.; McMillan, H.; Tukov, F.F.; Montgomery, K.; Kleyn, A.; Sun, R.; Tauscher-Wisniewski, S.; Kaufmann, P.; Kullak-Ublick, G. Hepatotoxicity following administration of onasemnogene abeparvovec (AVXS-101) for the treatment of spinal muscular atrophy. *J. Hepatol.* **2021**, *74*, 560–566. [CrossRef]
20. Finkel, R.S.; Darras, B.T.; Mendell, J.R.; Day, J.W.; Kuntz, N.L.; Connolly, A.M.; Zaidman, C.; Crawford, T.O.; Butterfield, R.J.; Shieh, P.B.; et al. Intrathecal Onasemnogene Abeparvovec for Sitting, Nonambulatory Patients with Spinal Muscular Atrophy: Phase I Ascending-Dose Study (STRONG). *J. Neuromuscul. Dis.* **2023**, *10*, 389–404. [CrossRef]
21. Mendell, J.R.; Al-Zaidy, S.; Shell, R.; Arnold, W.D.; Rodino-Klapac, L.R.; Prior, T.W.; Lowes, L.; Alfano, L.; Berry, K.; Church, K.; et al. Single-Dose Gene-Replacement Therapy for Spinal Muscular Atrophy. *N. Engl. J. Med.* **2017**, *377*, 1713–1722. [CrossRef] [PubMed]
22. Mendell, J.R.; Al-Zaidy, S.A.; Lehman, K.J.; McColly, M.; Lowes, L.P.; Alfano, L.N.; Reash, N.F.; Iammarino, M.A.; Church, K.R.; Kleyn, A.; et al. Five-Year Extension Results of the Phase 1 START Trial of Onasemnogene Abeparvovec in Spinal Muscular Atrophy. *JAMA Neurol.* **2021**, *78*, 834–841. [CrossRef]
23. Novartis. Novartis Shares Zolgensma Long-Term Data Demonstrating Sustained Durability up to 7.5 Years Post-Dosing; 100% Achievement of All Assessed Milestones in Children Treated Prior to SMA Symptom Onset. 2023. Available online: https://www.novartis.com/news/media-releases/novartis-shares-zolgensma-long-term-data-demonstrating-sustained-durability-75-years-post-dosing-100-achievement-all-assessed-milestones-children-treated-prior-sma-symptom-onset (accessed on 25 March 2023).
24. Kolb, S.J.; Coffey, C.S.; Yankey, J.W.; Krosschell, K.; Arnold, W.D.; Rutkove, S.B.; Swoboda, K.J.; Reyna, S.P.; Sakonju, A.; Darras, B.T.; et al. Natural history of infantile-onset spinal muscular atrophy. *Ann. Neurol.* **2017**, *82*, 883–891. [CrossRef]
25. Finkel, R.S.; McDermott, M.P.; Kaufmann, P.; Darras, B.T.; Chung, W.K.; Sproule, D.M.; Kang, P.B.; Foley, A.R.; Yang, M.L.; Martens, W.B.; et al. Observational study of spinal muscular atrophy type I and implications for clinical trials. *Neurology* **2014**, *83*, 810–817. [CrossRef] [PubMed]
26. Day, J.W.; Finkel, R.S.; Chiriboga, C.A.; Connolly, A.M.; Crawford, T.O.; Darras, B.T.; Iannaccone, S.T.; Kuntz, N.L.; Peña, L.D.M.; Shieh, P.B.; et al. Onasemnogene abeparvovec gene therapy for symptomatic infantile-onset spinal muscular atrophy in patients with two copies of SMN2 (STR1VE): An open-label, single-arm, multicentre, phase 3 trial. *Lancet Neurol.* **2021**, *20*, 284–293. [CrossRef]
27. Mercuri, E.; Muntoni, F.; Baranello, G.; Masson, R.; Boespflug-Tanguy, O.; Bruno, C.; Corti, S.; Daron, A.; Deconinck, N.; Servais, L.; et al. Onasemnogene abeparvovec gene therapy for symptomatic infantile-onset spinal muscular atrophy type 1 (STR1VE-EU): An open-label, single-arm, multicentre, phase 3 trial. *Lancet Neurol.* **2021**, *20*, 832–841. [CrossRef] [PubMed]
28. Strauss, K.A.; Farrar, M.A.; Muntoni, F.; Saito, K.; Mendell, J.R.; Servais, L.; McMillan, H.J.; Finkel, R.S.; Swoboda, K.J.; Kwon, J.M.; et al. Onasemnogene abeparvovec for presymptomatic infants with two copies of SMN2 at risk for spinal muscular atrophy type 1: The Phase III SPR1NT trial. *Nat. Med.* **2022**, *28*, 1381–1389. [CrossRef] [PubMed]
29. Strauss, K.A.; Farrar, M.A.; Muntoni, F.; Saito, K.; Mendell, J.R.; Servais, L.; McMillan, H.J.; Finkel, R.S.; Swoboda, K.J.; Kwon, J.M.; et al. Onasemnogene abeparvovec for presymptomatic infants with three copies of SMN2 at risk for spinal muscular atrophy: The Phase III SPR1NT trial. *Nat. Med.* **2022**, *28*, 1390–1397. [CrossRef] [PubMed]

30. Chand, D.H.; Mitchell, S.; Sun, R.; LaMarca, N.; Reyna, S.P.; Sutter, T. Safety of Onasemnogene Abeparvovec for Patients With Spinal Muscular Atrophy 8.5 kg or Heavier in a Global Managed Access Program. *Pediatr. Neurol.* **2022**, *132*, 27–32. [CrossRef]
31. Novartis. Zolgensma Global Managed Access Program in 2023. 2023. Available online: https://www.novartis.com/news/zolgensma-global-managed-access-program-2023 (accessed on 25 March 2023).
32. European-Medicines-Agency. Summary of the Risk Management Plan for Zolgensma®.(*Onasemnogene abeparvovec*). 2023. Available online: https://www.ema.europa.eu/en/documents/rmp-summary/zolgensma-epar-risk-management-plan-summary_en.pdf (accessed on 18 April 2023).
33. De Amicis, R.; Baranello, G.; Foppiani, A.; Leone, A.; Battezzati, A.; Bedogni, G.; Ravella, S.; Giaquinto, E.; Mastella, C.; Agosto, C.; et al. Growth patterns in children with spinal muscular atrophy. *Orphanet J. Rare Dis.* **2021**, *16*, 375. [CrossRef]
34. Hinderer, C.; Katz, N.; Buza, E.L.; Dyer, C.; Goode, T.; Bell, P.; Richman, L.K.; Wilson, J.M. Severe Toxicity in Nonhuman Primates and Piglets Following High-Dose Intravenous Administration of an Adeno-Associated Virus Vector Expressing Human SMN. *Hum. Gene Ther.* **2018**, *29*, 285–298. [CrossRef]
35. René, C.A.; Parks, R.J. Delivery of Therapeutic Agents to the Central Nervous System and the Promise of Extracellular Vesicles. *Pharmaceutics* **2021**, *13*, 492. [CrossRef]
36. Thomsen, G.; Burghes, A.H.M.; Hsieh, C.; Do, J.; Chu, B.T.T.; Perry, S.; Barkho, B.; Kaufmann, P.; Sproule, D.M.; Feltner, D.E.; et al. Biodistribution of onasemnogene abeparvovec DNA, mRNA and SMN protein in human tissue. *Nat. Med.* **2021**, *27*, 1701–1711. [CrossRef]
37. Yazaki, K.; Sakuma, S.; Hikita, N.; Fujimaru, R.; Hamazaki, T. Child Neurology: Pathologically Confirmed Thrombotic Microangiopathy Caused by Onasemnogene Abeparvovec Treatment for SMA. *Neurology* **2022**, *98*, 808–813. [CrossRef]
38. Waldrop, M.A.; Karingada, C.; Storey, M.A.; Powers, B.; Iammarino, M.A.; Miller, N.F.; Alfano, L.N.; Noritz, G.; Rossman, I.; Ginsberg, M.; et al. Gene Therapy for Spinal Muscular Atrophy: Safety and Early Outcomes. *Pediatrics* **2020**, *146*, e20200729. [CrossRef]
39. Weiß, C.; Ziegler, A.; Becker, L.L.; Johannsen, J.; Brennenstuhl, H.; Schreiber, G.; Flotats-Bastardas, M.; Stoltenburg, C.; Hartmann, H.; Illsinger, S.; et al. Gene replacement therapy with onasemnogene abeparvovec in children with spinal muscular atrophy aged 24 months or younger and bodyweight up to 15 kg: An observational cohort study. *Lancet Child Adolesc. Health* **2022**, *6*, 17–27. [CrossRef] [PubMed]
40. Silverman, E. Novartis Reports Two Children Died from Acute Liver Failure after Treatment with Zolgensma Gene Therapy. 2022. Available online: https://www.statnews.com/pharmalot/2022/08/11/novartis-zolgensma-liver-failure-gene-therapy-death/ (accessed on 11 October 2022).
41. Novartis. Zolgensma Acute Liver Failure Update. 2022. Available online: https://www.novartis.com/news/zolgensma-acute-liver-failure-update (accessed on 11 October 2022).
42. Astellas. Astellas Reports Update to September 1 Announcement on the ASPIRO Clinical Trial of AT132 in Patients with X-Linked Myotubular Myopathy. 2021. Available online: https://www.astellas.com/en/news/17161 (accessed on 19 October 2022).
43. Astellas. Audentes Therapeutics Provides Update on the ASPIRO Clinical Trial Evaluating AT132 in Patients with X-linked Myotubular Myopathy. 2020. Available online: https://www.astellas.com/en/news/22726 (accessed on 19 October 2022).
44. Philippidis, A. Fourth Boy Dies in Trial of Astellas Gene Therapy Candidate. 2021. Available online: https://www.genengnews.com/news/fourth-boy-dies-in-trial-of-astellas-gene-therapy-candidate/ (accessed on 19 October 2022).
45. Morales, L.; Gambhir, Y.; Bennett, J.; Stedman, H.H. Broader Implications of Progressive Liver Dysfunction and Lethal Sepsis in Two Boys following Systemic High-Dose AAV. *Mol. Ther.* **2020**, *28*, 1753–1755. [CrossRef]
46. Molera, C.; Sarishvili, T.; Nascimento, A.; Rtskhiladze, I.; Muñoz Bartolo, G.; Fernández Cebrián, S.; Valverde Fernández, J.; Muñoz Cabello, B.; Graham, R.J.; Miller, W.; et al. Intrahepatic Cholestasis Is a Clinically Significant Feature Associated with Natural History of X-Linked Myotubular Myopathy (XLMTM): A Case Series and Biopsy Report. *J. Neuromuscul. Dis.* **2022**, *9*, 73–82. [CrossRef]
47. Nault, J.C.; Datta, S.; Imbeaud, S.; Franconi, A.; Mallet, M.; Couchy, G.; Letouzé, E.; Pilati, C.; Verret, B.; Blanc, J.F.; et al. Recurrent AAV2-related insertional mutagenesis in human hepatocellular carcinomas. *Nat. Genet.* **2015**, *47*, 1187–1193. [CrossRef]
48. Zhong, L.; Malani, N.; Li, M.; Brady, T.; Xie, J.; Bell, P.; Li, S.; Jones, H.; Wilson, J.M.; Flotte, T.R.; et al. Recombinant adeno-associated virus integration sites in murine liver after ornithine transcarbamylase gene correction. *Hum. Gene Ther.* **2013**, *24*, 520–525. [CrossRef]
49. Donsante, A.; Vogler, C.; Muzyczka, N.; Crawford, J.M.; Barker, J.; Flotte, T.; Campbell-Thompson, M.; Daly, T.; Sands, M.S. Observed incidence of tumorigenesis in long-term rodent studies of rAAV vectors. *Gene. Ther.* **2001**, *8*, 1343–1346. [CrossRef]
50. Dalwadi, D.A.; Torrens, L.; Abril-Fornaguera, J.; Pinyol, R.; Willoughby, C.; Posey, J.; Llovet, J.M.; Lanciault, C.; Russell, D.W.; Grompe, M.; et al. Liver Injury Increases the Incidence of HCC following AAV Gene Therapy in Mice. *Mol. Ther.* **2021**, *29*, 680–690. [CrossRef]
51. Bell, P.; Moscioni, A.D.; McCarter, R.J.; Wu, D.; Gao, G.; Hoang, A.; Sanmiguel, J.C.; Sun, X.; Wivel, N.A.; Raper, S.E.; et al. Analysis of tumors arising in male B6C3F1 mice with and without AAV vector delivery to liver. *Mol. Ther.* **2006**, *14*, 34–44. [CrossRef]
52. Bell, P.; Wang, L.; Lebherz, C.; Flieder, D.B.; Bove, M.S.; Wu, D.; Gao, G.P.; Wilson, J.M.; Wivel, N.A. No evidence for tumorigenesis of AAV vectors in a large-scale study in mice. *Mol. Ther.* **2005**, *12*, 299–306. [CrossRef]

53. Gil-Farina, I.; Fronza, R.; Kaeppel, C.; Lopez-Franco, E.; Ferreira, V.; D'Avola, D.; Benito, A.; Prieto, J.; Petry, H.; Gonzalez-Aseguinolaza, G.; et al. Recombinant AAV Integration Is Not Associated With Hepatic Genotoxicity in Nonhuman Primates and Patients. *Mol. Ther.* **2016**, *24*, 1100–1105. [CrossRef]
54. Sabatino, D.E.; Bushman, F.D.; Chandler, R.J.; Crystal, R.G.; Davidson, B.L.; Dolmetsch, R.; Eggan, K.C.; Gao, G.; Gil-Farina, I.; Kay, M.A.; et al. Evaluating the state of the science for adeno-associated virus integration: An integrated perspective. *Mol. Ther.* **2022**, *30*, 2646–2663. [CrossRef] [PubMed]
55. Meyer, K.; Ferraiuolo, L.; Schmelzer, L.; Braun, L.; McGovern, V.; Likhite, S.; Michels, O.; Govoni, A.; Fitzgerald, J.; Morales, P.; et al. Improving single injection CSF delivery of AAV9-mediated gene therapy for SMA: A dose-response study in mice and nonhuman primates. *Mol. Ther.* **2015**, *23*, 477–487. [CrossRef] [PubMed]
56. Tukov, F.F.; Mansfield, K.; Milton, M.; Meseck, E.; Penraat, K.; Chand, D.; Hartmann, A. Single-Dose Intrathecal Dorsal Root Ganglia Toxicity of Onasemnogene Abeparvovec in Cynomolgus Monkeys. *Hum. Gene Ther.* **2022**, *33*, 740–756. [CrossRef]
57. Novartis. Novartis Announces AVXS-101 Intrathecal Study Update. 2019. Available online: https://www.novartis.com/news/media-releases/novartis-announces-avxs-101-intrathecal-study-update (accessed on 11 October 2022).
58. Novartis. Novartis Announces Lift of Partial Clinical Trial Hold and Plans to Initiate a New, Pivotal Phase 3 Study of Intrathecal OAV-101 in Older Patients with SMA. 2021. Available online: https://www.novartis.com/news/media-releases/novartis-announces-lift-partial-clinical-trial-hold-and-plans-initiate-new-pivotal-phase-3-study-intrathecal-oav-101-older-patients-sma (accessed on 11 October 2022).
59. Connolly, A.M.; Mercuri, E.; Strauss, K.A.; Day, J.W.; Chien, Y.-H.; Masson, R.; Widgerson, M.; Alecu, I.; Ballarini, N.; Mehl, L.; et al. Intravenous and Intrathecal Onasemnogene Abeparvovec Gene Therapy in Symptomatic and Presymptomatic Spinal Muscular Atrophy: Long-Term Follow-Up Study. In Proceedings of the 2023 MDA Clinical & Scientific Conference, Dallas, TX, USA, 19–23 March 2023.
60. Dangouloff, T.; Vrščaj, E.; Servais, L.; Osredkar, D.; Group, S.N.W.S. Newborn screening programs for spinal muscular atrophy worldwide: Where we stand and where to go. *Neuromuscul. Disord.* **2021**, *31*, 574–582. [CrossRef]
61. Finkel, R.S.; Mercuri, E.; Darras, B.T.; Connolly, A.M.; Kuntz, N.L.; Kirschner, J.; Chiriboga, C.A.; Saito, K.; Servais, L.; Tizzano, E.; et al. Nusinersen versus Sham Control in Infantile-Onset Spinal Muscular Atrophy. *N. Engl. J. Med.* **2017**, *377*, 1723–1732. [CrossRef]
62. Passini, M.A.; Bu, J.; Richards, A.M.; Kinnecom, C.; Sardi, S.P.; Stanek, L.M.; Hua, Y.; Rigo, F.; Matson, J.; Hung, G.; et al. Antisense oligonucleotides delivered to the mouse CNS ameliorate symptoms of severe spinal muscular atrophy. *Sci. Transl. Med.* **2011**, *3*, 72ra18. [CrossRef]
63. Biogen. Spinraza Prescribing Information. 2020. Available online: https://www.spinraza.com/content/dam/commercial/spinraza/caregiver/en_us/pdf/spinraza-prescribing-information.pdf (accessed on 20 October 2022).
64. Mercuri, E.; Darras, B.T.; Chiriboga, C.A.; Day, J.W.; Campbell, C.; Connolly, A.M.; Iannaccone, S.T.; Kirschner, J.; Kuntz, N.L.; Saito, K.; et al. Nusinersen versus Sham Control in Later-Onset Spinal Muscular Atrophy. *N. Engl. J. Med.* **2018**, *378*, 625–635. [CrossRef]
65. Jia, C.; Lei Mon, S.S.; Yang, Y.; Katsuyama, M.; Yoshida-Tanaka, K.; Nagata, T.; Yoshioka, K.; Yokota, T. Change of intracellular calcium level causes acute neurotoxicity by antisense oligonucleotides via CSF route. *Mol. Ther. Nucleic Acids* **2023**, *31*, 182–196. [CrossRef]
66. Southwell, A.L.; Skotte, N.H.; Kordasiewicz, H.B.; Østergaard, M.E.; Watt, A.T.; Carroll, J.B.; Doty, C.N.; Villanueva, E.B.; Petoukhov, E.; Vaid, K.; et al. In vivo evaluation of candidate allele-specific mutant huntingtin gene silencing antisense oligonucleotides. *Mol. Ther.* **2014**, *22*, 2093–2106. [CrossRef]
67. Toonen, L.J.A.; Casaca-Carreira, J.; Pellisé-Tintoré, M.; Mei, H.; Temel, Y.; Jahanshahi, A.; van Roon-Mom, W.M.C. Intracerebroventricular Administration of a 2′-O-Methyl Phosphorothioate Antisense Oligonucleotide Results in Activation of the Innate Immune System in Mouse Brain. *Nucleic Acid Ther.* **2018**, *28*, 63–73. [CrossRef] [PubMed]
68. Hagedorn, P.H.; Brown, J.M.; Easton, A.; Pierdomenico, M.; Jones, K.; Olson, R.E.; Mercer, S.E.; Li, D.; Loy, J.; Høg, A.M.; et al. Acute Neurotoxicity of Antisense Oligonucleotides after Intracerebroventricular Injection into Mouse Brain Can Be Predicted from Sequence Features. *Nucleic Acid Ther.* **2022**, *32*, 151–162. [CrossRef]
69. Pechmann, A.; Behrens, M.; Dörnbrack, K.; Tassoni, A.; Wenzel, F.; Stein, S.; Vogt, S.; Zöller, D.; Bernert, G.; Hagenacker, T.; et al. Improvements in Walking Distance during Nusinersen Treatment—A Prospective 3-year SMArtCARE Registry Study. *J. Neuromuscul. Dis.* **2023**, *10*, 29–40. [CrossRef]
70. Arslan, D.; Inan, B.; Kilinc, M.; Bekircan-Kurt, C.E.; Erdem-Ozdamar, S.; Tan, E. Nusinersen for adults with spinal muscular atrophy. *Neurol. Sci.* **2023**, *44*, 2393–2400. [CrossRef]
71. Dhillon, S. Risdiplam: First Approval. *Drugs* **2020**, *80*, 1853–1858. [CrossRef]
72. Wire, B. FDA Approves Genentech's Evrysdi (Risdiplam) for Use in Babies under Two Months with Spinal Muscular Atrophy (SMA). 2022. Available online: https://www.businesswire.com/news/home/20220530005033/en/FDA-Approves-Genentech (accessed on 11 October 2022).
73. Genentech. Evrysdi Prescribing Information. 2022. Available online: https://www.gene.com/download/pdf/evrysdi_prescribing.pdf (accessed on 3 April 2023)

74. Mercuri, E.; Baranello, G.; Boespflug-Tanguy, O.; De Waele, L.; Goemans, N.; Kirschner, J.; Masson, R.; Mazzone, E.S.; Pechmann, A.; Pera, M.C.; et al. Risdiplam in types 2 and 3 spinal muscular atrophy: A randomised, placebo-controlled, dose-finding trial followed by 24 months of treatment. *Eur. J. Neurol.* **2022**, *30*, 1945–1956. [CrossRef]
75. Mercuri, E.; Deconinck, N.; Mazzone, E.S.; Nascimento, A.; Oskoui, M.; Saito, K.; Vuillerot, C.; Baranello, G.; Boespflug-Tanguy, O.; Goemans, N.; et al. Safety and efficacy of once-daily risdiplam in type 2 and non-ambulant type 3 spinal muscular atrophy (SUNFISH part 2): A phase 3, double-blind, randomised, placebo-controlled trial. *Lancet Neurol.* **2022**, *21*, 42–52. [CrossRef]
76. Glanzman, A.M.; O'Hagen, J.M.; McDermott, M.P.; Martens, W.B.; Flickinger, J.; Riley, S.; Quigley, J.; Montes, J.; Dunaway, S.; Deng, L.; et al. Validation of the Expanded Hammersmith Functional Motor Scale in spinal muscular atrophy type II and III. *J. Child Neurol.* **2011**, *26*, 1499–1507. [CrossRef]
77. O'Hagen, J.M.; Glanzman, A.M.; McDermott, M.P.; Ryan, P.A.; Flickinger, J.; Quigley, J.; Riley, S.; Sanborn, E.; Irvine, C.; Martens, W.B.; et al. An expanded version of the Hammersmith Functional Motor Scale for SMA II and III patients. *Neuromuscul. Disord.* **2007**, *17*, 693–697. [CrossRef]
78. Malone, D.C.; Dean, R.; Arjunji, R.; Jensen, I.; Cyr, P.; Miller, B.; Maru, B.; Sproule, D.M.; Feltner, D.E.; Dabbous, O. Cost-effectiveness analysis of using onasemnogene abeparvocec (AVXS-101) in spinal muscular atrophy type 1 patients. *J. Mark. Access Health Policy* **2019**, *7*, 1601484. [CrossRef]
79. Oechsel, K.F.; Cartwright, M.S. Combination therapy with onasemnogene and risdiplam in spinal muscular atrophy type 1. *Muscle Nerve* **2021**, *64*, 487–490. [CrossRef] [PubMed]
80. Mirea, A.; Shelby, E.S.; Axente, M.; Badina, M.; Padure, L.; Leanca, M.; Dima, V.; Sporea, C. Combination Therapy with Nusinersen and Onasemnogene Abeparvovec-xioi in Spinal Muscular Atrophy Type I. *J. Clin. Med.* **2021**, *10*, 5540. [CrossRef] [PubMed]
81. Chiriboga, C.A.; Bruno, C.; Duong, T.; Fischer, D.; Mercuri, E.; Kirschner, J.; Kostera-Pruszczyk, A.; Jaber, B.; Gorni, K.; Kletzl, H.; et al. Risdiplam in Patients Previously Treated with Other Therapies for Spinal Muscular Atrophy: An Interim Analysis from the JEWELFISH Study. *Neurol. Ther.* **2023**, *12*, 543–557. [CrossRef]

pharmaceutics

Systematic Review

Intranasal Corticosteroids and Oral Montelukast for Paediatric Obstructive Sleep Apnoea: A Systematic Review

Marco Zaffanello [1,*], Angelo Pietrobelli [1], Luana Nosetti [2], Franco Antoniazzi [1], Rossella Frassoldati [3] and Giorgio Piacentini [1]

1 Department of Surgical Sciences, Dentistry, Gynecology and Pediatrics, University of Verona, 37126 Verona, Italy; angelo.pietrobelli@univr.it (A.P.); franco.antoniazzi@univr.it (F.A.); giorgio.piacentini@univr.it (G.P.)
2 Pediatric Department, Department of Medicine and Technological Innovation, Insubria University, F del Ponte Hospital, 21100 Varese, Italy; luana.nosetti@uninsubria.it
3 Department of Pediatrics, Women's & Child's University Hospital, 37126 Verona, Italy; rossella.frassoldati@aovr.veneto.it
* Correspondence: marco.zaffanello@univr.it

Abstract: Background/Objectives: Paediatric Obstructive Sleep Apnoea (OSA) is characterised by recurrent episodes of upper airway obstruction during sleep, manifesting as snoring, intermittent oxygen desaturation, and frequent nocturnal awakenings. Standard treatments include surgical interventions, pharmacological therapies, intranasal corticosteroids, and oral montelukast. However, significant variability exists across studies regarding dosage and outcome assessment. This literature review systematically evaluated clinical evidence regarding the efficacy and safety of intranasal corticosteroids and oral montelukast for treating sleep-disordered breathing and its primary underlying condition, adenoid hypertrophy, in otherwise healthy children. **Methods:** The MEDLINE (PubMed), Scopus, and Web of Science databases were systematically searched up to 13 February 2025, using tailored search terms combining keywords and synonyms related to paediatric OSA, adenoidal hypertrophy, corticosteroids, montelukast, and randomised controlled trials. Owing to variability in outcome measures, Fisher's method for p-value combination was employed to enable a comprehensive comparison of drug effects. **Results:** Available evidence shows that intranasal corticosteroids (mometasone, beclometasone, budesonide, fluticasone, and flunisolide), either as monotherapy or in combination with other agents, consistently lead to clinical and instrumental improvements in adenoid hypertrophy and related respiratory symptoms, with a generally favourable safety profile. Combining montelukast with intranasal corticosteroids appears to offer superior benefits compared with monotherapy. Nevertheless, the reviewed studies varied widely in dosage, treatment duration, design, and sample size. The reported side effects are mostly mild; however, long-term studies are lacking to establish the complete safety of these treatments in children. **Conclusions:** Intranasal corticosteroids and oral montelukast effectively and safely manage adenoid hypertrophy and mild-to-moderate OSA symptoms in children. Nonetheless, the heterogeneity of study designs necessitates larger prospective trials with standardised protocols and more extended follow-up periods to draw more robust conclusions. Future studies should aim to stratify treatment outcomes based on OSA severity and duration to tailor therapeutic approaches better.

Keywords: adenoid hypertrophy; children; corticosteroid; infant; montelukast; obstructive sleep apnoea; sleep-disordered breathing

1. Introduction

Obstructive Sleep Apnoea (OSA) is a disorder characterised by recurrent episodes of upper airway obstruction during sleep, associated with snoring, noisy breathing, intermittent desaturation, and nocturnal awakenings [1]. OSA affects approximately 3% of preschool- and school-aged children [2]. The most common cause is adenotonsillar hypertrophy (ATH) [2]. Other risk factors include obesity, craniofacial abnormalities, and neuromuscular diseases, although they are less common [2]. Children with OSA may present with habitual snoring, restless sleep, mouth breathing, and attention and mood disorders more frequently [3].

The gold standard for diagnosis is overnight Polysomnography (PSG). However, owing to the limited availability of paediatric sleep laboratories, screening questionnaires have been developed to identify children at risk of OSA, such as the Paediatric Sleep Questionnaire (PSQ) and OSA-18 [4,5]. An anatomical evaluation of the upper airway is required to complete the diagnostic assessment. In particular, adenoid size is assessed through nasopharyngeal endoscopy and/or radiological imaging [6,7].

The treatment of paediatric OSA is selected based on the severity of the clinical polysomnographic profile and the underlying causes [8]. In moderate-to-severe forms, adenotonsillectomy is the first-line treatment for significant ATH [9]. Medical treatment is available in mild-to-moderate cases, or when surgery is contraindicated. Specifically, local and systemic anti-inflammatory therapies may have therapeutic roles in paediatric OSA [9,10]. Intranasal corticosteroids and leukotriene antagonists, such as oral montelukast, may improve symptoms and reduce polysomnographic severity indices [11].

Intranasal corticosteroids reduce nasal mucosal oedema and inflammatory mediator production (IL-6, IL-1β, and TNF-α) [12] and decrease adenoid volume [12]. Montelukast inhibits the cysLT1 receptor, reduces eosinophilic infiltration and oedema in lymphoid tissues [13], decreases the expression of COX-2 and 5-lipoxygenase, and reduces circulating levels of IL-8 and high-sensitivity CRP [14,15].

Literature from the past decade suggests that intranasal corticosteroids can improve symptoms related to adenoid hypertrophy (AH). A meta-analysis of eight RCTs demonstrated that mometasone significantly reduced nasal obstruction and the adenoid-to-choana ratio (A/C ratio) [16]. Another meta-analysis, which included five trials (mometasone furoate, fluticasone propionate, and budesonide), also conducted on adults, revealed a high risk of bias and considerable methodological heterogeneity [17].

Oral montelukast, evaluated in four RCTs involving children with mild to moderate OSA, significantly improved polysomnographic parameters [15]. However, a review of five trials, three on intranasal corticosteroids and two on montelukast, with the Apnoea–Hypopnea index (AHI) as the primary outcome, demonstrated insufficient evidence supporting corticosteroid efficacy and only short-term benefits for montelukast, without long-term safety data [9]. Another study involving children aged 1 to 16 years confirmed the short-term positive effects of intranasal corticosteroids and montelukast on desaturation indices and oxygen saturation [18].

The combined use of montelukast and intranasal corticosteroids, as well as montelukast monotherapy, also appears effective in the short-term management of paediatric OSA (reduction in AHI) [11] and in the treatment of AH [19]. In an analysis of 17 RCTs involving children aged 2–14 years with OSA, mometasone combined with montelukast, budesonide, and montelukast monotherapy showed superiority over placebo in improving AHI [20]. Similarly, combined treatment with mometasone and montelukast was more effective than mometasone alone in improving symptoms and adenoid-to-nasopharynx ratio (A/N ratio) [21].

A traditional meta-analysis approach may be complex or less informative because of the significant heterogeneity in the primary outcomes reported in previous studies. Fisher's Combined Probability Test enables aggregating results based on p-values, avoiding methodological issues associated with data transformation into a single standard measure. Moreover, this method determines the overall significance of the association between the intervention and outcome [22,23].

2. Materials and Methods

2.1. Search Strategy and Study Selection

We searched three major databases—MEDLINE (PubMed), Scopus, and Web of Science—for English-language studies published up to 13 February 2025. MeSH terms and text words (and their combinations and truncated synonyms) were used. Customised search terms were adapted for each database, combining keywords and synonyms: (children OR pediatric) AND (obstructive sleep apnoea OR sleep-disordered breathing OR adenoidal hypertrophy) AND (corticosteroids OR montelukast) AND (randomised controlled study). The search terms used are presented in Appendix A.

Studies were eligible for inclusion if they were

(1) The paediatric population.
(2) Assessed the effects of intranasal corticosteroids and/or montelukast in treating Obstructive Sleep Apnoea (OSA), sleep disordered breathing (SDB), and adenoid hypertrophy (AH).
(3) Employed a randomised controlled design.
(4) Reported the clinical and/or instrumental outcomes.

We excluded studies that did not meet these criteria, non-English publications, animal studies, and studies involving surgical or non-pharmacological interventions. No restrictions were placed on geographical region, sex, or specific age ranges within the paediatric population. No particular outcome domains were predefined to allow the inclusion of all clinically relevant findings compatible with the scope of the review.

Duplicate articles were removed before screening the abstracts. Two authors (MZ and LN) reviewed the titles and abstracts independently, followed by full-text assessments. Discrepancies were resolved through discussion or adjudication by a third reviewer (AP). The reference lists of the included studies were screened for additional eligible articles. Ethical approval was not required because the study did not involve human participants. The systematic review followed the PRISMA guidelines [24].

2.2. Statistics

The AI tools (QUADAS-2 and QUADAS-C, ASReview, Abstrackr, RobotAnalyst, EPPI-Reviewer, and DistillerSR) are a promising innovation for systematic review practices [25,26]. During the revision process, Generative AI (ChatGPT 4 and 4o, Plus plan, OpenAI) [27,28] was used to explore appropriate statistical approaches for synthesising heterogeneous p-values derived from RCT.

To comprehensively compare the effect of the drug versus control across these studies, considering the variety of outcome measures and the predominant availability of p-values, we employed the probability combination method known as Fisher's [22,23].

Using Fisher's method, the statistic $X^2_{2k} = -2\sum_{i=1}^{k} \ln(p_i)$, where p_i is the p-value from the ith test, and k is the total number of combined tests. The resulting variables X^2 approximately follow a chi-square distribution with $2k$ degrees of freedom, calculated as twice the number of studies included. By comparing this X^2 value against critical values from the chi-square distribution with 2*k* degrees of freedom (as found in the chi-square distribution tables), an overall combined *p*-value was obtained [29].

The AI tool also assisted in designing a datasheet for applying Fisher's method of *p*-value combinations. The detailed procedure for calculating the combined *p*-values using Fisher's method in Microsoft® Excel® for Microsoft 365 MSO (Version 2503) is provided in Appendix B, Table A1.

The main *p*-values reported by each study were selected by identifying the value(s) representing the primary endpoint or the most directly comparable outcome across the trials. For each study, at least one *p*-value for the difference between the treatment and control groups was considered. This approach allowed for an overall estimation of treatment effectiveness, even when individual studies reported distinct *p*-values without sufficiently homogeneous data. The authors critically reviewed and approved all the analyses, decisions, and interpretations.

3. Results

In total, 170 articles were identified, of which 46 were duplicates. Consequently, 124 studies were included (Figure 1). After the selection process, 40 articles were included in the final analysis. After full-text analysis, an additional 10 studies were examined and excluded. Overall, 30 studies met the inclusion criteria.

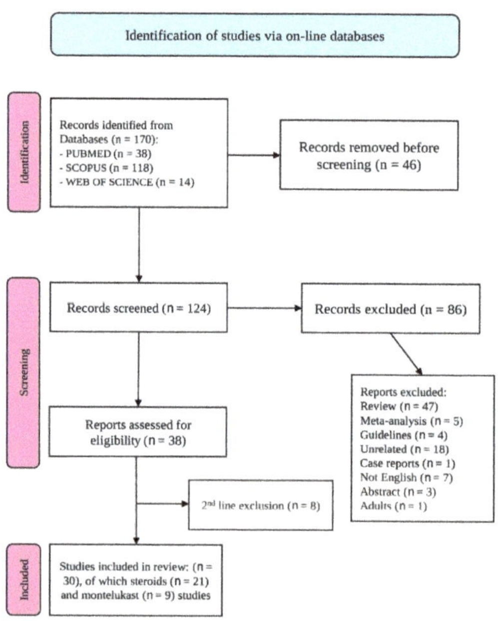

Figure 1. The PRISMA flow diagram [24] visually represents the study selection process and number of studies included at each stage. For more information, visit: http://www.prisma-statement.org/ (accessed on 16 February 2025).

Table 1 summarises the controlled clinical trials, including randomised [30–33], double-blind (placebo-controlled) [30–32], crossover [34], and multi-centre studies [31]. Some studies included larger sample sizes (*n* > 200) [31], whereas others enrolled fewer than 30 participants [34]. Inclusion criteria were clearly defined, targeting children with AH [30,34–36] associated with obstructive respiratory symptoms [31,32] and otitis media with effusion (OME) [35,36].

Table 1. Clinical studies on treating adenoid hypertrophy and sleep-disordered breathing symptoms with mometasone furoate (MF).

Reference	Design	Pop (Age)	N	In/Ex	Tx vs. Ctrl	Dur	O1	O2	Out (Tx)	Out (Ctrl)	Stat
Bhargava (2014) [35]	DB-RCT	Child. 2–12 yrs, AH ± OME	100 (30 vs. 32)	In: AH G3–4 ≥ 3 mo, no resp. prev. treatments Ex: prev. adenoidect., ster. < 1 yr, craniofacial disord., Down synd., recurr. acute inf.	MF 200 μg/day (2 puffs/nostril /day) vs. Saline	24 wks	OME resol., adenoid size reduct.	PTA, sympt., QoL	OME resol. 93%	OME resol. 50%	$p = 0.04$ sympt.; $p = 0.0001$ (adenoid reduct. Tx, NS in Ctrl); $p = 0.0004$ (OME); $p < 0.0001$ (PTA); $p = 0.0001$ (QoL)
Berlucchi (2007) [30]	RCT	Child. 3–7 yrs, AH ≥75%	60 tot (27 vs. 30; 57 compl.)	In: choan. obstruct. ≥75%, 3–7 yrs Ex: tonsil hypert., allergies, ster. < 4 wks, acute inf. < 2 wks, craniofacial disord.	MF 50 μg/day (1 puff/nostril /day) vs. Placebo	40 days + 3 mo maint.	Adenoid pad reduct. (avoid ade-noidect.)	Obstr. sympt. (obstruct., rhinor-rhea, cough, snoring, apnoea), AE	Choan. obstr. 88.5%→64% Tot sympt. 11→3	76.5%→76% Tot sympt. 10→9	$p < 0.001$ (choan. obstr., total sympt., nas. obstr.), $p = 0.00005$ (snor.), $p = 0.00034$ (apnoea)
Cengel (2006) [36]	CRS	Child. 3–15 yrs, AH ± OME ≥3 mo	122 tot (67 vs. 55)	In: AH/OME ≥ 3 mo, ≥2 ATB courses Ex: ster. < 4 wks, immunodef., MF allergy, craniofacial disord.	MF 100 μg/day (1 puff/nostril /day) vs. No Tx	6 wks	AH reduct. (choan. %), OME resol.	Sympt. improv. (snoring, obstr., mouth breath., apnoea)	OME resol. 42.2%, A/C ratio 80→40	OME resol. 14.5%, A/C ratio 70→80	$p < 0.001$ (OME, A/C ratio, sympt.)
Yilmaz (2013) [34]	DB-RXO	Adolesc. 12–18 yrs, AH	28 (30 init., 2 lost)	In: nasal obstruct. ≥ 6 mo Ex: ster. < 1 yr, immunodef., prev. adenoidect.	MF 200 μg/day (6 wks) vs. Saline, 3-wk wash-out, Tx crossover	6 wks + 6 wks	Adenoid vol. (NS)	Total sympt., QoL	TSS: 6.56→4.31	TSS: 6.50→5.33	$p = 0.000$ (total sympt.), $p = 0.428$ (adenoid vol.)
Baker (2023) [31]	MC-DB-RCT	Child. 3–12 yrs, SDB ≥ 2 wks	276 tot (138 vs. 138) 9.4% lost	In: SDB score ≥ −1, No prev. adenotonsillect., BMI <97th perc., no ster. < 6 wks	MF 100 μg/day (1 puff/nostril /day) vs. Saline	6 wks	SDB sympt. resol.	ENT eval., QoL (PedsQL), PSQ-SDB, OSA-5, parental satisf.	SDB resol. 44%, PSQ-SDB 0.51→0.38, OSA-5 6.2→3.6	SDB resol. 41%, PSQ-SDB 0.53→0.40, OSA-5 5.5→3.8	$p = 0.51$ (SDB), $p = 0.00$ (PSQ-SDB, OSA-5, QoL, satisf.)
Chan (2015) [32]	RCT	Child. 6–18 yrs, mild OSA	62 tot (31 vs. 31; 50 compl.)	In: OAHI 1–5, snoring ≥ 3 nights/wk Ex: craniofacial disord., elev. BMI, nasal/phar. surg.	MF 200 μg/day (2 puff/nostril /day) vs Placebo	4 mo	OAHI change (PSG pre/post)	ODI, snoring freq., ade-noid/tonsil size (endosc.), sleep param.	OAHI 2.7→1.7, ODI −0.6, snoring 75%→54.5%	OAHI 2.5→2.9, ODI +0.7, snoring un-changed	$p = 0.039$ (OAHI), $p = 0.037$ (ODI), $p = 0.031$ (snoring)
Sobhy (2013) [33]	RCT	Child. 3–13 yrs post-adenoidect.	200 tot (100 vs. 100)	In: post-adenoidect. with persistent sympt. Ex: ster. < 1 yr, epistaxis, immunodef., ge-netic/neuromusc. disord.	MF 40 μg/day vs. Saline	12 mo	Sympt. re-currence prev. (nasal obstruct., rhinor-rhea, snoring)	QoL, reduct. reinter-vention	Obstr. 2.31→0.73, Nasal secr. 2.16→0.67, Snor. 2.27→0.79	Obstr. 2.33→1.49, Nasal secr. 2.12→1.53, Snor. 2.25→1.44	$p = 0.001$ (obstr.), $p = 0.0001$ (secr./snor.), $p = 0.003$ (X-ray)

Legend: A/C ratio: Adenoid/Choana ratio; AE: adverse events; compl.: completed; CRS: Controlled Retrospective Study; DB-RCT: Double-Blind Randomised Controlled Trial; DB-RXO: Double-Blind Randomised Crossover; ENT: ear–nose–throat; freq.: frequency; init.: initial; MC: multi-centre; MF: Mometasone Furoate; mo: months; nas.: nasal; NS, not significant; obstr.: obstruction; ODI: Oxygen Desaturation Index; OSA-5: Obstructive Sleep Apnoea-5; PSQ-SDB: Paediatric Sleep Questionnaire; PTA: Pure Tone Audiometry; QoL: quality of life; resol.: resolution; satisf.: satisfaction; SDB: Sleep-disordered breathing; secr.: secretion; snor.: snoring; ster.: steroids; surg.: surgery; sympt.: symptoms; tot: total; wks: weeks; yrs: years.

The exclusion criteria were recent steroid use [30–36], craniofacial anomalies or malformations [30–33,35,36], and allergic or immunodeficiency conditions [30,33,34,36].

All studies measured at least one objective parameter (e.g., adenoid volume reduction via endoscopy, radiography, A/C ratio), obstructive AHI—oAHI—on PSG (etc.), and subjective symptoms (snoring and mouth breathing). Many studies have employed validated tools such as the PedsQL or the Glasgow Children's Benefit Inventory [31]. One study extensively analysed polysomnographic parameters (AHI and ODI) [32]. Studies with greater methodological robustness (multi-centre, large sample size, double-blind) and others that were smaller [34] or shorter in duration [36].

The dosage of mometasone furoate typically ranges from 50 to 100 µg per nostril per day (100–200 µg/day total), administered once or twice daily. Some protocols begin with two puffs per nostril per day [35], others with a single puff [30], occasionally followed by alternate-day maintenance or reduced dosing [30,35]. The treatment duration varied from 6 weeks [36] to 3–4 months [30], 6 months [35], or a one-year follow-up [33]. Some studies have reported reduced sample sizes and significant dropout rates [32]. Most comparisons were between mometasone furoate and placebo (saline solution) [30–35].

The most significant studies [30] showed decreased endoscopic or radiological obstruction (A/C ratio). One study did not find statistically significant differences in adenoid volume, but noted symptomatic improvement [34]. Most studies reported reduced severity scores for symptoms (apnoea, snoring, and nasal obstruction) in the mometasone group compared to controls [30,32,35,36]. One study documented a significant reduction in polysomnographic parameters (oAHI and ODI) [32]. In cases of OME, some studies demonstrated quicker radiological and clinical resolution/improvement in patients treated with mometasone [35,36]. Other studies reported decreased symptom severity scores and reduced perceived need for adenoidectomy [31]. Relevant adverse events were rare; one study noted mild epistaxis [30], but mometasone use was generally tolerated.

Considering the statistical analysis of p-values reported, due to the very small individual p-values (except for one study with $p = 0.51$) [33], the sum of log-transformed p-values was extremely low. The resulting χ^2 statistic far exceeded the critical threshold of a χ^2 distribution with 2k degrees of freedom. Notably, one study reporting a non-significant p-value for the 'resolution of SDB symptoms' ($p = 0.51$) still indicated significant differences in other outcomes, such as quality of life scores ($p = 0.001$) [33].

The studies presented in Table 2 [37–39] aimed to evaluate the effectiveness of nasal beclomethasone spray in reducing AH and associated obstructive symptoms such as nasal obstruction, snoring, and related issues (e.g., OME). All studies were randomised and double-blind, with some including a crossover study component.

Despite some differences in the study design (duration, dosage, and outcome measures), there is a general trend toward moderate methodological quality. Specifically, the enrolled sample sizes were relatively small, ranging from a minimum of 20 children [39] to a maximum of 60 children [38], with notable dropout rates during follow-up [39].

Regarding therapeutic protocols, all three studies used nasal beclomethasone (generally 200–400 µg/day) for periods ranging from 8 weeks [37] to 24 weeks [38]. One study began with a higher initial dose, followed by a maintenance phase at a reduced dose [38]. The follow-up durations varied from 8 weeks [37] to 24 weeks [39]. In one case, the authors followed the children for up to 100 weeks [38]. However, only a part of the protocol was double-blind and controlled.

Table 2. Clinical studies on the treatment of adenoid hypertrophy and sleep-related breathing disorder symptoms with beclometasone.

Reference	Design	Pop (Age)	N	In/Ex	Tx vs. Ctrl	Dur	O1	O2	Out (Tx)	Out (Ctrl)	Stat
Lepcha (2002) [37]	DB-RCT	Child. 3–12 yrs	31 tot (5 lost)	In: AH (clinical + X-ray), no ster. < 1 yr, no nasal spray < 2 wks, no immunodef./epistaxis. Ex: see inclusion criteria	Beclom. 200 μg/day vs. Placebo	8 wks	Improv. obstruct. sympt. + adenoid size reduct. (X-ray/endosc.)	Eval. nasal secretion, OME, AE	Nasal Block: −1.54 ± 0.97; Snoring: −1.31 ± 1.18; Endosc.: −0.38 ± 0.51	Nasal Block: −1.69 ± 1.11; Snoring: −1.77 ± 1.01; Endosc.: −0.08 ± 0.28	p = NS symptom scores ($p \geq 0.07$)
Criscuoli (2003) [38]	Rnd single-blind, crossover	Child. ~3.8 yrs	60 tot (53 compl.)	In: obstruct. ≥ 6 mo, AH/NF > 0.5, planned A-T. Ex: ster. < 1 yr, epistaxis, immunodef., URTI < 2 wks	Beclom. 400 μg/day vs Saline (2-wk cross.), then 200 μg/day "open" 24 wks	4 wks (cross.) + 24 wks (open) (total ~28 wks); follow-up 100 wks	≥50% reduct. nasal obstruction index (NOI) score	Freq. adenotonsillect., AE, obstruct. meas. at 24, 52, and 100 wks	Nasal Block: −1.54 ± 0.97; Snoring: −1.31 ± 1.18; Mild improv. X-ray/endosc. (NS)	N/A (placebo 2 wks), then all open-label beclom.	$p > 0.05$ for radiogr. and endosc. diff.; no severe AE reported
Demain (1995) [39]	DB-PC-RXO	Child. 5–11 yrs	20 tot (17 compl. 8 wks, 14 compl. 24 wks)	In: Chron. nasal obstruct. sympt., A/C ratio ~90%, no ster. < 12 mo, no immunodef./epistaxis	Beclom. 336 μg/day (2 puff x2/day) vs. Placebo (8 wks), then "open" 168 μg/day for 16 wks	8-wk cross + 16 wks open (total 24 wks)	Adenoid size reduct. (rhinoscopy: −29% at 24 wks) Obstruct. sympt. reduct. (−82% score)	Reduct. snoring, rhinolalia, enuresis in 8/9, fewer ATB, improv. OME pressures	A/C ratio 91%→−14/−15% at 4 wks, −29% at 24 wks; sympt. score: −82%	Ctrl: minimal ratio changes (0%→−2%); sympt. scores essentially unchanged	p = 0.0002 and 0.0006 (A/C reduct.), $p \approx 0.05$ (sympt.); carryover eff. in RXO

Legend: A/C ratio: Adenoid-to-Choana ratio; AE: adverse events; AH: Adenoid Hypertrophy; ATB: antibiotics; compl.: completed; DB-PC-RXO: Double-Blind Placebo-Controlled Randomised Crossover; DB-RCT: Double-Blind Randomised Controlled Trial; diff.: difference; endosc.: endoscopic; Improv.: improvement; In/Ex: Inclusion/Exclusion criteria; immunodef.: immunodeficiency; mo: months; NF: Nasopharynx; NOI: Nasal Obstruction Index; NS: not significant; OME: Otitis Media with Effusion; obstruct.: obstruction; radiogr.: radiographic; reduct.: reduction; Rnd: Randomised; ster.: steroids; sympt.: symptoms; tot: total; Tx vs. Ctrl: Treatment vs. Control; URTI: Upper Respiratory Tract Infection; wks: weeks; yrs: years.

Concerning efficacy, one study reported modest and sometimes non-significant reductions in adenoid size documented through instrumental examinations [37]. Another study demonstrated a 29% reduction in the adenoid area after 24 weeks of therapy [39], significantly improving obstructive symptoms.

In the study by Lepcha et al. [37], p-values ranged from 0.71 to 1.00 for most variables, with the lowest value of 0.07 for endoscopy; thus, a p-value of 0.07 was selected for the endoscopic endpoint. Criscuoli et al. [38] reported p-values of 0.71 (nasal obstruction), 0.30 (snoring), and 0.39 (nasal discharge), along with values greater than 0.05 for endoscopic and radiographic findings. Since all values exceeded 0.05, a representative p-value of 0.30 (snoring) was selected. Demain and Goetz [39] reported significantly lower p-values for the A/C ratio reduction (p = 0.0002 right, p = 0.0006 left) and around 0.05 for symptomatic scores. The smallest and most statistically significant p-value for adenoid reduction was 0.0002.

Although two studies reported non-statistically significant results for the primary endpoints [37,38], the pronounced effect observed by Demain and Goetz [39] (p = 0.0002) strongly influenced Fisher's combined analysis, resulting in a highly significant global p-value ($p < 0.001$). Fisher's combined p-value analysis suggested an overall benefit of beclometasone compared to controls ($p < 0.001$). However, discrepancies among studies (two showing no significant differences [37,38]), one demonstrating significance [39], and the variability of outcomes warrant caution in clinical interpretation.

The studies presented in Table 3 evaluate the effects of beclometasone on AH and symptoms related to SDB [40–42]. These studies exhibited good methodological quality: prospective, randomised, placebo-controlled, and double blind. Inclusion and exclusion criteria were clearly defined, with sufficiently large populations ranging from 60 [40] to 100 children [41]. However, not all studies have provided long-term follow-up [40,42].

Table 3. Clinical studies on treating adenoid hypertrophy and sleep-related breathing disorder symptoms with budesonide.

Reference	Design	Pop (Age)	N	In/Ex	Tx vs. Ctrl	Dur	O1	O2	Out (Tx)	Out (Ctrl)	Stat
Gudnadottir (2018) [40]	Pros, Rnd, DB, PC	Child. 4–10 yrs with SDB	60 tot (30 vs. 30)	In: SDB ≥ 3 mo, no steroids < 4 wks, no prev. AT surgery, no craniofacial disorders. Ex: acute infections, severe SDB	Budesonide 128 μg/day vs. Placebo	6 wks	OSA-18 reduction (QoL in SDB)	Snoring, apnoeas, nasal obstruction, QoL (VAS), adenoid size	OSA-18: 65.2→45.7 (Δ −19.5)	OSA-18: 54.8→47.3 (Δ −7.5)	OSA-18: $p = 0.0014$ Snoring: $p = 0.0020$ Caregiver concern: $p = 0.0057$ QoL (VAS): $p < 0.001$
Hong (2017) [41]	Rnd, DB	Prepubertal child. 6–8 yrs	100 tot (92 compl.)	In: nasal obstruction + snoring ≥ 6 mo, A/N ratio > 0.5, AHI ≥ 2, scheduled adenoidectomy. Ex: steroids < 6 mo, epistaxis, immunodef., URTI < 2 wks, required tonsillectomy	Nebulised budesonide (1 mg/2 mL/day, 2 wks) + subsequent nasal spray 64 μg/nostril /day vs. Saline 2 mL/day for 2 wks	Tot 26 wks (2 wks DB + 12 wks open-label + follow-up)	NOI reduction ≥ 2 + reduced adenoidectomy rate	Snoring, nasal secretion, OME, AE, growth	NOI: 3.41→1.92 Snoring: 3.39→2.01 Adenoidectomy: 30.77%	NOI: 3.37→3.32 Snoring: 3.42→3.38 Adenoidectomy: 73.33%	NOI, snoring, secretion: $p < 0.001$ Adenoidectomy: $p = 0.002$
Kheirandish-Gozal (2008) [42]	DB, Rnd, crossover	Child. 6–12 yrs with mild OSAS	62 tot (48 vs. 32)	In: mild OSAS (AHI 2–7), habitual snoring, hypertrophic AH Ex: asthma with prev. therapy, recent steroids, immunodef., nasal surg., craniofacial abnormalities	Budesonide 64 μg/day vs. Placebo (saline)	6 wks	AHI and N/P ratio reduction	Sleep architecture, SpO_2	OAHI: 3.7→1.3 N/P: 0.71→0.57 Nadir SpO_2: 88.9%→91.4%	OAHI: 2.9→4.0 N/P: 0.77→0.77 Nadir SpO_2: 90.1%→88.5%	$p < 0.0001$ (AHI, N/P) $p = 0.004$ (SpO_2)

Legend: AE: Adverse Events; AHI: Apnoea–Hypopnea Index; AT: Adenotonsillar; compl.: completed; DB: Double-Blind; freq.: frequency; immunodef.: immunodeficiency; In/Ex: Inclusion/Exclusion criteria; mo: months; N/P: Nasopharyngeal/Oropharyngeal ratio; NOI: Nasal Obstruction Index; OAHI: Obstructive Apnoea–Hypopnea Index; OME: Otitis Media with Effusion; OSA-18: Obstructive Sleep Apnoea-18 questionnaire; OSAS: Obstructive Sleep Apnoea Syndrome; param.: parameters; PC: Placebo-Controlled; prev.: previous; Pros: Prospective; QoL: Quality of Life; Rnd: Randomised; reduct.: reduction; SDB: Sleep-Disordered Breathing; SpO_2: Oxygen Saturation; surg.: surgery; tot: total; Tx vs. Ctrl: Treatment vs. Control; URTI: Upper Respiratory Tract Infection; VAS: Visual Analogue Scale; wks: weeks; yrs: years; Δ: delta (change).

Budesonide was administered at dosages between 64 μg [41] and 128 μg [40] per day via nasal spraying [41] or transnasal nebulisation. The treatment duration ranged from six weeks [40] to approximately 14 weeks [41]. One study included additional observation weeks to monitor potential recurrence [41]. In one case, a two-week double-blind phase (with nebulised budesonide or placebo) was followed by a twelve-week open-label phase using a nasal spray [41].

Clinically, the results confirmed significant improvement in SDB, including reduced nasal obstruction and snoring [40] and decreased AHI scores in mild-to-moderate OSA cases [42]. Positive impacts on the quality of life of patients and their families have also been reported [40]. Additionally, some studies have documented a reduction in the adenoid-to-nasopharynx ratio [42].

From a safety and tolerability perspective, the adverse events reported were mild and clinically insignificant. The study by Gudnadottir et al. included various outcome measures, such as OSA-18, sleep disturbances, caregiver concerns, and quality of life, reporting a p-value of 0.0014 for the OSA-18 score (considered the most comprehensive variable) [40].

Hong et al. reported p-values < 0.001 for the nasal obstruction index (NOI), snoring, and nasal discharge, while the adenoidectomy rate had a p-value of 0.002 [41]. Considering NOI as the primary endpoint, we assumed an indicative p value of 0.0005 (between 0.0001 and 0.001, representing $p < 0.001$). Kheirandish-Gozal and Gozal reported p-values of <0.0001 for oAHI, 0.001 for the arousal index (RAI), 0.004 for Nadir SpO_2, and again <0.0001 for the adenoid/nasopharynx (N/P) ratio. Typically, oAHI is the primary endpoint in OSA studies; hence, a reference value of $p = 0.0001$ (equivalent to $p < 0.0001$) was selected for calculations [42]. For a χ^2 distribution with 6 degrees of freedom, a value of approximately 46.76 corresponds to a p-value of <0.0001, favouring budesonide efficacy compared to placebo in the considered studies.

The three clinical trials presented in Table 4 investigate the treatment of AH and related symptoms of SDB using fluticasone [43–45]. Each of these studies follows an RCT methodology, but differs in design (open-label [43] vs. blinded [44]).

In the study by Esteitie et al., conducted on 24 children aged 2 to 12 years diagnosed with OSA (AHI ≥ 5/hour), nasal spray fluticasone furoate (55 µg per nostril, once daily) was administered for only two weeks compared to an untreated control group [43]. Although prospective, this study was not blinded, introducing potential observer bias. The primary outcome was evaluating an inflammatory marker (IL-6) in adenoid tissue. Children treated with steroids showed a significant reduction in IL-6 compared to untreated controls, while other mediators (IL-10, TGF-β, TNF, etc.) showed no relevant changes [43].

The study by Brouillette et al. is a triple-blind randomised trial involving 25 children with mild-to-moderate OSA [44]. Treatment consisted of nasal fluticasone at 200 µg/day for one week, reduced to 100 µg/day for the subsequent five weeks, compared to a placebo. Results showed a significant reduction in AHI and ODI in the steroid-treated group [44].

Demirhan et al. evaluated the efficacy of fluticasone propionate (400 µg/day) nasal drops for eight weeks compared to saline solution in 45 children aged 4 to 16 years with indications for adenoidectomy [45]. The primary objective parameter was the A/C ratio measured endoscopically and an obstructive symptom index. After eight weeks, the steroid-treated group showed substantial improvement in the A/C ratio and symptoms, with three-quarters of patients avoiding surgery compared to 80% progressing to surgery in the control group.

Overall, methodological quality appears heterogeneous. Sample sizes were modest [43,44], and observation periods were relatively brief [43]. However, the rigorous triple-blind design of Brouillette's study lends credibility to its findings [44]. Demirhan's study supports the potential utility of intranasal steroids in quickly reducing AH [45]. Esteitie's conclusions are limited, focusing on local inflammatory markers rather than long-term clinical effects [43].

Esteitie et al. reported p-values for various inflammatory markers (IL-6, IL-10, etc.), with the lowest, potentially significant value being $p = 0.05$ for IL-6. Despite being marginally significant, this value is chosen as a reference [43]. Brouillette et al. reported severity indices for OSA with p-values: AHI ($p = 0.04$), ODI ($p = 0.03$), arousal index

($p = 0.05$), and desaturation frequency ($p = 0.030$). As AHI is typically the primary endpoint in OSA studies, $p = 0.04$ was selected [44].

Table 4. Clinical studies on the treatment of adenoid hypertrophy and sleep breathing disorder symptoms with fluticasone.

Reference	Design	Pop (Age)	n	In/Ex	Tx vs. Ctrl	Dur	O1	O2	Out (Tx)	Out (Ctrl)	Stat
Esteitie (2011) [43]	Rnd, prosp., open-label, parallel-group	Child. 2–12 yrs OSA (AHI ≥5/h)	24 tot (11 vs. 13)	In: OSAS (PSG), scheduled for A-T, BMI < 95th perc., no recent steroids, no uncontrolled asthma Ex: craniofacial anomalies, systemic disorders	Fluticasone furoate 55 µg/nostril /day vs. No Tx	2 wks	Adenoid tissue IL-6 reduction	Other inflamm. markers (IL-10, TGF-β, etc.)	IL-6: 44 (13–311) pg/mL	IL-6: 133 (10–674) pg/mL	$p = 0.05$ (IL-6); NS other cytokines
Brouillette (2001) [44]	Rnd, triple-blind, PC, parallel	Child. 1–10 yrs mild-mod. OSA	25 tot (13 vs. 12)	In: OSA (AHI > 1/h), hypertrophic AH/tonsils, no acute inf., no steroids < 3 wks Ex: severe OSA, craniofacial anomalies, steroid allergies	Nasal Fluticasone: 200 µg/day (1st wk), then 100 µg/day (5 wks) vs. Placebo	6 wks	AHI reduction	ODI, arousal, SpO_2 desat., adenoid/tonsil size, parental sympt. score	AHI: 10.7→5.8 ODI: 7.0→2.9 Arousal: 6.1→2.7	AHI: 10.9→13.1 ODI: 5.6→5.4 Arousal: 4.1→3.9	AHI: $p = 0.04$ ODI: $p = 0.03$ Arousal: $p = 0.05$
Demirhan (2010) [45]	Prosp., Rnd, PC	Child. 4–16 yrs AH	45 tot (25 vs. 20)	In: AH with indication for A-T, sympt. > 6 mo, no recent steroids, no allergies Ex: allergic rhinitis, turbinate hypertrophy, chronic disorders	Fluticasone Prop. nasal drops 400 µg/day vs Saline	8 wks	Reduction A/C ratio, obstr. sympt., apnoeas, snoring	Total sympt. score, tonsil size, otologic parameters	Total sympt.: 13.72→2.96 A/C: 86.9%→56.2% Surgery avoided ~76%	Total sympt.: 14.85→14.65 A/C: 87.2%→85.2% Surgery 80%	$p < 0.05$ (sympt., A/C) No OR/RR data

Legend: AH: Adenoid Hypertrophy; AHI: Apnoea–Hypopnea Index; A-T: Adenotonsillectomy; BMI: Body Mass Index; desat.: desaturation; IL-6: Interleukin-6; IL-10: Interleukin-10; In/Ex: Inclusion/Exclusion criteria; inf.: infections; inflamm.: inflammatory; mo: months; NS: not significant; obstr.: obstruction; ODI: Oxygen Desaturation Index; OR: Odds Ratio; OSA: Obstructive Sleep Apnoea; OSAS: Obstructive Sleep Apnoea Syndrome; PC: Placebo-Controlled; perc.: percentile; Prop.: Propionate; Prosp.: Prospective; PSG: Polysomnography; Rnd: Randomised; RR: Relative Risk; SpO_2: Oxygen saturation; sympt.: symptoms; TGF-β: Transforming Growth Factor-beta; tot: total; Tx vs. Ctrl: Treatment vs. Control; wks: weeks; yrs: years.

Demirhan et al. reported $p < 0.05$ for total symptom reduction and A/C ratio improvement without exact values provided. For calculation purposes, a conservative intermediate value of $p = 0.02$ was assumed [45]. A χ^2 value of approximately 20.25 with 6 degrees of freedom corresponds to $p \approx 0.002$. Thus, Fisher's combined analysis indicates a significant overall effect ($p < 0.01$) favouring fluticasone treatment compared to control.

The two studies mentioned in Table 5 [46,47], while sharing the goal of evaluating the effectiveness of intranasal flunisolide in reducing AH and related obstructive symptoms, present differing methodological features.

The study by Ciprandi et al. involved a sample of 178 children aged between 3 and 6 years, divided into a larger group treated with flunisolide (n = 139) and a control group receiving saline solution (n = 39) [46]. The treatment duration was eight weeks, with flunisolide dosage based on body weight, specifically 0.5 drops × kg per nostril, twice daily, administered via an aerosolisation device (Rinowash).

Table 5. Clinical studies on treating adenoid hypertrophy and sleep-related breathing disorder symptoms with flunisolide.

Reference	Design	Pop (Age)	N	In/Ex	Tx vs. Ctrl	Dur	O1	O2	Out (Tx)	Out (Ctrl)	Stat
Ciprandi (2007) [46]	Prosp., parallel-group	Child. 3–6 yrs (mean 4.5)	178 tot (139 vs. 39)	In: AH GIII/IV, surgical indication. No steroids < 1 yr, no acute conditions < 2 wks	Nasal Flunisolide (dose in drops per weight, 2×/day, Rinowash) vs. Saline solution	8 wks	AH grade reduction (I–IV), avoid adenoidectomy	Nasal obstruction sympt., potential surgery prevention, NS AE	AH reduction in 72.6% (AH IV: 41.7% →8.6%; Surgery avoided in 46/58)	AH reduction in 30.7% (AH IV: 15.4% →12.8%)	$p < 0.02$ (overall AH reduction); $p < 0.04$ (GIV reduction)
Varricchio (2009) [47]	[abstract] (Possibly Prosp. study)	Child. with AH GIII/IV (age n.r.)	178 tot (group details n.r.)	In: AH GIII/IV (endoscopic); Exclusions not specified	Nasal Flunisolide (dose n.r.) 8 wks vs. Saline, 12-mo follow-up	8 wks + 6–12 mo follow-up	AH grade reduction (endoscopic)	Maintenance of AH reduction (especially in allergic subjects), need for surgery, NS AE	Significant AH reduction at 8 wks ($p < 0.01$), maintained in allergic subjects ($p < 0.05$)	n.d.	$p < 0.01$ (initial AH reduction), $p < 0.05$ (maintenance in allergic subjects)

Legend: AE: Adverse events; AH: Adenoid Hypertrophy; GIII/IV: Grade III/IV; In/Ex: Inclusion/Exclusion criteria; mo: months; n.d.: Not determined; n.r.: Not reported; NS: not significant; Prosp.: Prospective; Rinowash: Nasal irrigation device; tot: total; Tx vs. Ctrl: Treatment vs. Control; wks: weeks; yrs: years.

More than 70% of subjects in the treatment arm showed a significant reduction of adenoid tissue, compared to approximately 30% in the placebo group. Many children with grade IV AH improved to lower levels, thus avoiding surgery. However, randomisation appeared imbalanced, and it was unclear whether a genuine blinding procedure was applied [46].

The study by Varricchio et al., for which only the abstract is available, refers to a sample of 178 children with grade III or IV AH. The duration of flunisolide treatment was also eight weeks, with a longer follow-up (at 6 and 12 months post-treatment). Reported data indicate a statistically significant reduction in AH severity by the end of treatment ($p < 0.01$) [47]. The maintenance of benefit was more stable in allergic children ($p < 0.05$).

Each study reported multiple outcomes. We selected $p_1 = 0.02$ [46] and $p_2 = 0.01$ [47]. For a χ^2 distribution with 4 degrees of freedom, a value of 17.03 corresponds to $p < 0.001$. The combination of these p-values derived from the two studies indicates a highly significant effect of flunisolide in reducing AH compared to controls [46,47].

Several clinical studies have focused on the treatment of AH and SDB with steroids in combination with other drugs (Table A2).

One study utilised a double-blind, double-dummy design involving 240 children, initially divided into two groups: mometasone furoate vs. placebo. Subsequently, non-responders were assigned to four combination groups with or without oxymetazoline. The results provide evidence of a significant reduction in the A/C ratio and an improvement in symptom scores (snoring, nasal congestion, rhinorrhoea) [48]. The efficacy appears to be enhanced in the presence of the nasal vasoconstrictor.

Another study compared the use of fluticasone spray with a repeated course of azithromycin in 39 children with AH and OSA symptoms [49]. Although a placebo group was lacking, the study design included two randomised active treatments. Overall efficacy was similar between the two treatments, with a slight advantage for the fluticasone-treated group in residual apnoea parameters (p = 0.020) [49]. However, the study had a small sample size (n = 39) and an open-label design. Therefore, while the data are encouraging, they should be interpreted cautiously.

Finally, Evangelisti et al. evaluated the effect of combined therapy with oral betamethasone and intranasal beclomethasone for one week, compared to intranasal beclomethasone alone in 28 children with severe OSAS [50]. The results showed significant differences in the improvement of oxygenation (mean and minimum SpO_2) and acute symptoms, favouring the group receiving systemic steroids [50]. However, the absence of a placebo group reduces the experimental rigour.

The studies listed in Table 6 focus on the use of montelukast in children with AH and/or mild-to-moderate OSAS. These studies predominantly follow a randomised, placebo-controlled methodological design [13,51,52], sometimes with a double-blind approach [13,14,52,53]. The recruited samples are not always large [14,53], and the follow-up duration varies from one month [53] to three to four months [13,14,51,52].

Some research focuses on reducing AH and nasal obstruction symptoms [51,52]. Other studies have conducted polysomnographic assessments: AHI and ODI were decreased significantly in children treated with montelukast [13,14]. However, in Goldbart et al.'s study, the reduction in AHI did not reach full statistical significance (p = 0.07) [14], while the OAI and adenoid size showed significant improvement (p = 0.01). Conversely, in Kheirandish-Gozal et al.'s study [13], montelukast was associated with a marked reduction in AHI, with $p < 0.0001$, along with benefits in tonsillar and adenoidal size [13].

The double-blind, placebo-controlled study by Wang et al., conducted over four weeks, histopathologically assessed adenoid tissue. The group treated with montelukast showed reduced inflammatory infiltration. The limitations of these studies mainly lie in the small sample sizes (treated patients ranged from n = 23 to n = 30) [14,53] and relatively short follow-up periods (minimum four weeks and maximum three months) [14,52,53].

Naqi et al.'s study included several outcomes (endoscopy, radiography, snoring, mouth breathing, etc.) with $p \leq 0.0001$ [51]. We select $p = 0.0001$ (endoscopy score or radiography). Goldbart et al.'s study reported $p < 0.001$ for the A/N ratio (the lowest) and $p < 0.01$ for OAI, while AHI, desaturation, and SaO_2 showed $p > 0.05$ [14]. We choose $p = 0.001$ (A/N ratio). Kheirandish-Gozal et al.'s study reported $p < 0.0001$ for AHI and SpO_2 nadir, $p = 0.001$ for ODI3%, etc. [13]. We take the most classical endpoint (AHI) with $p = 0.0001$. Shokouhi et al.'s study reported $p < 0.0001$ for total symptoms, mouth breathing, and sleep discomfort and $p = 0.007$ for snoring [52]. We use $p = 0.0001$ (total symptom score). Wang et al.'s study reported $p = 0.029$ (number of germinal centres), $p = 0.024$ (cystic cavities), and $p = 0.040$ (inflammatory infiltration) [53]. We select the lowest value, $p = 0.024$ (cystic cavities). With 10 degrees of freedom (2×5 studies), a χ^2 value of 76.55 corresponds to a p-value < 0.0001.

The data suggest that, in paediatric settings (AH, OSAS, OME, etc.), the use of montelukast is associated with significant improvements in various parameters compared to placebo or control treatment.

The studies in Table 7 focus on administering montelukast with mometasone furoate, compared with using each drug alone or with a placebo. The studies exhibit some heterogeneity regarding experimental design, sample size, and the evaluation tools [54–57].

Yang et al.'s study involved 195 children with mild-to-moderate OSAS, who were randomised into three groups: montelukast, mometasone, or a combination of both [54]. The study shows that after 12 weeks, all treated groups experienced a significant reduction in AHI and an improvement in minimum SpO_2, with the most important benefit observed in the combination therapy group.

Table 6. Clinical studies on treating adenoid hypertrophy and sleep-related breathing disorder symptoms with montelukast.

Reference	Design	Pop (Age)	N	In/Ex	Tx vs. Ctrl	Dur	O1	O2	Out (Tx)	Out (Ctrl)	Stat
Naqi (2021) [51]	RCT	Child. 4–12 yrs AH	60 tot (30 vs. 30)	In: Symptomatic AH (snoring, apnoea, mouth breathing) + endoscopic /X-ray confirmation Ex: Obesity, acute infections, prev. A-T, recent ster./ATB	Montelukast 5 mg/day vs. Placebo	3 mo	Adenoid reduction (endoscopy, X-ray)	Improvement in snoring, apnoea, mouth breathing	Endoscopy 3.77→2.37, X-ray 87.23% →51.33%	Endoscopy 3.57→3.43, X-ray 81.16 % →77.83%	$p \leq 0.0001$ (endo, X-ray), $p = 0.007$ (snoring), $p \leq 0.0001$ (mouth breathing, sleep)
Goldbart (2012) [14]	DB-PC	Child. 2–10 yrs Mild-mod. OSAS	46 tot (23 vs. 23)	In: AHI < 10, habitual snoring, AH Ex: Obesity, craniofacial anomalies, recent ster./mont.	Montelukast 4 or 5 mg/day (12 wks) vs. Placebo	12 wks	AHI reduction, adenoid size reduction	OSAS symptom improvement, saturation	A/N ratio 0.81→0.57, AHI 6.0→3.6, OAI 3.9→1.7	N/A	$p < 0.001$ (A/N ratio), $p = 0.07$ (AHI), $p < 0.01$ (OAI)
Kheirandish-Gozal (2016) [13]	DB-RCT-PC	Child. 2–10 yrs Mild-mod. OSA	64 tot (28 vs. 29; 57 compl.)	In: AHI > 2, no prev. A-T, no recent ster./mont. Ex: Severe OSA, chronic conditions, craniofacial anomalies	Montelukast 4 mg/day <6 yrs, 5 mg/day ≥6 yrs (16 wks) vs. Placebo	16 wks	AHI and OSA severity reduction (PSG)	Improvement in ODI3%, min. SpO_2, arousal index	AHI 9.2→4.2, ODI3 7.2→2.8, Ad. size 2.4→2.0, SpO_2 nadir 85.2→91.0	AHI 8.2→8.7, ODI3 7.0→6.8, Ad. size 2.5→2.4, SpO_2 nadir 84.8→86.1	$p < 0.0001$ (AHI, SpO_2), $p = 0.001$ (ODI3), $p < 0.001$ (Ad. size), $p = 0.01$ (arousal)
Shokouhi (2015) [52]	DB-RCT-PC	Child. 4–12 yrs AH ≥75%	60 tot (30 vs. 30)	In: AH ≥ 75% (endo), nasal obstr. (snoring, apnoea, mouth breathing) Ex: Prev. A-T, ster./mont. < 4 wks, genetic/systemic disorders	Montelukast 5 mg/day vs. Placebo (12 wks)	12 wks	Adenoid reduction (endo, A/N ratio)	Symptom improvement (snoring, mouth breathing, sleep)	76% adenoid reduction, Sympt. 7.7→3.3	3% adenoid reduction, Sympt. 7.4→6.7	$p < 0.0001$ (total sympt., mouth breathing), $p < 0.007$ (snoring)
Wang (2023) [53]	DB-RCT prosp.	Child. 3–8 yrs Mod-sev. AH	20 tot (10 vs. 10)	In: AH ≥ 50%, no mont. allergy, no acute infections Ex: Tonsillar hypertrophy, OME, sinusitis, recent ster./ATB	Montelukast 5 mg/day vs. Placebo (4 wks)	4 wks	Histopathological evaluation of adenoids (germinal centres, inflammatory infiltration)	Blood lymphocyte count, epithelial cysts, inflammation grade	Germ centres: 8.7, Cysts: 0.0, Inflamm. infiltration: 1.1	Germ centres: 16.5, Cysts: 0.6, Inflamm. infiltration: 2.0	$p = 0.029$ (germ centres), $p = 0.024$ (cysts), $p = 0.040$ (infiltration)

Legend: A-T: Adenotonsillectomy; AH: Adenoid Hypertrophy; AHI: Apnoea–Hypopnea Index; A/N ratio: Adenoid/Nasopharynx ratio; ATB: Antibiotics; compl.: completed; DB: Double-Blind; endo: Endoscopy; germ centre: Germinal Centre; In/Ex: Inclusion/Exclusion criteria; inflam.: Inflammation; mo: months; mont.: montelukast; N/A: not available; OAI: Obstructive Apnoea Index; ODI3: Oxygen Desaturation Index (≥3% desaturation); obstr.: Obstruction; OSA: Obstructive Sleep Apnoea; OSAS: Obstructive Sleep Apnoea Syndrome; PC: Placebo-Controlled; prosp.: Prospective; PSG: Polysomnography; RCT: Randomised Controlled Trial; SpO_2: Oxygen Saturation; sympt.: Symptoms; tot: total; Tx vs. Ctrl: Treatment vs Control; wks: weeks; yrs: years.

In the prospective randomised study by Ras et al., the researchers divided 100 patients into montelukast plus mometasone and mometasone alone [55]. The study did not include a placebo group. After three months of treatment and an additional three-month follow-up, the montelukast–mometasone combination resulted in a more marked reduction in adenoid volume than nasal steroid treatment alone.

The studies by TuhanıOğLu and Erkan and Ras et al., which assessed AH control through symptom scores, reported similar findings [55,57]. The combination of montelukast and mometasone significantly reduced adenoid volume and associated symptoms (snoring, obstruction, mouth breathing) compared to mometasone alone. TuhanıOğLu and Erkan also included groups treated with montelukast alone or receiving no treatment. Their findings indicate that any therapeutic option provides benefits compared to the absence of treatment [56].

Table 7. Clinical studies on treating adenoid hypertrophy and sleep-related breathing disorder symptoms with montelukast and mometasone.

Reference	Design	Pop (Age)	n	In/Ex	Tx vs. Ctrl	Dur	O1	O2	Out (Tx)	Out (Ctrl)	Stat
Yang (2017) [54]	RCT	Child. 2–8 yrs, Mild-mod. OSAS	195 tot (65 Mont., 61 Mom., 57 Comb.)	In: AHI 5–10/h, snoring, obstruct. apnoeas Ex: Prev. A-T, drug allergies, craniofacial anomalies, severe obesity	Montelukast 5 mg/day vs. Nasal Mometasone 50 µg/day vs. Comb. (Mont. + Mom.)	12 wks	AHI reduction, ↑ min SaO_2	Reduction in symptom scores (snoring, hyperventilation, restless sleep)	AHI: baseline 6.9→1.61, Min SaO_2: 90.16→94.8, A/N ratio: 0.75→0.50, Snoring: 3.59→1.51 (Data across 3 groups: Mont. baseline 7.25→1.3, Mom. baseline 6.1→1.15)	N/A	$p < 0.01$ (AHI, snoring), $p < 0.05$ (min SaO_2, mouth br.), $p < 0.05$ (A/N ratio)
Ras (2020) [55]	Prosp. Rnd	Child. 3–10 yrs, AH G3/4	100 tot (50 vs 50)	In: A/N ratio > 50%, AH G3/4, no severe OSAS, no recent ster./mont. Ex: Chronic conditions, craniofacial anomalies, allergies	Nasal Mom. (100 µg/day) + Mont. (4/5 mg/day) vs. Mom. alone	3 mo + 3 mo follow-up	Adenoid volume reduction (A/N ratio), endoscopic improvement	VAS symptom score, recurrence rate	A/N ratio: 52.8 ± 11.3, Endoscopic improvement 68%, Recurrence 23.5%	A/N ratio: 62.88 ± 12.1, Endoscopic improvement 36%, Recurrence 55.5%	p = 0.001–0.02 (rhino, mouth br., snore, A/N ratio, endosc., recurrence)
Jafari (2024) [56]	Rnd, DB, PC	Child. 2–14 yrs, AH	96 tot (51 vs. 45)	In: AH diagnosis (clinical + X-ray), obstruct. symptoms Ex: Drug allergies, genetic/neuromusc. conditions, recurrent infections, ster./ATB < 2 wks	Mont. 5 mg/day + Nasal Mom. (50 µg/puff /na/day) vs. Mom. (50 µg/puff /na/day) + placebo	2 mo	Clinical score reduction (snoring, mouth br., nasal voice)	Reduced need for adenoidectomy, QoL	Clinical score 9.1→6.4, A/N ratio 0.80→0.74	Clinical score 8.9→6.6, A/N ratio 0.80→0.75	$p = 0.117$ (clinical score), $p = 0.161$ (A/N ratio); no significant difference between groups
Tuhanioglu and Erkan (2017) [57]	Rnd, prosp.	Child. 4–10 yrs, AH 3–4	120 tot (4 groups of 30)	In: AH ≥ 50%, obstruct. sympt., no immediate adenoidectomy Ex: Acute infections, craniofacial anomalies, ster. <3 wks, allergies	G1 Nasal Mom. (50 µg/day) G2 Mont. (4/5 mg/day) G3 Mom. + Mont. G4 No Tx (Ctrl)	3 mo	Adenoid size reduction (X-ray, endoscopy)	Symptom improvement (scale 0–10)	Airway clearance: Mont. −22.51%, Mom. −21.76%, Comb. −21.79%; Obstr. sympt. −14.77 /−17.03 /−17.54%	Ctrl: −12.46% (adenoid), −8.8% (obstr. sympt.)	$p < 0.05$ (vs. control); no significant difference among the 3 Tx

Legend: ↑: increased; AH: Adenoid Hypertrophy; AHI: Apnoea–Hypopnea Index; A/N ratio: Adenoid/Nasopharynx ratio; A-T: Adenotonsillectomy; ATB: Antibiotics; compl.: completed; DB: Double-Blind; endo: Endoscopy; germ centre: Germinal Centre; In/Ex: Inclusion/Exclusion criteria; inflam.: Inflammation; mont.: montelukast; Mom.: Mometasone; mo: months; N/A: not available; obstr.: Obstruction; OAI: Obstructive Apnoea Index; ODI3: Oxygen Desaturation Index (≥3% desaturation); OSA: Obstructive Sleep Apnoea; OSAS: Obstructive Sleep Apnoea Syndrome; PC: Placebo-Controlled; prosp.: Prospective; PSG: Polysomnography; RCT: Randomised Controlled Trial; SpO_2: Oxygen Saturation; sympt.: Symptoms; tot: total; Tx vs. Ctrl: Treatment vs. Control; wks: weeks; yrs: years.

Most studies propose a treatment duration of at least 8–12 weeks [54–57], sometimes extending follow-up to six months [55]. In Jafari et al.'s study, the analysis did not detect a statistically significant difference between the montelukast + mometasone group and the mometasone-alone group [56].

Yang et al.'s study reported $p < 0.01$ (AHI), $p < 0.05$ (Min SaO_2, A/N ratio, mouth breathing), and $p < 0.01$ (snoring). We select $p = 0.01$ [54]. Ras et al.'s study reported improvements with $p = 0.001$, $p = 0.008$, $p = 0.019$, and up to $p < 0.001$ for the A/N ratio [55]. We take the lowest value, $p = 0.0001$, as a conservative estimate of $p < 0.001$. Jafari et al. showed no significant differences between montelukast + mometasone and Mometasone alone (clinical score: $p = 0.117$; A/N ratio: $p = 0.161$) [56]. We select $p = 0.117$. TuhanıOğLu and Erkan reported $p < 0.05$ for all treatments (montelukast, mometasone, and combination) vs. control [57]. Since they did not provide a precise p-value, we adopt $p = 0.05$ as a reasonable estimate. For a χ^2 distribution with 10 degrees of freedom, approximately 42.83 corresponds to a p-value far below 0.0001.

From a statistical perspective, the combined results of the five studies strongly suggest that montelukast, mometasone, or their combination have a significant positive effect compared to controls. The presence of one study with a non-significant p-value ($p = 0.117$) does not invalidate the evidence provided by the other four, which report $p < 0.05$, some well below 0.001.

The studies reported in Table A3 differ from the previous ones in several aspects, making their inclusion in the study incompatible. Gelardi et al.'s study focuses on saline/iodine aerosol therapy [58]. In contrast, Tracy's study (1998) evaluates the role of antibiotics in combination with beclometasone (or placebo) for the treatment of OME rather than AH [59].

Hood et al.'s study involves populations with sickle cell anaemia [60], where the primary endpoint is improving cognitive performance rather than reducing adenoidal obstruction or OSAS. Sobhy et al.'s study is dedicated to children who have already undergone adenoidectomy and focuses on the prevention of post-surgical recurrences [33].

The publications by Bilgili et al. lack a proper control group, and their primary focus is on eustachian tube dysfunction associated with adenoids rather than simple AH or OSAS [61]. Wang et al.'s study consists of retrospective or descriptive analyses of steroid use [62].

4. Discussion

The results of the study converge in demonstrating that intranasal steroid therapy (mometasone, beclometasone, budesonide, fluticasone, flunisolide), whether as monotherapy or in combination with other drugs, leads to clinical and instrumental improvement in AH and related symptoms compared to the control population. The safety profile of the studies is generally reasonable.

An alternative to steroids for paediatric OSA is oral montelukast. Furthermore, combining montelukast and intranasal corticosteroids offers more significant benefits than treating mild OSA alone. The studies also report mild side effects; however, long-term studies are lacking to verify the safety of these treatments in paediatric patients. Overall, the variety of experimental designs and sample sizes suggests a degree of caution in the clinical interpretation of the results.

Although heterogeneity in study design, population characteristics, and outcome measures limits definitive conclusions, the available evidence suggests that intranasal corticosteroids and montelukast are particularly effective in cases of mild-to-moderate OSA [32]. Similarly, montelukast demonstrated efficacy in studies focusing on mild-to-moderate cases [13,14,51–53]. Furthermore, combination therapy with mometasone and montelukast appears particularly beneficial in this subgroup [54,55], although not all trials confirmed superiority over monotherapy [56]. In terms of treatment duration, studies with longer follow-up (≥12 weeks) tend to report more substantial clinical and instrumental improvements with mometasone therapy [63]. Similarly, positive outcomes were documented following 12–16 weeks of montelukast treatment [13,52,54,55]. These trends underscore the potential influence of baseline disease severity and treatment duration on therapeutic outcomes.

It is essential to highlight the variability in clinical outcomes across the different studies. In particular, the reduction in adenoidal volume assessed endoscopically or radiologically, exhibited a variable range. In trials involving mometasone furoate, the A/C ratio decreased from 80% to 40% over six weeks in one study [36], whereas other studies reported more modest or non-significant reductions [34]. Similarly, the improvement in the AHI varied considerably. In patients treated with budesonide, the AHI decreased from 3.7 to 1.3 [42], while in studies involving montelukast, reductions ranged from 9.2 to 4.2 [13] or were not statistically significant (e.g., from 6.0 to 3.6; $p = 0.07$) [14]. In addition, symptom scores also demonstrated considerable heterogeneity. In one study with mometasone furoate, the total symptom score decreased from 11 to 3 [30], whereas in other cases, the reduction was more limited (e.g., from 6.5 to 5.3) [34]. Finally, in some studies, the combination of mometasone and oral montelukast was associated with a more pronounced improvement than monotherapy, showing greater reductions in AHI and endoscopic obstruction [54,55]. However, other studies did not observe significant differences [56]. Although a formal meta-analysis was not performed due to the considerable variability in outcome measures, treatment durations, and study designs, we have extracted and summarised the effect sizes from key studies in Figure A1 shown in Appendix C.

These findings underscore clinical heterogeneity across studies. Therefore, clinical interpretation of results requires caution, and further standardised trials are needed to clarify the actual benefits in different paediatric subpopulations.

Intranasal steroids, treatment duration, and sample size.

The available studies on mometasone furoate have treatment durations ranging from a few weeks [31,36] to one year of follow-up [33]. Typical findings include a significant reduction in endoscopic or radiological obstruction (A/C ratio) [30,36], improvement in polysomnographic and clinical parameters (snoring and apnoea) [30,31,34,36], and a positive effect on patients' quality of life [35]. Statistical analysis reveals highly significant results.

Studies on beclometasone [37–39] are generally double-blind but involve small samples (20–60 children) [38,39]. The treatment duration can extend up to 24 weeks [39]. Two studies did not report statistically significant differences in AH [37,38], while one showed a marked reduction [39]. However, the overall statistical analysis result is substantial.

Similar results emerge from studies on budesonide [40–42], with sample sizes ranging from 60 [40] to 100 subjects [41] and follow-up durations of 6 [40,42] to 14 weeks [41]. These studies confirm improvements in respiratory symptoms [40,41] and a reduction in AHI [41].

For fluticasone [43–45], a reduction in the A/C ratio [42], a decrease in AHI [44], and an improvement in local inflammation [43] have been observed. The combination of p-values highlights a significantly positive overall effect.

For flunisolide [46,47], the results confirm a significant reduction in adenoid volume [46,47]. The available data indicate robust statistical significance ($p < 0.001$).

4.1. Intranasal Steroids and Dosages

The available studies show significant variability in the dosages used for intranasal corticosteroids in treating paediatric SDB. Mometasone furoate ranges from 40 μg/day [33] to 200 μg/day [32,34,35], beclometasone from 200 μg/day [37] to 400 μg/day [38], budesonide from 64 μg/day [42] to 1 mg/2 mL nebulised [41], fluticasone from 55 μg/day [43] to 400 μg/day [45], while flunisolide is administered based on body weight or through unspecified dosing regimens [46,47].

This heterogeneity limits the identification of an optimal therapeutic regimen and complicates efficacy comparisons between studies [44], particularly given differences in the study populations (age, severity, comorbidities). Furthermore, chronic use of intranasal steroids raises safety concerns, especially in young children. High-dose treatments require long-term monitoring to identify potential adverse effects [45], such as hypothalamic–pituitary–adrenal axis suppression or reduced growth. Therefore, a personalised therapeutic approach may be appropriate, tailored to the patient's age [34] and clinical severity, potentially including systemic steroid therapy in more severe cases [50].

Steroids in combination with other drugs (oxymetazoline, azithromycin, betamethasone).

Some studies have explored the use of steroids in combination with other drugs, such as oxymetazoline (mometasone vs. placebo) [48], azithromycin (comparison between fluticasone spray and a macrolide) [49], or oral betamethasone combined with intranasal beclometasone [50]. The addition of a nasal vasoconstrictor (oxymetazoline) or systemic therapy (betamethasone) is associated with an enhancement of the steroid effect.

Statistical analyses from individual studies confirm a significant advantage compared to control groups. However, while these studies provide encouraging preliminary data, methodological limitations—including the absence of placebo groups in two studies and small sample sizes—necessitate caution in interpreting the results.

4.2. Montelukast

The studies reviewed on montelukast, both as monotherapy [13,14,51–53] and in combination with mometasone [54–56], collectively present a positive outlook for treating mild-to-moderate AH and OSAS. Double-blind, placebo-controlled studies [13,51–53] offer high methodological evidence. However, one study did not demonstrate improvement across all variables [14]. The effects on specific parameters (e.g., AHI) may vary depending on the clinical presentation's initial complexity and severity.

The combination of montelukast and mometasone appears particularly beneficial, addressing both inflammatory/leukotriene mechanisms and obstructive components. Studies comparing monotherapy (either montelukast or mometasone) with their combination typically indicate superior outcomes with the combined therapy [54,55,57]. However, one study found no significant differences between mometasone monotherapy and combination treatment [56]. This suggests that synergistic effectiveness may depend on factors such as treatment duration and AH severity. Additionally, a significant proportion of the analysed studies involved small to moderate sample sizes [14,53], potentially limiting statistical power. Furthermore, follow-up durations often did not exceed three to four months [54–57]. More extended monitoring periods would allow a better assessment of the long-term clinical benefits.

Figure 2 shows a flowchart that outlines the pharmacologic treatment approach for paediatric OSA, particularly in cases of mild-to-moderate severity or when surgical intervention is not feasible. It integrates current evidence on using intranasal corticosteroids, oral montelukast, and their combination. The approach emphasises initial evaluation, stratified treatment selection, and reassessment after 8–12 weeks.

Given the reports of neuropsychiatric adverse effects, including agitation, depression, and suicidal thoughts, the U.S. Food and Drug Administration (FDA; 4 March 2020) has issued a boxed warning regarding the use of montelukast, particularly in children. Other regulatory agencies have echoed similar warnings (GOV.UK; 29 April 2024). Therefore, careful consideration is warranted when prescribing montelukast, with a preference for alternative therapies when appropriate. If used, close monitoring of neuropsychiatric symptoms is recommended [64].

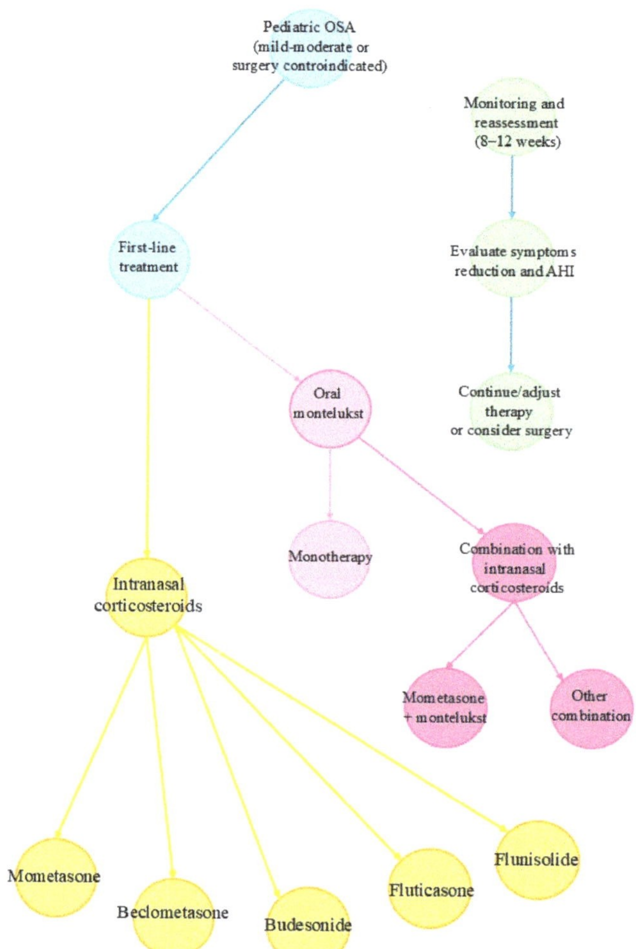

Figure 2. Clinical decision-making flowchart for pharmacologic treatment of paediatric OSA.

4.3. Study Limitations

The presence of trials with and without placebo groups and heterogeneous or sometimes absent control groups complicates direct comparisons across studies. Inclusion criteria were not consistently homogeneous. Some studies targeted children with mild OSAS, others included more moderate forms, while others focused on AH associated with diverse clinical scenarios (allergic rhinitis, recurrent otitis media with effusion, etc.). Such variability complicates the interpretation and practical clinical applicability of the findings.

To address this heterogeneity, we employed Fisher's combined probability test. Although this test does not offer quantitative effect estimates such as risk ratios or mean differences, it indicates the overall statistical significance of the available evidence. However, a more accurate clinical and quantitative evaluation would require meta-analytic analyses based on more homogeneous data, standardised outcomes, measurement units, and known variances. The available literature, however, demonstrates substantial heterogeneity among studies in terms of outcome measures and sample sizes, restricting the possibility of rigorous synthesis.

Another limitation of the current literature is the lack of stratification by OSA severity and treatment duration. Our review highlights that several studies suggest greater efficacy in cases of mild-to-moderate OSA and with longer treatment courses. However, these findings are not consistently reported or statistically stratified, which limits the ability to draw definitive conclusions regarding optimal treatment regimens and clinical indications.

5. Conclusions

Findings from this review confirm that intranasal corticosteroid therapy, whether as monotherapy or in combination with other medications, is an effective and safe option for managing AH and mild-to-moderate OSAS symptoms in children. Oral montelukast is validated as an alternative therapeutic option, demonstrating particular benefit when combined with intranasal corticosteroids. Nevertheless, variability in trial designs—including the use or absence of a placebo and the heterogeneity or lack of control groups—complicates direct comparisons across studies. Future prospective studies on larger scales, with longer follow-ups and standardised protocols, are essential to evaluate the effectiveness of different treatment durations and identify patient subgroups most likely to benefit from specific therapeutic strategies. Finally, future studies should adopt consistent criteria to classify OSA severity and evaluate these interventions' time-dependent efficacy.

Author Contributions: Conceptualisation, M.Z. and A.P.; methodology, M.Z.; software, M.Z.; validation, L.N., F.A. and R.F.; formal analysis, M.Z.; investigation, M.Z.; resources, A.P. and G.P.; data curation, R.F.; writing—original draft preparation, M.Z.; writing—review and editing, F.A.; visualisation, R.F.; supervision, G.P. All authors have read and agreed to the published version of the manuscript.

Funding: This research received no external funding.

Data Availability Statement: Data derived from public domain resources.

Acknowledgments: During the preparation of this manuscript, the authors reviewed the protocol development process and employed OpenAI's ChatGPT (versions GPT-4 and GPT-4o, OpenAI, March 2024) to support the identification of a suitable statistical method and to assist in structuring a spreadsheet for the calculation of combined *p*-values. The authors have reviewed, edited, and take full responsibility for the content of this publication.

Conflicts of Interest: The authors declare no conflicts of interest.

Abbreviations

The following abbreviations are used in this manuscript:

AH	Adenoid Hypertrophy
AHI	Apnoea–Hypopnea Index
ATH	Adenotonsillar Hypertrophy
ADI	Oxygen Desaturation Index
A/N ratio	Adenoid-to-Nasopharynx ratio

A/C ratio	Adenoid-to-Choana ratio
oAHI	Obstructive Apnoea–Hypopnea Index
OME	Otitis Media with Effusion
OSA	Obstructive Sleep Apnoea
PSQ	Paediatric Sleep Questionnaire
PSG	Polysomnography
RCS	Randomised Controlled Study
RCT	Randomised Controlled Trial
SDB	Sleep Disordered Breathing

Appendix A

Customised and database-specific search terms (MEDLINE (PubMed), Scopus, and Web of Science), combining keywords and synonyms.

PUBMED: ("children" OR "child" OR "infants" OR "infant" OR "pediatric" OR "paediatric") AND ("sleep disordered breathing" OR "sleep-disordered breathing" OR "sleep related breathing disorder" OR "SDB" OR "upper airway resistance syndrome" OR "UARS" OR "obstructive sleep apnea" OR "obstructive sleep apnoea" OR "OSA" OR "obstructive sleep apnea syndrome" OR "OSAS" OR "sleep apnea syndrome" OR "sleep apnoea" OR "adenoid hypertrophy" OR "adenoidal hypertrophy" OR "adenoid enlargement" OR "tonsillar hypertrophy" OR "tonsil hypertrophy" OR "tonsillar enlargement" OR "snoring" OR "snore") AND ("corticosteroid" OR "corticosteroids" OR "steroid" OR "steroids" OR "intranasal corticosteroid" OR "nasal corticosteroid" OR "mometasone" OR "fluticasone" OR "beclometasone" OR "budesonide" OR "prednisone" OR "prednisolone" OR "montelukast" OR "leukotriene receptor antagonist") AND ("Randomised, double-blind, placebo-controlled" OR "randomised controlled study" OR "randomised controlled trial" OR "randomised controlled study" OR "randomised controlled trial" OR "RCT" OR "randomised clinical trial" OR "randomised clinical trial") NOT review.

SCOPUS: TITLE-ABS-KEY(("children" OR "child" OR "infants" OR "infant" OR "pediatric" OR "paediatric")) AND TITLE-ABS-KEY(("sleep disordered breathing" OR "sleep-disordered breathing" OR "sleep related breathing disorder" OR "SDB" OR "upper airway resistance syndrome" OR "UARS" OR "obstructive sleep apnea" OR "obstructive sleep apnoea" OR "OSA" OR "obstructive sleep apnea syndrome" OR "OSAS" OR "sleep apnea syndrome" OR "sleep apnoea" OR "adenoid hypertrophy" OR "adenoidal hypertrophy" OR "adenoid enlargement" OR "tonsillar hypertrophy" OR "tonsil hypertrophy" OR "tonsillar enlargement" OR "snoring" OR "snore")) AND TITLE-ABS-KEY(("corticosteroid" OR "corticosteroids" OR "steroid" OR "steroids" OR "intranasal corticosteroid" OR "nasal corticosteroid" OR "mometasone" OR "fluticasone" OR "beclometasone" OR "budesonide" OR "prednisone" OR "prednisolone" OR "montelukast" OR "leukotriene receptor antagonist")) AND TITLE-ABS-KEY(("Randomised, double-blind, placebo-controlled" OR "randomised controlled study" OR "randomised controlled trial" OR "randomised controlled study" OR "randomised controlled trial" OR "RCT" OR "randomised clinical trial" OR "randomised clinical trial")) AND NOT (DOCTYPE(review))

WEB-OF-SCIENCE: TS = (("children" OR "child" OR "infants" OR "infant" OR "pediatric" OR "paediatric") AND ("sleep disordered breathing" OR "sleep-disordered breathing" OR "sleep related breathing disorder" OR "SDB" OR "upper airway resistance syndrome" OR "UARS" OR "obstructive sleep apnea" OR "obstructive sleep apnoea" OR "OSA" OR "obstructive sleep apnea syndrome" OR "OSAS" OR "sleep apnea syndrome" OR "sleep apnoea" OR "adenoid hypertrophy" OR "adenoidal hypertrophy" OR "adenoid enlargement" OR "tonsillar hypertrophy" OR "tonsil hypertrophy" OR "tonsillar enlargement" OR "snoring" OR "snore") AND ("corticosteroid" OR "corticosteroids" OR "steroid" OR "steroids" OR "intranasal corticosteroid" OR "nasal corticosteroid" OR "mometasone" OR "fluticasone" OR "beclometasone" OR "budesonide" OR "prednisone" OR "prednisolone" OR "montelukast" OR "leukotriene receptor antagonist") AND ("Randomised, double-blind, placebo-controlled" OR "randomised controlled study" OR "randomised controlled trial" OR "randomised controlled study" OR "randomised controlled trial" OR "RCT" OR "randomised clinical trial" OR "randomised clinical trial")) NOT DT = (Review).

Appendix B

Table A1. Procedure (Fisher's combined probability test) for calculating the combination of probabilities (*p*-values) in Microsoft Excel for Windows.

A	B
p-values	LN(*p*-value)
A2: *p*-value1	=LN(A2)
A3: *p*-value2	=LN(A3)
…	…
A11: *p*-value10	=LN(A11)
SUM:	=SUM(B2:B11)
$X^2 = -2 \times$ SUM:	$=-2 \times$ B12
combined *p*-value:	=CHISQ.DIST.RT(B13, 2 × COUNT(A2:A11))

Legend: LN, natural logarithm; LN(A2), natural logarithmic conversion; SUM(B2:B11), sum of logarithms; (=−2 × B12), Chi-square statistic calculation; 2 × COUNT(A2:A11), degrees of freedom; CHISQ.DIST.RT(B13, 2 × COUNT(A2:A11)), combined *p*-value calculation.

Table A2. Clinical studies on the treatment of adenoid hypertrophy and sleep-related breathing disorder symptoms with steroids in combination with other drugs.

Reference	Design	Pop (Age)	N	In/Ex	Tx vs. Ctrl	Dur	O1	O2	Out (Tx)	Out (Ctrl)	Stat
Liu (2017) [48]	Two-stage, parallel, Rnd, DB, DD	Child. 6–12 yrs AH + AR	240 tot (MF vs. Placebo; Stage 2: 4 groups)	In: AH ≥ 75% rhinoph., sympt. ≥ 12 mo, positive allergy tests Ex: Seasonal rhinitis, craniofacial anomalies, recent ster./ATB	Stage 1 (6 wks): MF 50 µg/nostril /day vs placebo Stage 2 (8 wks, non-responders): MF + Oxymet vs. MF + Placebo vs. Placebo + Oxymet vs. Placebo + Placebo	6 wks + 8 wks	A/C reduction, increased nasal volume	Symptom reduction (congestion, snoring, etc.)	A/C: 87.2→27.3; Nasal vol. 11.2→16.8; TSS: 16.5→4.8	A/C: 85.1→83.4; Nasal vol. 11.1→11.2; TSS: 15.3→14.9	$p < 0.05$ (A/C, nasal vol., TSS, congestion, snoring)
Hashemi Jazi (2011) [49]	Prosp., Rnd, longitudinal	Child. 2–10 yrs AH	39 tot (20 Flutic. vs. 19 Azithro)	In: AH + OSA sympt. (apnoea, snoring, hypernasality) Ex: Craniofacial, neuromusc. anomalies, recurrent infections, ster./ATB < 4 wks	Nasal Fluticasone (1 puff/nostril × 2/day ×1 wk, then 1/day × 5 wks) vs Azithromycin (12 mg/kg × 5 days in cycles × 6 wks)	6 wks	AH severity reduction, OSA sympt. reduction	Reduced nasal obstr., snoring, mouth breathing	Obstr. 51–100%: 70%→40%; Snoring: 85%→10%; Mouth Breathing: 60%→10%; Apnoea: 10%→5%	Obstr. 51–100%: 79%→47%; Snoring: 95%→5%; Mouth Breathing: 68%→5%; Apnoea: 15%→0%	Obstr. $p = 0.004$; Snoring /Mouth Breathing $p < 0.001$; Apnoea $p = 0.02$

Table A2. *Cont.*

Reference	Design	Pop (Age)	N	In/Ex	Tx vs. Ctrl	Dur	O1	O2	Out (Tx)	Out (Ctrl)	Stat
Evangelisti (2022) [50]	Unblinded, open-label	Child. 3–10 yrs Severe OSAS (AHI > 10)	28 tot (15 vs. 13)	In: Severe OSAS (PSG), awaiting A-T Ex: Chronic cardiopulm., craniofacial, genetic disorders, epilepsy, severe obesity	Oral Betamethasone (0.1 mg/kg/day × 7 days) + Nasal Beclometasone vs. Nasal Beclometasone alone	7 days	Improved SpO_2 (mean, min.), SCR reduction	ODI reduction, time < 90% SpO_2	SCR: 12.6→8.3; Mean SpO_2: 95.3→97.0; Min SpO_2: 78.8→89.2; ODI: 11.7→3.0; <90% time: 1.75→0.0	SCR: 12.2→12.3; Mean SpO_2: 95.6→95.5; Min SpO_2: 82.5→77.8; ODI: 12.3→11.3; <90% time: 1.35→2.0	$p = 0.0001$ (SCR, Mean SpO_2), $p = 0.001$ (Min SpO_2), $p < 0.0001$ (ODI, desaturation <90% time)

Legend: A/C: Adenoid/Choana ratio; AHI: Apnoea–Hypopnea Index; AH: Adenoid Hypertrophy; A-T: Adenotonsillectomy; ATB: Antibiotics; Azithro: Azithromycin; DB: Double-Blind; DD: Double Dummy; desatur.: Desaturation; Flutic.: Fluticasone; In/Ex: Inclusion/Exclusion criteria; Mom.: Mometasone; mo: months; Nasal vol.: Nasal Volume; Obstr.: Obstruction; ODI: Oxygen Desaturation Index; OAI: Obstructive Apnoea Index; OSA: Obstructive Sleep Apnoea; OSAS: Obstructive Sleep Apnoea Syndrome; PSG: Polysomnography; prosp.: Prospective; Rnd: Randomised; SCR: Sleep-Related Complaints; SpO_2: Oxygen Saturation; sympt.: Symptoms; TSS: Total Symptom Score; tot: total; Tx vs. Ctrl: Treatment vs. Control; wks: weeks; yrs: years.

Table A3. Clinical studies that were excluded from the review after a comprehensive assessment of the full manuscript.

Reference	Design	Pop (Age)	N	In/Ex	Tx vs. Ctrl	Dur	O1	O2	Out (Tx)	Out (Ctrl)	Stat
Gelardi (2013) [58]	Rnd, blinded, PC study	Child. 4–12 yrs AH/sub-obstr. tonsils	45 tot (27 vs. 18)	In: AH/sub-obstr. tonsils, SDB/OME > 6 mo, no immuno-suppr. < 3 mo Ex: Cardiac, bronch. disorders, iodine allergy, TB	Aerosal® (micronized NaCl + iodine) 10 sessions vs. Placebo (no aerosol)	~2 wks (10 sessions) + 3-mo follow-up	≥25% hypertrophy reduction (clinical-endoscopic)	Hearing (≥10 dB), tympanograms, SpO_2, nasal cytology	≥25% reduction: 44.4%; Hearing +5 dB; Tymp. improvement 29.6%	≥25% reduction: 22.2%; Hearing 0 dB; Tymp. 5.6%	$p = 0.204$ (hypertrophy), $p = 0.018$ (hearing), $p = 0.064$ (tymp.)
Hood (2021) [60]	MC, DB, Rnd, CT	Child. 3–7.99 yrs with SCA + SDB	Expected 200 tot	In: SCA (HbSS /HbSβ0), SDB, no current mont. Ex: Adverse mont. reactions, developmental disorders, participation in other trials	Montelukast 4 mg/day vs. Placebo	12 wks	Primary: ↑ cognitive processing speed (secondary: AH reduction)	Executive function, cerebral perfusion, SDB parameters	Mont. (n = 100): Processing speed +8 pts; A/N ratio 0.81→0.57	Ctrl (n = 100): No change; A/N ratio unchanged	Power 90% for $\Delta = 8$ pts cognitive; $\alpha = 0.025$; ITT analysis
Tracy (1998) [59]	DB-PC-Rnd	Child. 3–11 yrs Chronic OME	61 tot (20 vs. 19 vs. 20) (3 groups)	In: OME > 3 mo, >3 AOM episodes in 6 mo Ex: Systemic ster. <6 mo, tubes, beclom. allergy, nasal spray < 2 wks	1) ATB (amoxic. /sulf.) 2) ATB + nasal beclom. 336 µg/day 3) ATB + nasal placebo	12 wks	Middle ear effusion resolution (tympanometry /otoscopy)	Ear pain, hearing, tympanic mobility	G2 (ATB+bec.): Faster effusion resolution, improved tympanic /otoscopy scores ($p \leq 0.05$ at 4–8 wks)	G1/G3: Slower improvement, "catch-up" at 12 wks	$p \leq 0.01$ (right tymp. pressure), $p \leq 0.004$ (symptoms), $p \leq 0.05$ (effusion)
Wang (2017) [62]	Cross-sect.	Child. <18 yrs with OME	Data on 1.94×10^9 visits	In: OME diagnosis Ex: Acute otitis media, ATB use, recent surgery	Intranasal steroids (various) vs. No use	Retrosp. 2005–2012	Intranasal steroid prescription frequency in OME	QoC implications, appropriateness	Steroids 10.0% (95% CI 6.3–15.5) OR = 3.58	Steroids 3.5% (95% CI 3.1–3.9)	$p = 0.002$ (OR), $p < 0.001$ (risk diff.)

Table A3. *Cont.*

Reference	Design	Pop (Age)	N	In/Ex	Tx vs. Ctrl	Dur	O1	O2	Out (Tx)	Out (Ctrl)	Stat
Sobhy (2013) [33]	Rnd prosp. parallel	Child. 3–13 yrs Post-adenoidectomy	200 tot (100 vs. 100)	In: Adenoidectomy, residual symptoms, no ster. < 1 yr Ex: Epistaxis, immunodef., genetic /neuromusc. disorders	Mom. furoate 40 µg/nostril /day × 12 wks vs. Saline	12 mo	Prevention of nasal obstr., rhinorrhea, post-surg. snoring recurrence	QoL, re-surgery reduction	Nasal obstr.: 2.31→0.73; Discharge: 2.16→0.67; Snoring: 2.27→0.79	Nasal obstr.: 2.33→1.49; Discharge: 2.12→1.53; Snoring: 2.25→1.44	OR = 2.89 $p = 0.001$ (obstr.), OR = 3.21 $p = 0.0001$ (discharge), OR = 2.95 $p = 0.0001$ (snore)
Zhao (2023) [65]	Prosp. Rnd CT	Child. 2–9 yrs AH	93 tot (31 AAT, 32 Xiaoxian + AAT, 30 Montel.)	In: AH + nasal congestion, mouth br., snoring, high OSA-18 Ex: Prev. adenoidectomy, polyps, septal dev., recent ster.	AAT vs. Xiaoxian + AAT vs Mont. 4–5 mg/day	1 mo + 6-mo follow-up	Improvement in congestion, mouth br., snoring	QoL, recurrence rate	OSA-18: 69.56→53.47; Congestion: 1.63→0.50; Mouth br.: 1.56→0.47; Snoring: 1.88→0.38; Sec. sympt.: 3.0→0.72	OSA-18: 67.43→58.50; Congestion: 1.67→0.57; Snoring: 1.87→1.0; Sec. sympt.: 2.87→1.32	OSA-18: $p = 0.004$, Open-mouth $p = 0.006$, Snore $p = 0.008$, Sec. sympt. $p = 0.0014$
Bilgili (2023b) [61]	Prosp. Rnd longit.	Child. 4–14 yrs ET dysfunction + AH	100 tot	In: AH, ETD, snoring, mouth br., no prev. surgery Ex: Acute nas./otol. infections, craniofacial disorders, recent ster./ATB	Azelastine + Flutic. dipr. 2×/day (548 µg + 200 µg total/day)	3 mo, No Ctrl	A/C reduction (endoscopic), ETS-7, tubomanometry	OME resolution, nasal symptoms	A/C 82→37%, ETS-7: 6.36→9.72, OME resolved 66%	N/A (no ctrl)	$p < 0.01$ (A/C), $p = 0.001$ (ETS-7, adenoid volume)
Bilgili (2023a) [66]	Prosp. Rnd longit.	Child. 4–13 yrs AH	65 tot No Ctrl	In: AH > 6 mo, no ster. < 4 wks, no allergies/atopy Ex: Prev. surgery, craniofacial disorders	Azelastine+ Flutic. (MP-AzeFlu) 2×/day (548 µg azel. + 200 µg flutic.)	24 wks, No Ctrl	A/C reduction, symptom improvement (obstr., snoring, apnoea, etc.)	Need for surgery, QoL	A/C: 3.57→1.74, Total sympt.: 15.63→2.31, Snoring: 2.82→0.62, Apnoea: 2.52→0.22	N/A (no ctrl)	$p < 0.01$–< 0.001 (A/C, all symptoms)

Legend: ↑: increased; A/C ratio: Adenoid/Choana ratio; AH: Adenoid Hypertrophy; ATB: Antibiotics; Azel.: Azelastine; CI: Confidence Interval; Cross-sect.: Cross-Sectional; CT: Controlled Trial; DB: Double-Blind; Δ: Delta (Change); Endosc.: Endoscopy; ETD: Eustachian Tube Dysfunction; ETS-7: Eustachian Tube Score-7; Flutic.: Fluticasone; Immunsoppr.: Immunosuppression; In/Ex: Inclusion/Exclusion criteria; Longit.: Longitudinal; MC: Multi-Centre; Mom.: Mometasone; Mont.: Montelukast; MP-AzeFlu: Combination of Azelastine + Fluticasone; NaCl: Sodium Chloride (Saline); N/A: not available; NS: not significant; O1: Primary Outcome; O2: Secondary Outcome; OME: Otitis Media with Effusion; OR: Odds Ratio; OSA: Obstructive Sleep Apnoea; OSA-18: Paediatric Sleep Questionnaire for OSA; *p*: *p*-value (statistical significance); PC: Placebo-Controlled; Prosp.: Prospective; QoL: Quality of Life; Rnd: Randomised; RR: Relative Risk; SDB: Sleep-Disordered Breathing; Ster.: Steroids; tot: Total; TSS: Total Symptom Score; Tx vs. Ctrl: Treatment vs. Control; Tymp.: Tympanometry; VAS: Visual Analogue Scale; wks: Weeks; yrs: Years.

Appendix C

The descriptive forest plot illustrates the effect of intranasal corticosteroids and/or oral montelukast in paediatric patients with OSA or AH. As reported in individual studies, the horizontal bars represent the magnitude and direction of change in selected clinical outcomes (e.g., AHI, A/C, symptom scores). Negative values indicate improvement (i.e., reduction from baseline or compared to control).

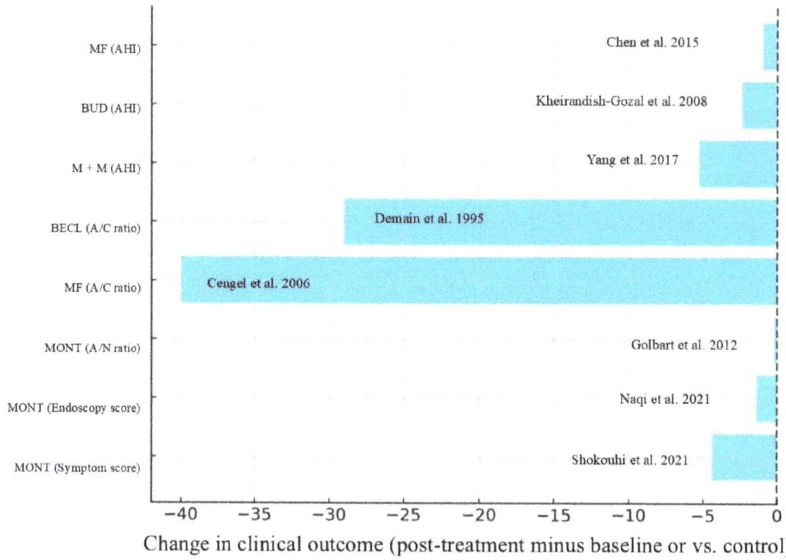

Figure A1. Descriptive forest plot grouped by outcome type [14,32,36,39,42,51,52,54]. Legend: A/C Ratio, Adenoid-to-Choana Ratio; A/N Ratio, Adenoid-to-Nasopharynx Ratio; AHI, Apnoea–Hypopnea Index; BECL, Beclometasone; BUD, budesonide; M+M, combined montelukast and mometasone; MF, mometasone furoate; MONT, montelukast.

References

1. Bitners, A.C.; Arens, R. Evaluation and Management of Children with Obstructive Sleep Apnea Syndrome. *Lung* **2020**, *198*, 257–270. [CrossRef] [PubMed]
2. Chang, S.J.; Chae, K.Y. Obstructive sleep apnea syndrome in children: Epidemiology, pathophysiology, diagnosis and sequelae. *Korean J. Pediatr.* **2010**, *53*, 863–871. [CrossRef] [PubMed]
3. Kaditis, A.G.; Alonso Alvarez, M.L.; Boudewyns, A.; Alexopoulos, E.I.; Ersu, R.; Joosten, K.; Larramona, H.; Miano, S.; Narang, I.; Trang, H.; et al. Obstructive sleep disordered breathing in 2- to 18-year-old children: Diagnosis and management. *Eur. Respir. J.* **2016**, *47*, 69–94. [CrossRef] [PubMed]
4. Cremonini, F.; Zucchini, L.; Pellitteri, F.; Palone, M.; Lombardo, L. Obstructive Sleep Apnea in Developmental Age: 22-Item Pediatric Sleep Questionnaire for an Observational Descriptive Investigation. *Children* **2023**, *10*, 1265. [CrossRef]
5. Nosetti, L.; Zaffanello, M.; Simoncini, D.; Dellea, G.; Vitali, M.; Amoudi, H.; Agosti, M. Prioritising Polysomnography in Children with Suspected Obstructive Sleep Apnoea: Key Roles of Symptom Onset and Sleep Questionnaire Scores. *Children* **2024**, *11*, 1228. [CrossRef]
6. Lein, A.; Altumbabic, H.; Đešević, M.; Baumgartner, W.D.; Salkic, A.; Umihanic, S.; Ramaš, A.; Harčinović, A.; Kosec, A.; Brkic, F.F. Association of adenoid hypertrophy and clinical parameters with preoperative polygraphy in pediatric patients undergoing adenoidectomy. *Eur. Arch. Otorhinolaryngol.* **2025**, *282*, 1075–1084. [CrossRef]
7. Sant'Ana, J.P.; Mastrandonakis, I.C.F.; Silva, R.S.B.; Duprat, A.C.; Floriano, C.G.; Miyake, M.M. Reliability of nasofibroscopy for the evaluation of adenoid hypertrophy and its correlation with clinical symptoms. *Braz. J. Otorhinolaryngol.* **2023**, *89*, 101307. [CrossRef]
8. Gupta, S.; Sharma, R. Pediatric Obstructive Sleep Apnea: Diagnostic Challenges and Management Strategies. *Cureus* **2024**, *16*, e75347. [CrossRef]
9. Kuhle, S.; Hoffmann, D.U.; Mitra, S.; Urschitz, M.S. Anti-inflammatory medications for obstructive sleep apnoea in children. *Cochrane Database Syst. Rev.* **2020**, *1*, Cd007074. [CrossRef]
10. Kheirandish-Gozal, L.; Bhattacharjee, R.; Bandla, H.P.R.; Gozal, D. Antiinflammatory therapy outcomes for mild OSA in children. *Chest* **2014**, *146*, 88–95. [CrossRef]
11. Liming, B.J.; Ryan, M.; Mack, D.; Ahmad, I.; Camacho, M. Montelukast and Nasal Corticosteroids to Treat Pediatric Obstructive Sleep Apnea: A Systematic Review and Meta-analysis. *Otolaryngol. Head. Neck Surg.* **2019**, *160*, 594–602. [CrossRef] [PubMed]

12. de Benedictis, F.M.; Bush, A. Corticosteroids in respiratory diseases in children. *Am. J. Respir. Crit. Care Med.* **2012**, *185*, 12–23. [CrossRef]
13. Kheirandish-Gozal, L.; Bandla, H.P.; Gozal, D. Montelukast for Children with Obstructive Sleep Apnea: Results of a Double-Blind, Randomized, Placebo-Controlled Trial. *Ann. Am. Thorac. Soc.* **2016**, *13*, 1736–1741. [CrossRef] [PubMed]
14. Goldbart, A.D.; Greenberg-Dotan, S.; Tal, A. Montelukast for children with obstructive sleep apnea: A double-blind, placebo-controlled study. *Pediatrics* **2012**, *130*, e575–e580. [CrossRef] [PubMed]
15. Ji, T.; Lu, T.; Qiu, Y.; Li, X.; Liu, Y.; Tai, J.; Guo, Y.; Zhang, J.; Wang, S.; Zhao, J.; et al. The efficacy and safety of montelukast in children with obstructive sleep apnea: A systematic review and meta-analysis. *Sleep. Med.* **2021**, *78*, 193–201. [CrossRef]
16. Chohan, A.; Lal, A.; Chohan, K.; Chakravarti, A.; Gomber, S. Systematic review and meta-analysis of randomized controlled trials on the role of mometasone in adenoid hypertrophy in children. *Int. J. Pediatr. Otorhinolaryngol.* **2015**, *79*, 1599–1608. [CrossRef]
17. Liu, H.T.; Lin, Y.C.; Kuan, Y.C.; Huang, Y.H.; Hou, W.H.; Liou, T.H.; Chen, H.C. Intranasal corticosteroid therapy in the treatment of obstructive sleep apnea: A meta-analysis of randomized controlled trials. *Am. J. Rhinol. Allergy* **2016**, *30*, 215–221. [CrossRef] [PubMed]
18. Chidambaram, A.G.; Chervoneva, I.; Cielo, C.M.; Bradford, R.; Cornaglia, M.A.; Tapia, I. Secondary Analysis of a Randomized Controlled Trial of Intranasal Corticosteroids in the Treatment of Mild to Moderate Pediatric Obstructive Sleep Apnea. In *TP73. TP073 PEDIATRIC SLEEP*; American Thoracic Society International Conference Abstracts; American Thoracic Society: New York, NY, USA, 2021; p. A3345.
19. Alanazi, F.; Alruwaili, M.; Alanazy, S.; Alenezi, M. Efficacy of montelukast for adenoid hypertrophy in paediatrics: A systematic review and meta-analysis. *Clin. Otolaryngol.* **2024**, *49*, 417–428. [CrossRef] [PubMed]
20. Zhang, Y.; Leng, S.; Hu, Q.; Li, Y.; Wei, Y.; Lu, Y.; Qie, D.; Yang, F. Pharmacological interventions for pediatric obstructive sleep apnea (OSA): Network meta-analysis. *Sleep. Med.* **2024**, *116*, 129–137. [CrossRef] [PubMed]
21. Joseph, M.; Krishna, M.M.; Franco, A.J.; Jekov, L.; Sudo, R.Y.U.; Cabral, T.D.D. Efficacy of combination therapy with mometasone and montelukast versus mometasone alone in treatment of adenoid hypertrophy in children: A systematic review and meta-analysis. *Am. J. Otolaryngol.* **2025**, *46*, 104566. [CrossRef]
22. Yoon, S.; Baik, B.; Park, T.; Nam, D. Powerful *p*-value combination methods to detect incomplete association. *Sci. Rep.* **2021**, *11*, 6980. [CrossRef] [PubMed]
23. Wilson, D.J. The harmonic mean *p*-value for combining dependent tests. *Proc. Natl. Acad. Sci. USA* **2019**, *116*, 1195–1200. [CrossRef] [PubMed]
24. Page, M.J.; McKenzie, J.E.; Bossuyt, P.M.; Boutron, I.; Hoffmann, T.C.; Mulrow, C.D.; Shamseer, L.; Tetzlaff, J.M.; Akl, E.A.; Brennan, S.E.; et al. The PRISMA 2020 statement: An updated guideline for reporting systematic reviews. *BMJ* **2021**, *372*, n71. [CrossRef]
25. van Dijk, S.H.B.; Brusse-Keizer, M.G.J.; Bucsán, C.C.; van der Palen, J.; Doggen, C.J.M.; Lenferink, A. Artificial intelligence in systematic reviews: Promising when appropriately used. *BMJ Open* **2023**, *13*, e072254. [CrossRef] [PubMed]
26. Yao, X.; Kumar, M.V.; Su, E.; Flores Miranda, A.; Saha, A.; Sussman, J. Evaluating the efficacy of artificial intelligence tools for the automation of systematic reviews in cancer research: A systematic review. *Cancer Epidemiol.* **2024**, *88*, 102511. [CrossRef]
27. Islam, N.; van der Schaar, M. Use of generative artificial intelligence in medical research. *BMJ* **2024**, *384*, q119. [CrossRef]
28. Ganjavi, C.; Eppler, M.B.; Pekcan, A.; Biedermann, B.; Abreu, A.; Collins, G.S.; Gill, I.S.; Cacciamani, G.E. Publishers' and journals' instructions to authors on use of generative artificial intelligence in academic and scientific publishing: Bibliometric analysis. *BMJ* **2024**, *384*, e077192. [CrossRef]
29. Won, S.; Morris, N.; Lu, Q.; Elston, R.C. Choosing an optimal method to combine P-values. *Stat. Med.* **2009**, *28*, 1537–1553. [CrossRef]
30. Berlucchi, M.; Salsi, D.; Valetti, L.; Parrinello, G.; Nicolai, P. The role of mometasone furoate aqueous nasal spray in the treatment of adenoidal hypertrophy in the pediatric age group: Preliminary results of a prospective, randomized study. *Pediatrics* **2007**, *119*, e1392–e1397. [CrossRef]
31. Baker, A.; Grobler, A.; Davies, K.; Griffiths, A.; Hiscock, H.; Kubba, H.; Peters, R.L.; Ranganathan, S.; Rimmer, J.; Rose, E.; et al. Effectiveness of Intranasal Mometasone Furoate vs Saline for Sleep-Disordered Breathing in Children: A Randomized Clinical Trial. *JAMA Pediatr.* **2023**, *177*, 240–247. [CrossRef]
32. Chan, C.C.; Au, C.T.; Lam, H.S.; Lee, D.L.; Wing, Y.K.; Li, A.M. Intranasal corticosteroids for mild childhood obstructive sleep apnea--a randomized, placebo-controlled study. *Sleep. Med.* **2015**, *16*, 358–363. [CrossRef] [PubMed]
33. Sobhy, T.S. Role of intranasal steroid in the prevention of recurrent nasal symptoms after adenoidectomy. *Int. J. Otolaryngol.* **2013**, *2013*, 603493. [CrossRef]

34. Yilmaz, H.B.; Celebi, S.; Sahin-Yilmaz, A.; Oysu, C. The role of mometasone furoate nasal spray in the treatment of adenoidal hypertrophy in the adolescents: A prospective, randomized, cross-over study. *Eur. Arch. Otorhinolaryngol.* **2013**, *270*, 2657–2661. [CrossRef] [PubMed]
35. Bhargava, R.; Chakravarti, A. A double-blind randomized placebo-controlled trial of topical intranasal mometasone furoate nasal spray in children of adenoidal hypertrophy with otitis media with effusion. *Am. J. Otolaryngol.* **2014**, *35*, 766–770. [CrossRef]
36. Cengel, S.; Akyol, M.U. The role of topical nasal steroids in the treatment of children with otitis media with effusion and/or adenoid hypertrophy. *Int. J. Pediatr. Otorhinolaryngol.* **2006**, *70*, 639–645. [CrossRef] [PubMed]
37. Lepcha, A.; Kurien, M.; Job, A.; Jeyaseelan, L.; Thomas, K. Chronic adenoid hypertrophy in children-is steroid nasal spray beneficial? *Indian. J. Otolaryngol. Head. Neck Surg.* **2002**, *54*, 280–284. [CrossRef]
38. Criscuoli, G.; D'Amora, S.; Ripa, G.; Cinquegrana, G.; Mansi, N.; Impagliazzo, N.; Pisacane, A. Frequency of surgery among children who have adenotonsillar hypertrophy and improve after treatment with nasal beclomethasone. *Pediatrics* **2003**, *111*, e236–e238. [CrossRef]
39. Demain, J.G.; Goetz, D.W. Pediatric adenoidal hypertrophy and nasal airway obstruction: Reduction with aqueous nasal beclomethasone. *Pediatrics* **1995**, *95*, 355–364. [CrossRef]
40. Gudnadottir, G.; Ellegård, E.; Hellgren, J. Intranasal Budesonide and Quality of Life in Pediatric Sleep-Disordered Breathing: A Randomized Controlled Trial. *Otolaryngol. Head. Neck Surg.* **2018**, *158*, 752–759. [CrossRef]
41. Hong, H.; Chen, F.; Zheng, X.; Liao, W.; Liao, Z.; Cao, Y.; He, H.; Zhu, Z.; Fan, Y. Decreased frequency of adenoidectomy by a 12-week nasal budesonide treatment. *Ther. Clin. Risk Manag.* **2017**, *13*, 1309–1316. [CrossRef]
42. Kheirandish-Gozal, L.; Gozal, D. Intranasal budesonide treatment for children with mild obstructive sleep apnea syndrome. *Pediatrics* **2008**, *122*, e149–e155. [CrossRef]
43. Esteitie, R.; Emani, J.; Sharma, S.; Suskind, D.L.; Baroody, F.M. Effect of fluticasone furoate on interleukin 6 secretion from adenoid tissues in children with obstructive sleep apnea. *Arch. Otolaryngol. Head. Neck Surg.* **2011**, *137*, 576–582. [CrossRef] [PubMed]
44. Brouillette, R.T.; Manoukian, J.J.; Ducharme, F.M.; Oudjhane, K.; Earle, L.G.; Ladan, S.; Morielli, A. Efficacy of fluticasone nasal spray for pediatric obstructive sleep apnea. *J. Pediatr.* **2001**, *138*, 838–844. [CrossRef]
45. Demirhan, H.; Aksoy, F.; Ozturan, O.; Yildirim, Y.S.; Veyseller, B. Medical treatment of adenoid hypertrophy with "fluticasone propionate nasal drops". *Int. J. Pediatr. Otorhinolaryngol.* **2010**, *74*, 773–776. [CrossRef]
46. Ciprandi, G.; Varricchio, A.; Capasso, M.; Varricchio, A.M.; De Lucia, A.; Ascione, E.; Avvisati, F.; Capristo, C.; Marseglia, G.L.; Barillari, U. Intranasal flunisolide treatment in children with adenoidal hypertrophy. *Int. J. Immunopathol. Pharmacol.* **2007**, *20*, 833–836. [CrossRef] [PubMed]
47. Varricchio, A.; Tortoriello, G.; Capasso, M.; De Lucia, A.; Marchisio, P.; Varricchio, A.M.; Mansi, N.; Giordano, L.; Liberatore, G.; Di Gioacchino, M.; et al. Prevention of surgery in children with adenoidal hypertrophy treated with intranasal flunisolide: A 12-month follow-up. *J. Biol. Regul. Homeost. Agents* **2009**, *23*, 95–101. [PubMed]
48. Liu, W.; Zhou, L.; Zeng, Q.; Luo, R. Combination of mometasone furoate and oxymetazoline for the treatment of adenoid hypertrophy concomitant with allergic rhinitis: A randomized controlled trial. *Sci. Rep.* **2017**, *7*, 40425. [CrossRef]
49. Jazi, S.M.; Barati, B.; Kheradmand, A. Treatment of adenotonsillar hypertrophy: A prospective randomized trial comparing azithromycin vs. fluticasone. *J. Res. Med. Sci.* **2011**, *16*, 1590–1597.
50. Evangelisti, M.; Barreto, M.; Di Nardo, G.; Del Pozzo, M.; Parisi, P.; Villa, M.P. Systemic corticosteroids could be used as bridge treatment in children with obstructive sleep apnea syndrome waiting for surgery. *Sleep. Breath.* **2022**, *26*, 879–885. [CrossRef]
51. Naqi, S.A.; Ashfaq, A.H.; Umar, M.A.; Karmani, J.K.; Arshad, N. Clinical outcome of Montelukast Sodium in Children with Adenoid Hypertrophy. *Pak. J. Med. Sci.* **2021**, *37*, 362–366. [CrossRef]
52. Shokouhi, F.; Meymaneh Jahromi, A.; Majidi, M.R.; Salehi, M. Montelukast in Adenoid Hypertrophy: Its Effect on Size and Symptoms. *Iran. J. Otorhinolaryngol.* **2015**, *27*, 443–448. [PubMed]
53. Wang, Z.; Wu, X.; Liu, J.; Wang, Y.; Zhang, Y.; Wu, Y.; Kang, Y.; Zhang, R.; Li, J.; Liu, D. Effects of oral cysteine leukotriene receptor antagonist-montelukast on adenoid lymphoid tissue: A histopathological study under light microscope. *Front. Pharmacol.* **2023**, *14*, 1285647. [CrossRef]
54. Yang, D.Z.; Liang, J.; Zhang, F.; Yao, H.B.; Shu, Y. Clinical effect of montelukast sodium combined with inhaled corticosteroids in the treatment of OSAS children. *Medicine* **2017**, *96*, e6628. [CrossRef]
55. Ras, A.E.; Hamed, M.H.; Abdelalim, A.A. Montelukast combined with intranasal mometasone furoate versus intranasal mometasone furoate; a comparative study in treatment of adenoid hypertrophy. *Am. J. Otolaryngol.* **2020**, *41*, 102723. [CrossRef] [PubMed]
56. Jafari, M.; Pourroshani, B.; Eftekhari, K.; Malekiantaghi, A.; Ashournia, P.; Shafiei, A. Effect of Combination Montelukast and Nasal Mometasone on Childhood Adenoid Hypertrophy. *Iran. J. Otorhinolaryngol.* **2024**, *36*, 391–397. [CrossRef]

57. Tuhanıoğlu, B.; Erkan, S.O. Evaluation of the effects of montelukast, mometasone furoate, and combined therapyon adenoid size: A randomized, prospective, clinical trial with objective data. *Turk. J. Med. Sci.* **2017**, *47*, 1736–1743. [CrossRef] [PubMed]
58. Gelardi, M.; Iannuzzi, L.; Greco Miani, A.; Cazzaniga, S.; Naldi, L.; De Luca, C.; Quaranta, N. Double-blind placebo-controlled randomized clinical trial on the efficacy of Aerosal in the treatment of sub-obstructive adenotonsillar hypertrophy and related diseases. *Int. J. Pediatr. Otorhinolaryngol.* **2013**, *77*, 1818–1824. [CrossRef]
59. Tracy, J.M.; Demain, J.G.; Hoffman, K.M.; Goetz, D.W. Intranasal beclomethasone as an adjunct to treatment of chronic middle ear effusion. *Ann. Allergy Asthma Immunol.* **1998**, *80*, 198–206. [CrossRef]
60. Hood, A.M.; Stotesbury, H.; Kölbel, M.; DeHaan, M.; Downes, M.; Kawadler, J.M.; Sahota, S.; Dimitriou, D.; Inusa, B.; Wilkey, O.; et al. Study of montelukast in children with sickle cell disease (SMILES): A study protocol for a randomised controlled trial. *Trials* **2021**, *22*, 690. [CrossRef]
61. Bilgili, A.M.; Durmaz, H.; Dilber, M. Eustachian Tube Dysfunction in Children with Adenoid Hypertrophy: The Effect of Intranasal Azelastine-Fluticasone Spray Treatment on Middle Ear Ventilation and Adenoid Tissue. *Ear Nose Throat J.* **2023**, *102*, 198–203. [CrossRef]
62. Wang, D.E.; Lam, D.J.; Bellmunt, A.M.; Rosenfeld, R.M.; Ikeda, A.K.; Shin, J.J. Intranasal Steroid Use for Otitis Media with Effusion: Ongoing Opportunities for Quality Improvement. *Otolaryngol. Head. Neck Surg.* **2017**, *157*, 289–296. [CrossRef] [PubMed]
63. Bhargava, R.; Chakravarti, A. Role of mometasone furoate aqueous nasal spray for management of adenoidal hypertrophy in children. *J. Laryngol. Otol.* **2014**, *128*, 1060–1066. [CrossRef] [PubMed]
64. Lo, C.W.H.; Pathadka, S.; Qin, S.X.; Fung, L.W.Y.; Yan, V.K.C.; Yiu, H.H.E.; Bloom, C.I.; Wong, I.C.K.; Chan, E.W.Y. Neuropsychiatric events associated with montelukast in patients with asthma: A systematic review. *Eur. Respir. Rev.* **2023**, *32*, 230079. [CrossRef]
65. Zhao, X.; Xu, J.; Wang, M.Y.; Hou, Z.W.; Shi, H.S.; Zhang, X.X. Effect of oral Xiao-xian decoction combined with acupoint application therapy on pediatric adenoid hypertrophy: A randomized trial. *Medicine* **2023**, *102*, e32804. [CrossRef] [PubMed]
66. Bilgili, A.M.; Durmaz, H.; Dilber, M. Efficacy of Topical Azelastine and Fluticasone Dipropionate Combination in Children with Adenoid Hypertrophy. *Ear Nose Throat J.* **2023**, *102*, 28–34. [CrossRef]

MDPI AG
Grosspeteranlage 5
4052 Basel
Switzerland
Tel.: +41 61 683 77 34

Pharmaceutics Editorial Office
E-mail: pharmaceutics@mdpi.com
www.mdpi.com/journal/pharmaceutics